GW01459006

CROSS SECTIONAL
ANATOMY
CT & MRI

CROSS SECTIONAL
ANATOMY
CT & MRI

Govind Chavhan MD DNB

Pediatric Radiologist
The Hospital for Sick Children
Assistant Professor, University of Toronto, Canada

Bhavin Jankharia MD

Consultant Radiologist
Jankharia Imaging Center, Mumbai, Maharashtra, India
Trustee, Radiology Education Foundation

JAYPEE BROTHERS MEDICAL PUBLISHERS (P) LTD

New Delhi • Panama City • London

Jaypee Brothers Medical Publishers (P) Ltd.

Headquarter

Jaypee Brothers Medical Publishers (P) Ltd
4838/24, Ansari Road, Daryaganj
New Delhi 110 002, India
Phone: +91-11-43574357
Fax: +91-11-43574314
Email: jaypee@jaypeebrothers.com

Overseas Offices

J.P. Medical Ltd.,
83 Victoria Street London
SW1H 0HW (UK)
Phone: +44-2031708910
Fax: +02-03-0086180
Email: info@jpmedpub.com

Jaypee-Highlights Medical Publishers Inc.
City of Knowledge, Bld. 237, Clayton
Panama City, Panama
Phone: +507-301-0496
Fax: +507-301-0499
Email: cservice@jphmedical.com

Website: www.jaypeebrothers.com
Website: www.jaypeedigital.com

Inquiries for bulk sales may be solicited at: jaypee@jaypeebrothers.com

This book has been published in good faith that the contents provided by the authors contained herein are original, and is intended for educational purposes only. While every effort is made to ensure accuracy of information, the publisher and the authors specifically disclaim any damage, liability, or loss incurred, directly or indirectly, from the use or application of any of the contents of this work. If not specifically stated, all figures and tables are courtesy of the authors. Where appropriate, the readers should consult with a specialist or contact the manufacturer of the drug or device. The authors have no financial interest in any procedure or product mentioned in this book.

Cross Sectional Anatomy CT and MRI

First Edition : **2012**

ISBN 978-93-5025-046-4

Printed at: Ajanta Offset & Packagings Ltd., New Delhi

Dedicated to

My wife Barakha
and
son Yash
for their love, support and time

—**Govind Chavhan**

Sana, Sach, Bijal and my parents
for their unstinting support

—**Bhavin Jankharia**

Preface

Cross sectional imaging like CT and MRI is the mainstay of medical imaging. Radiologists interpreting these images need to be thorough in human anatomy. Because of the vastness of the subject, it is difficult to remember anatomy. This atlas is our attempt to provide the quick reference for imaging anatomy to the radiologist while reporting. It will also be helpful to the radiology residents and those who need to understand the human anatomy.

CT and MR images of all body parts are given in all three planes. These images are accompanied by color diagrams for better understanding of the anatomy. The structures are labeled on these color images. We have also given CT and MRI angiographic images with labeling of all relevant branches.

We hope that in the era of Internet and 'Professor Google', where everything is available, this atlas will still serve as a handy, convenient and quick reference for reporting radiologists.

Your suggestions, criticism and queries will make this atlas better. They are most welcome at k.space@yahoo.com

Best Wishes and Happy Reporting!

Govind Chavhan
Bhavin Jankharia

Acknowledgments

Authors would like to thank the following:

- The high resolution CT and MRI images used in this atlas were obtained at Jankharia Imaging, Mumbai. Authors would like to thank entire team at Jankharia Imaging for their help in this.

- Reshma Dalvi (Consultant Radiologist, Goa, India) for her significant contribution in chapters on Upper and Lower Extremities.

- Shri Jitendar P Vij (Chairman and Managing Director) and Mr Tarun Vij of M/s Jaypee Brothers Medical Publishers (P) Ltd., New Delhi for publishing this atlas.

- Mr Tarun Duneja (Director–Publishing) and his team of Graphics for the excellent work on color images.

Contents

Section 1

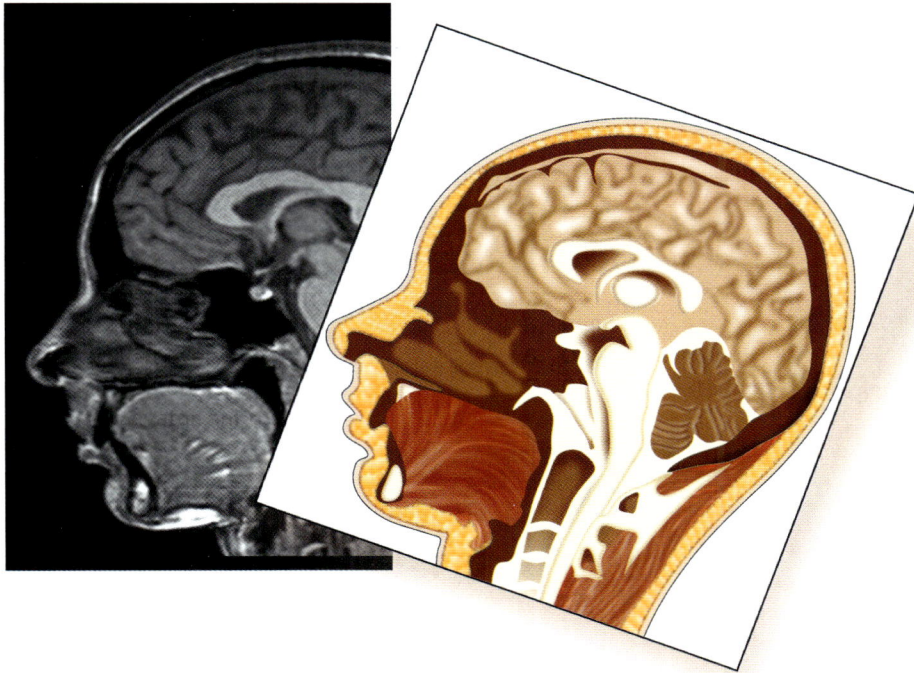

Head and Neck

- Brain
- Orbit
- PNS and Skull Base
- Temporal Bones and TM Joint
- Neck

CHAPTER 1

Brain

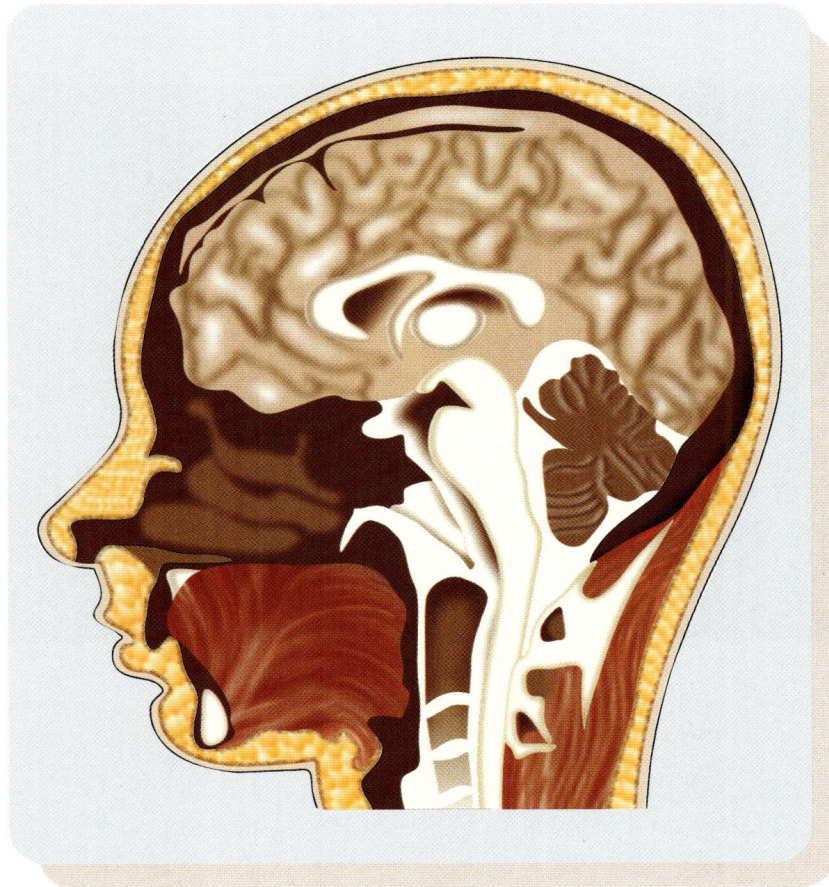

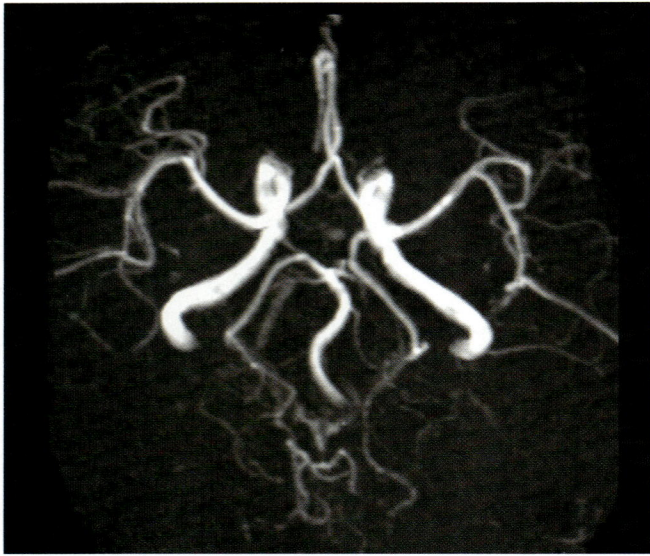

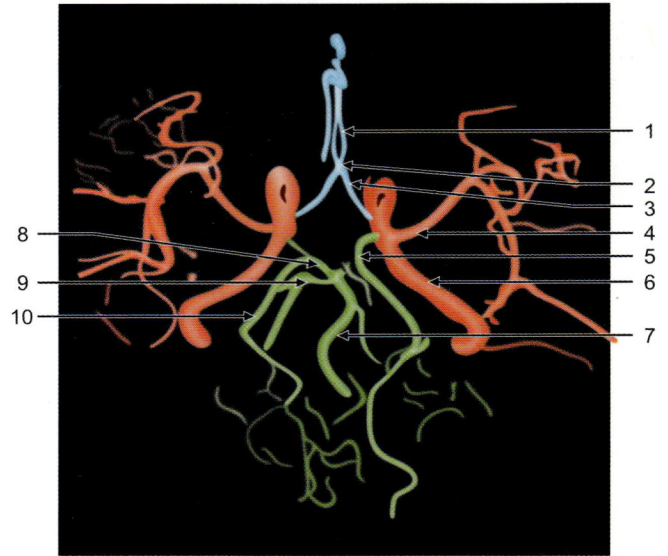

Figure 1.1

1. A2, anterior cerebral artery
2. Anterior communicating artery
3. A1 ACA
4. M1, Middle cerebral artery
5. Posterior communicating artery
6. Internal carotid artery
7. Basilar artery
8. P1, PCA
9. Superior cerebral artery
10. P2, Posterior cerebral artery

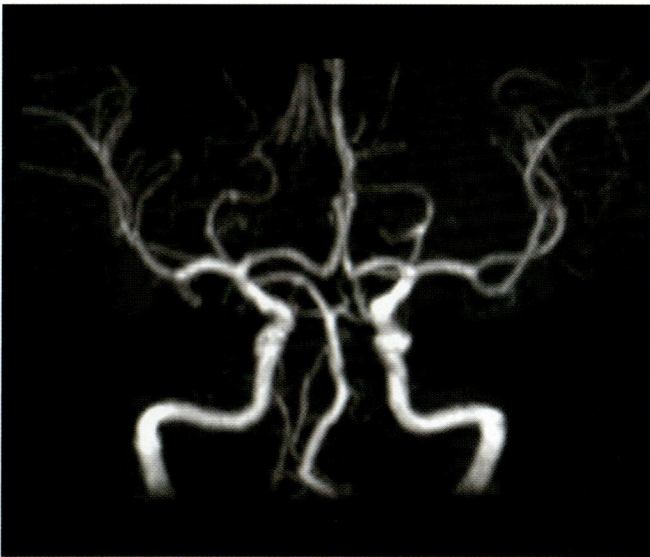

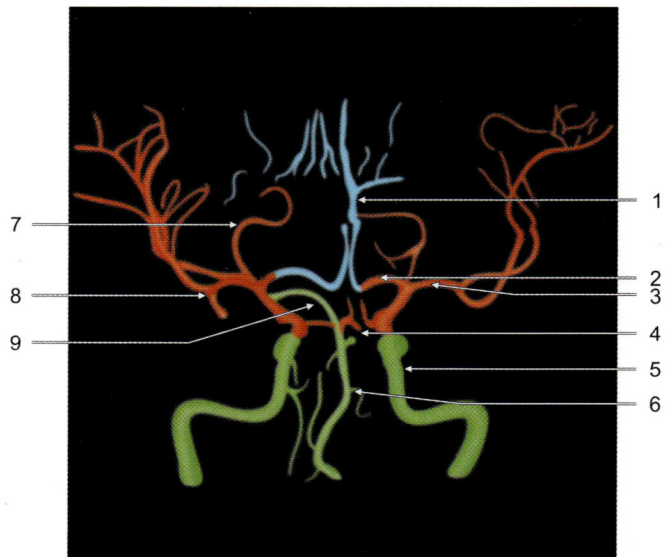

Figure 1.2

1. A2, anterior cerebral artery
2. A1, ACA
3. M1, middle cerebral artery
4. Superior cerebellar artery
5. Internal carotid artery
6. Basilar artery
7. PCA
8. MCA, genu
9. Posterior cerebral artery

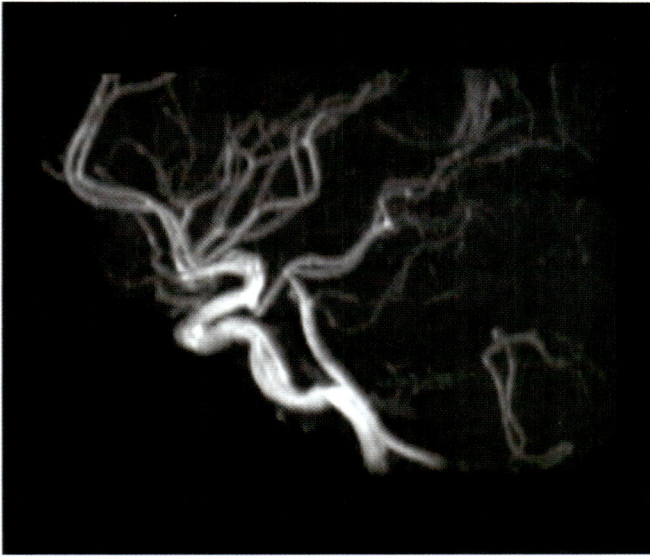
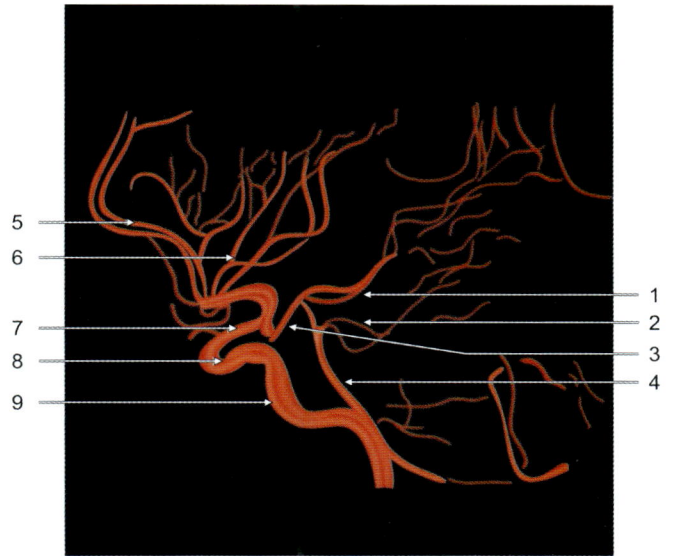

Figure 1.3

1. Posterior cerebral artery	6. Middle cerebral artery
2. Superior cerebellar artery	7. ICA, supraclinoid
3. Posterior communicating artery	8. ICA, cavernous
4. Basilar artery	9. Internal carotid artery, petrous part
5. Anterior cerebral artery	

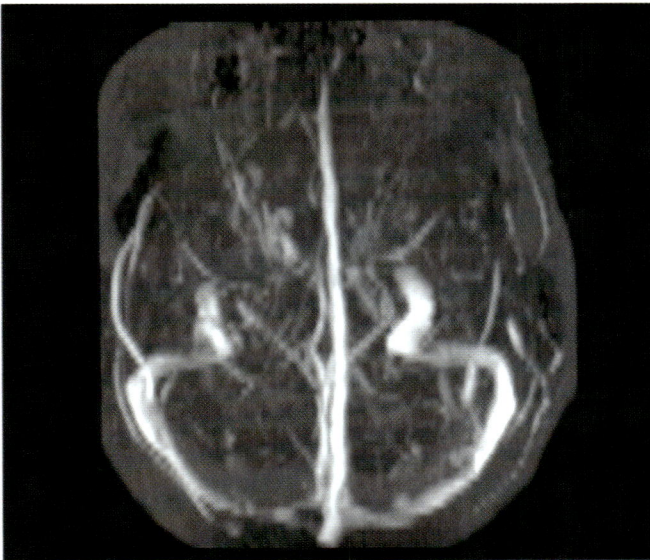
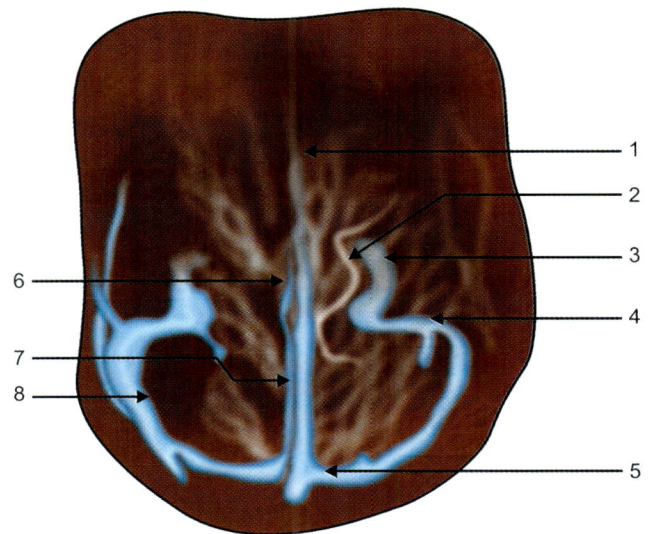

Figure 1.4

1. Superior sagittal sinus	5. Torcular herophili
2. Basal vein of Rosenthal	6. Internal cerebral vein
3. Internal jugular vein	7. Straight sinus
4. Sigmoid sinus	8. Transverse sinus

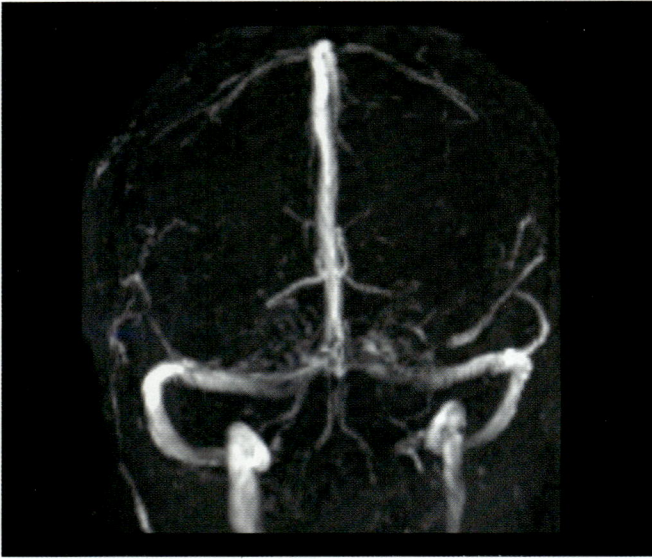
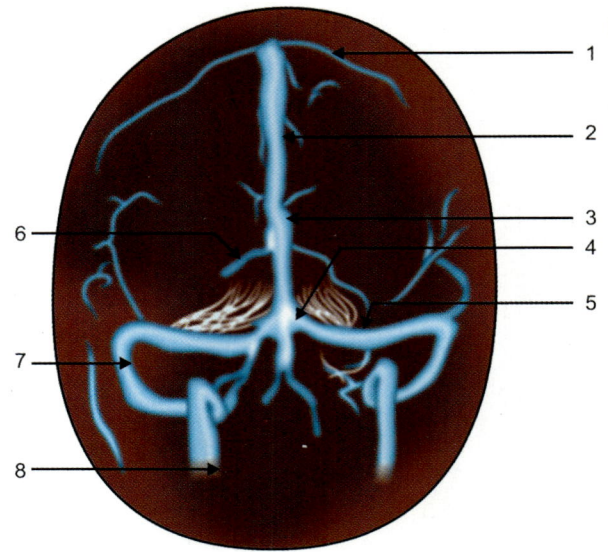

Figure 1.5

1. Cortical veins	5. Transverse sinus
2. Superior sagittal sinus	6. Basal vein of Rosenthal
3. Internal cerebral vein	7. Sigmoid sinus
4. Torcular herophili	8. Internal jugular vein

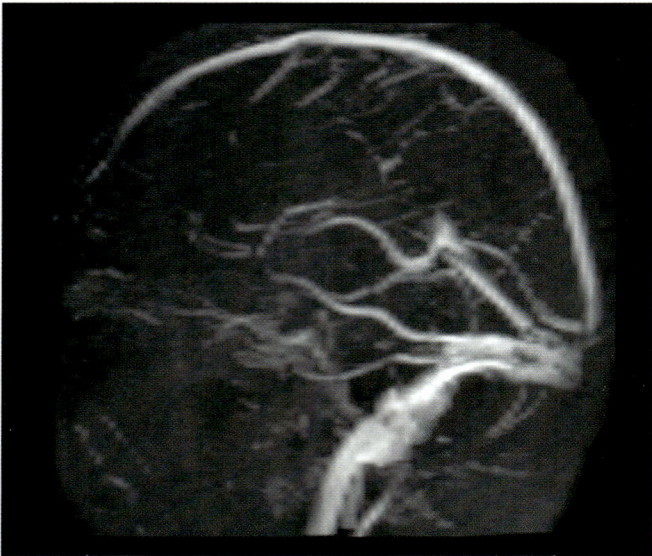
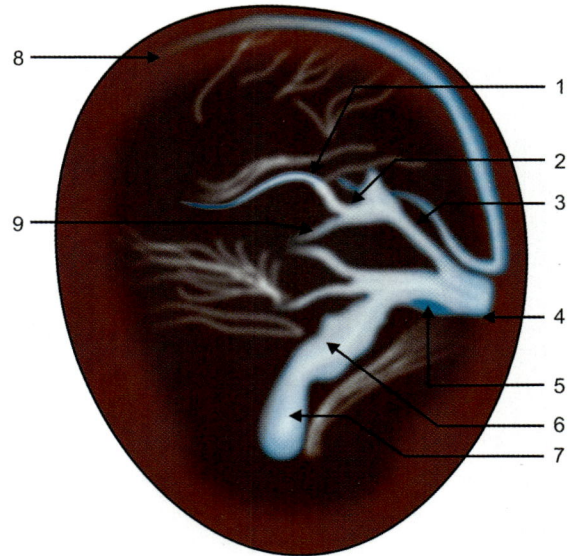

Figure 1.6

1. Internal cerebral vein	6. Sigmoid sinus
2. Vein of Galen	7. Internal jugular vein
3. Straight sinus	8. Superior sagittal sinus
4. Torcular herophili	9. Basal vein of Rosenthal
5. Transverse sinus	

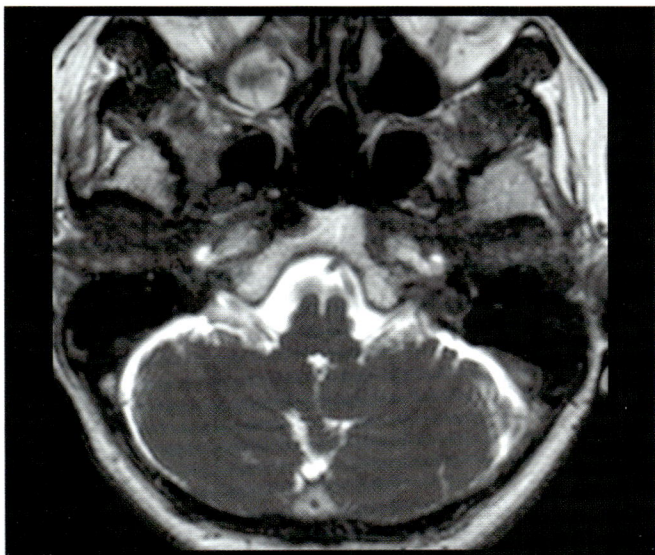

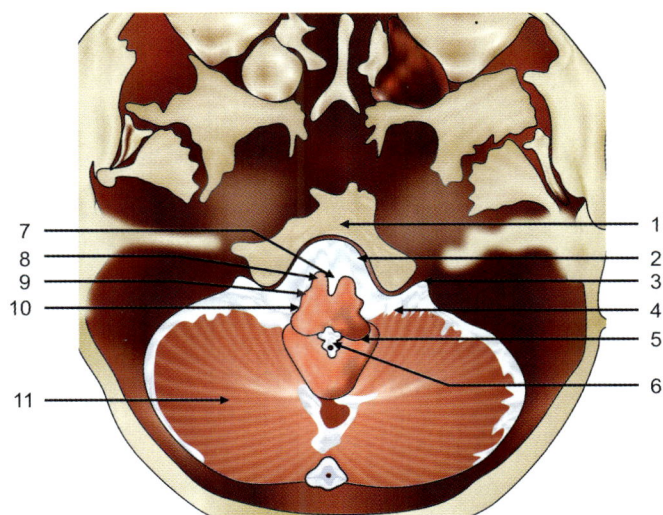

Figure 1.7

1. Clivus	7. Anterior median sulcus
2. Left vertebral artery	8. Pyramid
3. Jugular foramen	9. Olive
4. IX, X XI cranial nerves	10. Postolivary sulcus
5. Restiform body	11. Cerebellum
6. Obex	

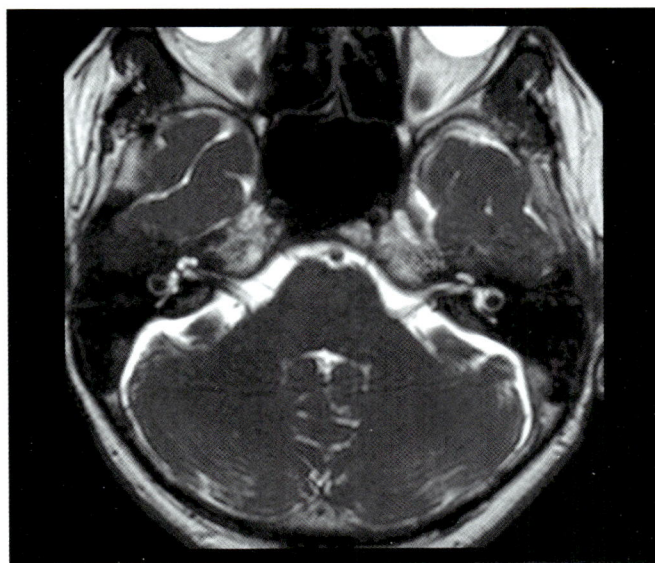

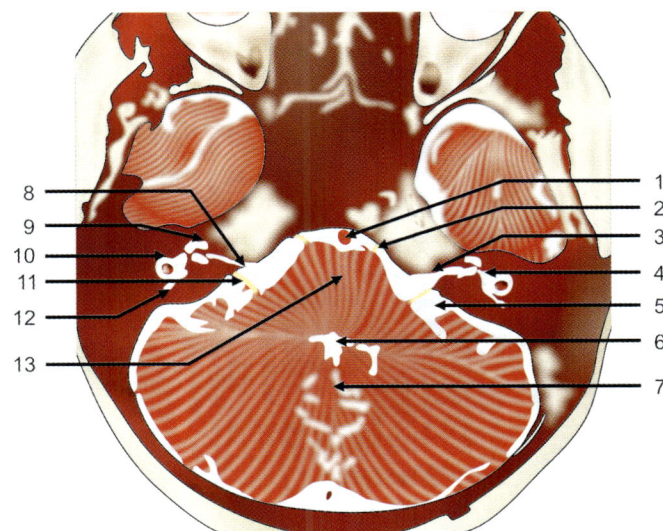

Figure 1.8

1. Basilar artery	6. Fourth ventricle	11. Vestibular nerve
2. Abducent nerve	7. Vermis	12. Posterior semicircular canal
3. Internal auditory canal	8. Facial nerve	13. Pons
4. Vestibule	9. Cochlea	
5. CP angle cistern	10. Lateral semicircular canal	

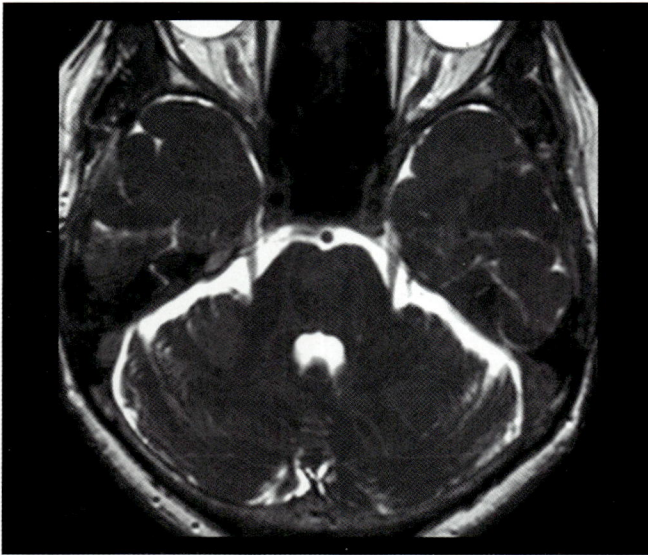

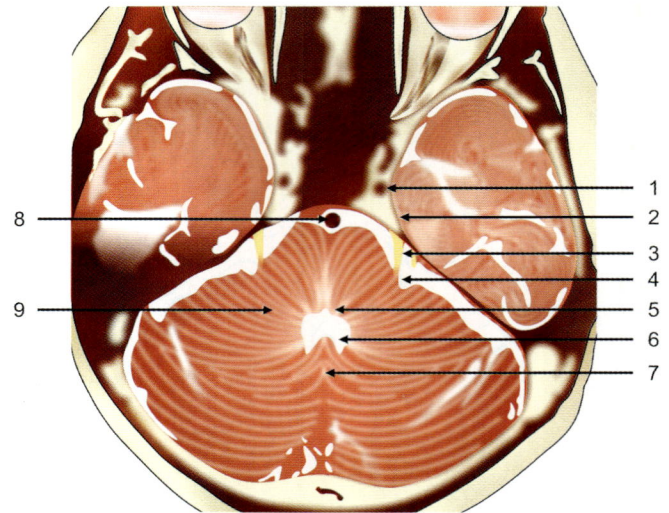

Figure 1.9

1. ICA	6. Fourth ventricle
2. Meckel's cave	7. Vermis
3. Trigeminal nerve	8. Basilar artery
4. Root entry zone	9. Middle cerebellar peduncle
5. Facial colliculus	

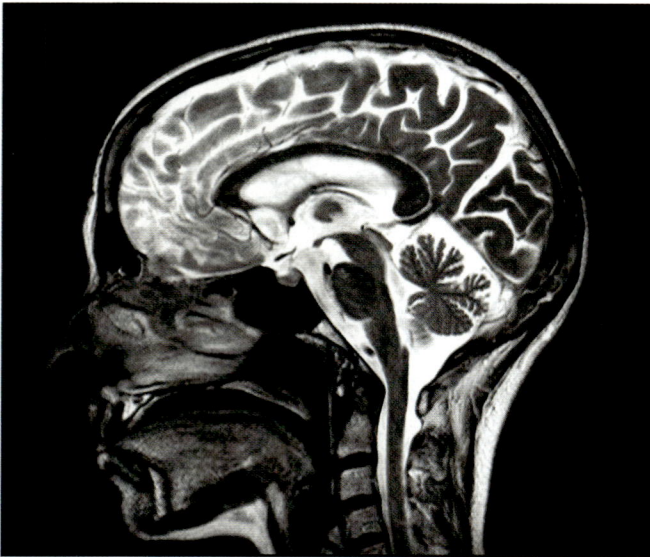

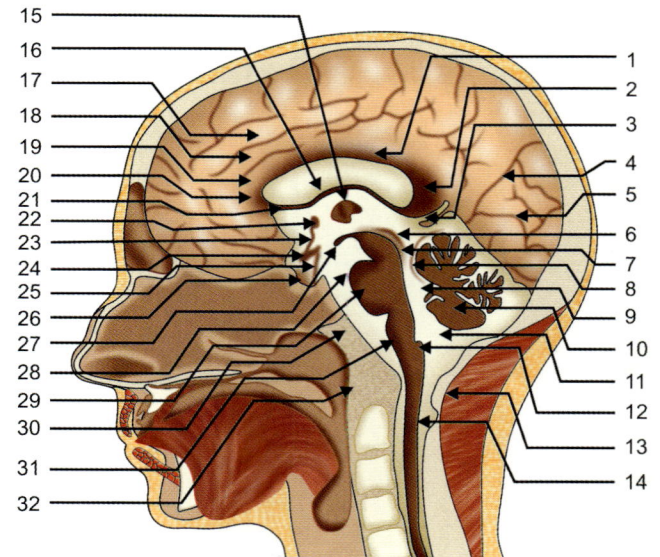

Figure 1.10

1. Corpus callosum body	9. Fourth ventricle	17. Cingulate sulcus	25. Pituitary stalk
2. Splenium	10. Cerebellum	18. Cingulate gyrus	26. Pituitary gland
3. Vein of Galen	11. Cerebellar tonsil	19. Pericallosal sulcus	27. Mammillary body
4. Parieto-occipital sulcus	12. Obex	20. Genu, corpus callosum	28. Basilar artery
5. Calcarine sulcus	13. Posterior tubercle, C1	21. Rostrum, corpus callosum	29. Pons
6. Tectum	14. Spinal cord	22. Anterior commissure	30. Clivus
7. Aqueduct of sylvius	15. Massa intermedia, thalamus	23. Anterior lamina	31. Medulla oblongata
8. Superior medullary velum	16. Fornix	24. Optic chiasm	32. Anterior tubercle C1

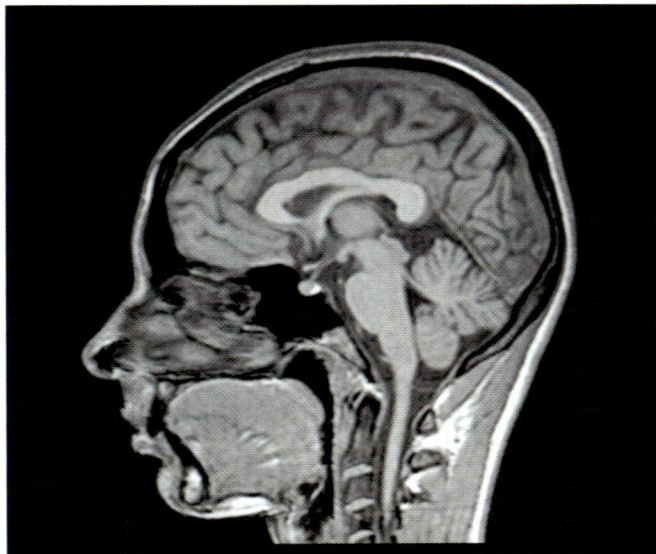

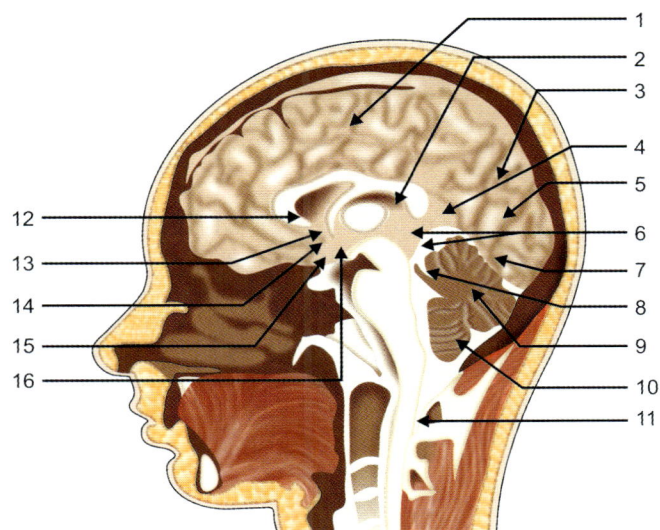

Figure 1.11

1. Cingulate sulcus	7. Straight sinus	13. Anterior commissure
2. Internal cerebral vein	8. Superior medullary velum	14. Lamina terminalis
3. Parieto-occipital sulcus	9. Vermis	15. Tuber cinereum
4. Superior cerebellar cistern	10. Tonsil	16. Third ventricle chiasmatic, infundibular recesses
5. Calcarine sulcus	11. Spinal cord	
6. Superior, inferior colliculi	12. Rostrum	

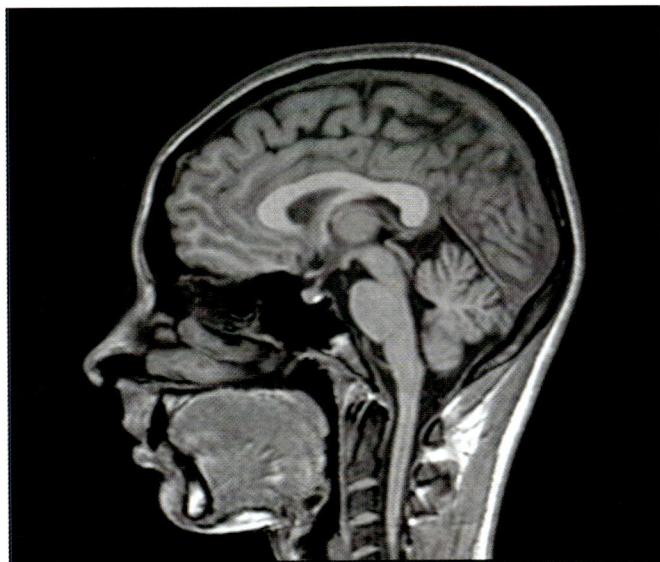

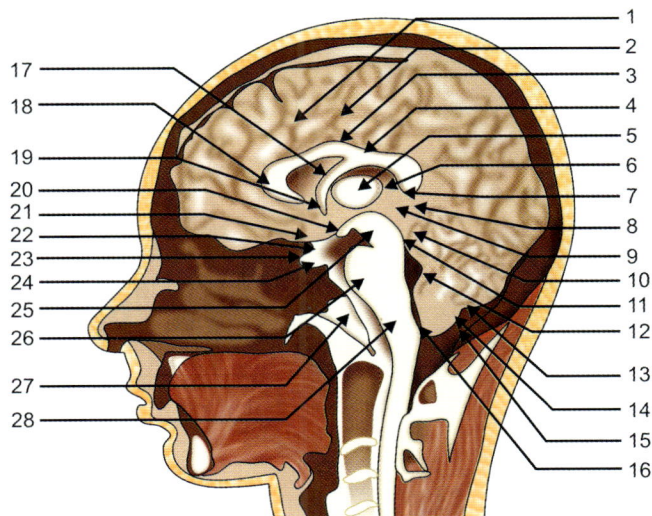

Figure 1.12

1. Cingulate gyrus	8. Pineal gland	15. Cisterna magna	22. Pituitary stalk
2. Cingulate sulcus	9. Posterior commissure	16. Foramen of Magendie	23. Anterior pituitary
3. Pericallosal sulcus	10. Tectum-midbrain	17. Fornix	24. Posterior pituitary
4. Corpus callosum	11. Aqueduct of sylvius	18. Genu	25. Midbrain
5. Massa intermedia	12. Fourth ventricle	19. Anterior commissure	26. Pons
6. Stria medullaris thalami	13. Vermis	20. Mammillary body	27. Clivus
7. Habenular commissure	14. Tonsil	21. Optic chiasm	28. Medulla oblongata

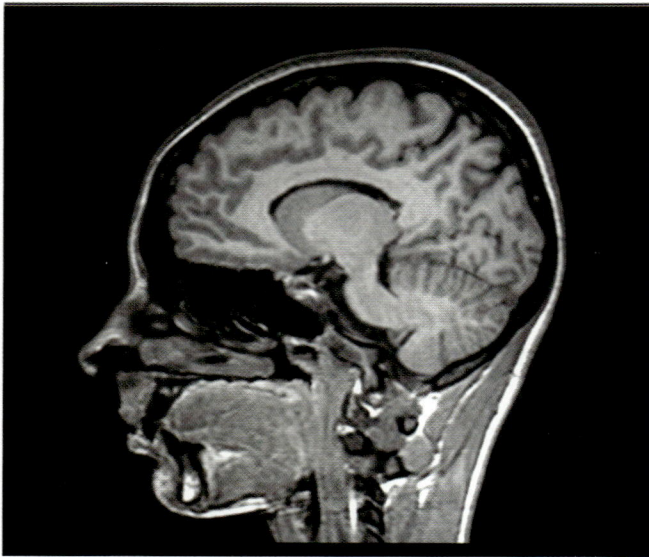

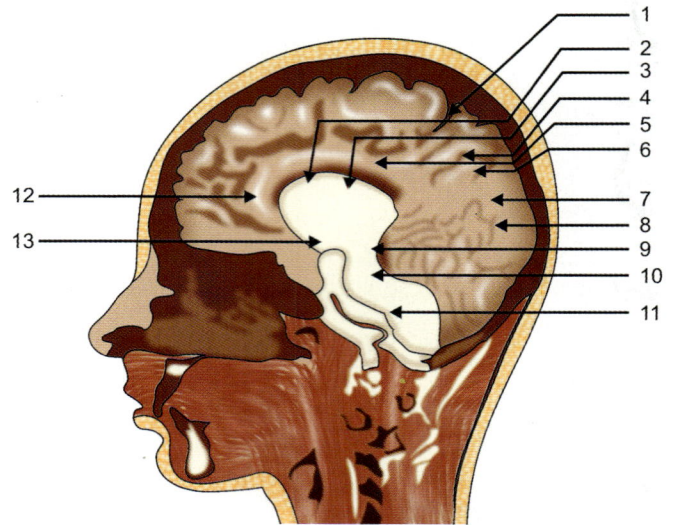

Figure 1.13

1. Cingulate sulcus	8. Calcarine sulcus
2. Caudate nucleus	9. Cerebral peduncle
3. Thalamus	10. Middle cerebellar peduncle
4. Precuneus	11. Cerebellar hemisphere
5. Lateral ventricle	12. Genu
6. Parieto-occipital sulcus	13. Optic tract
7. Cuneus	

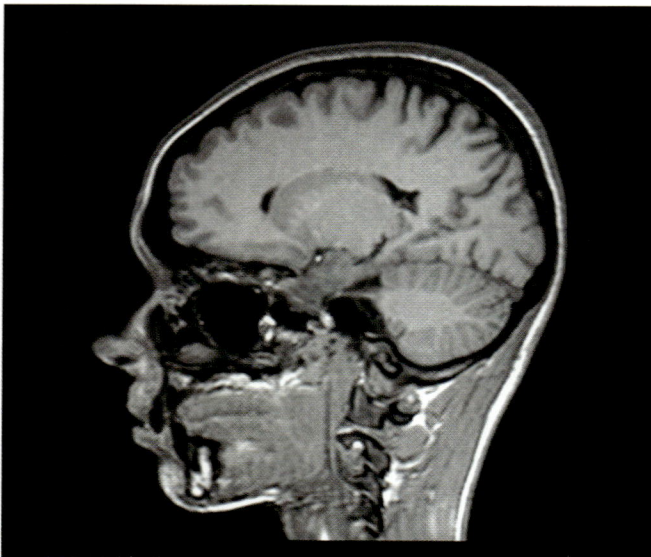

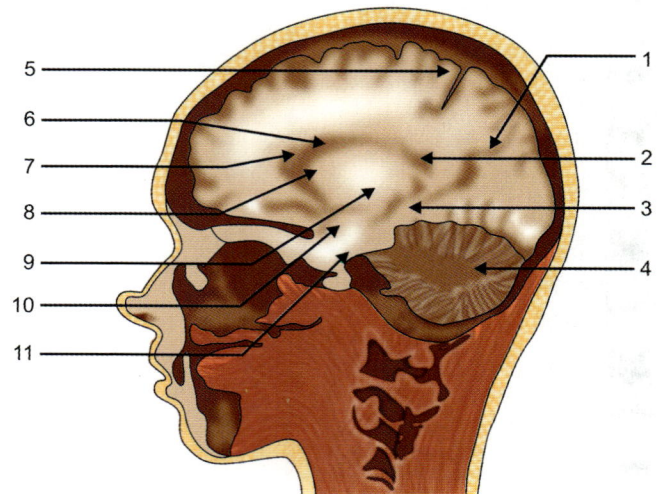

Figure 1.14

1. Parieto-occipital sulcus	7. Lateral ventricle
2. Atrium of lateral ventricle	8. Internal capsule
3. Parahippocampal gyrus	9. Thalamus
4. Cerebellar hemisphere	10. Uncus
5. Cingulate sulcus, marginal branch	11. Trigeminal nerve
6. Caudate nucleus body	

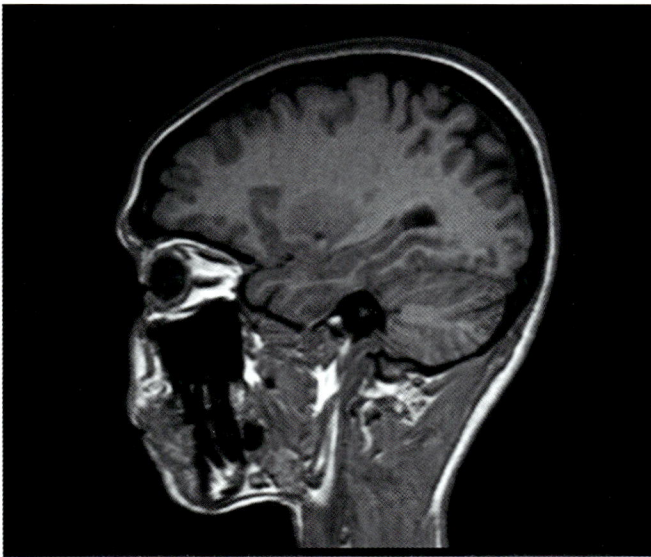

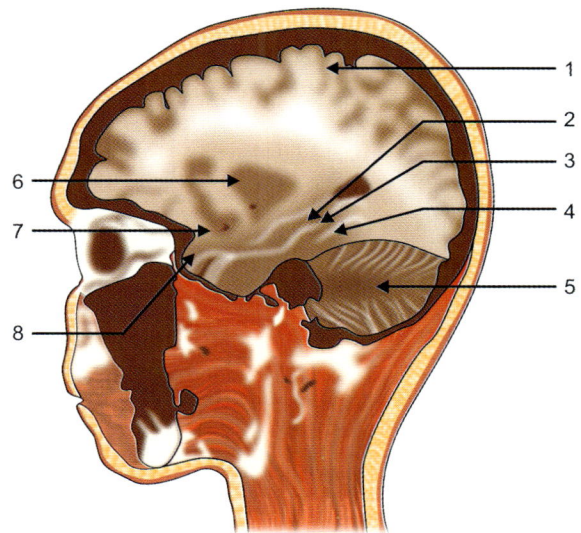

Figure 1.15

1. Central sulcus	5. Cerebellar hemisphere
2. Hippocampus	6. Putamen
3. Parahippocampal gyrus	7. Stem of lateral sulcus
4. Occipitotemporal gyrus	8. Superior temporal gyrus

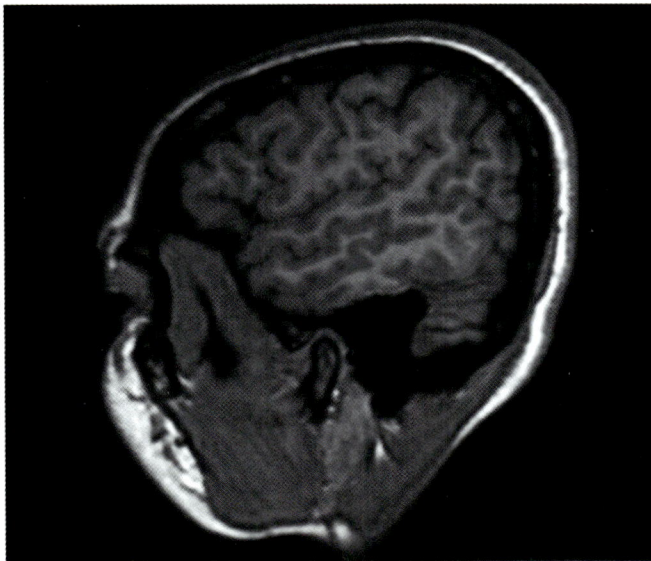

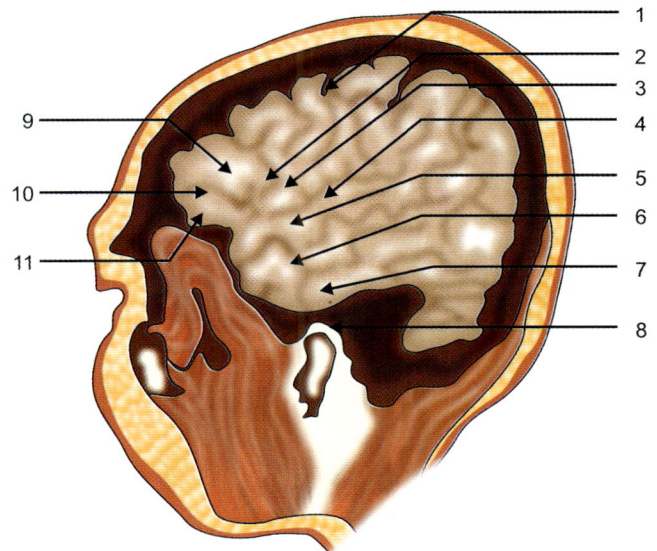

Figure 1.16

1. Central sulcus	7. Inferior temporal gyrus
2. Ascending ramus-lateral sulcus	8. TM joint
3. Pars opercularis	9. Pars triangularis
4. Lateral sulcus	10. Anterior ramus-lateral sulcus
5. Superior temporal gyrus	11. Pars orbitalis
6. Middle temporal gyrus	

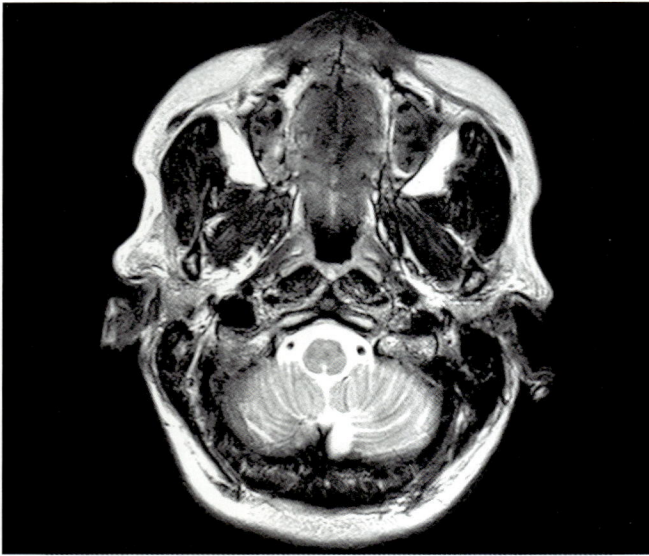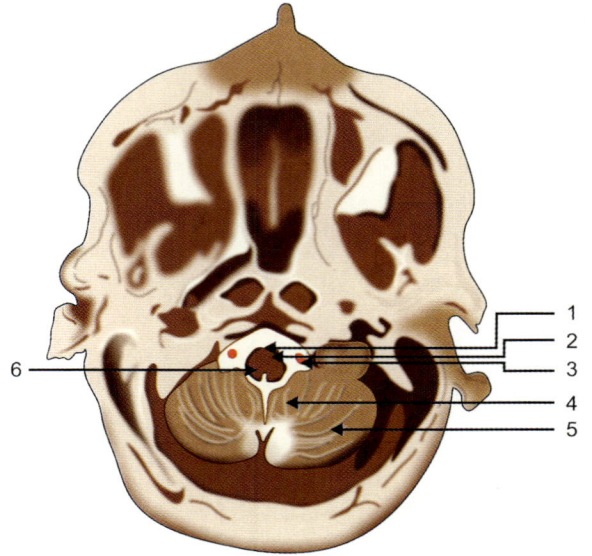

Figure 1.17

1. Median sulcus of medulla	4. Tonsil
2. Pyramid	5. Cerebellum
3. Vertebral artery	6. Medulla

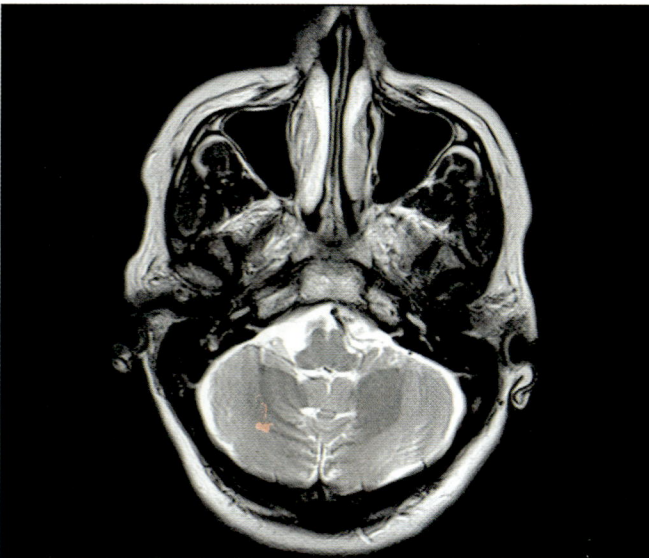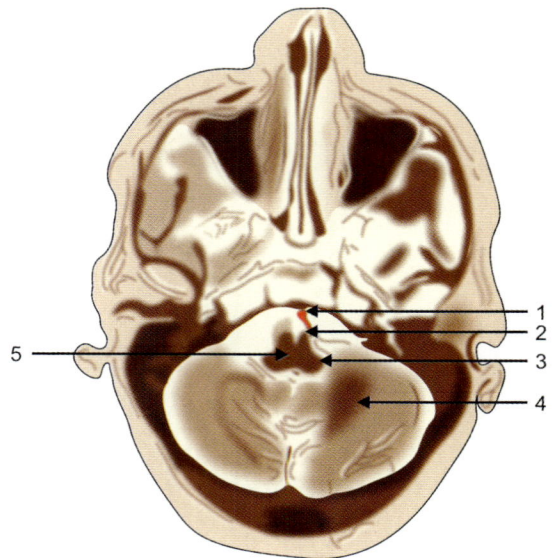

Figure 1.18

1. Basilar artery	4. Cerebellar white matter
2. Pyramid	5. Medulla
3. Inferior cerebellar peduncle	

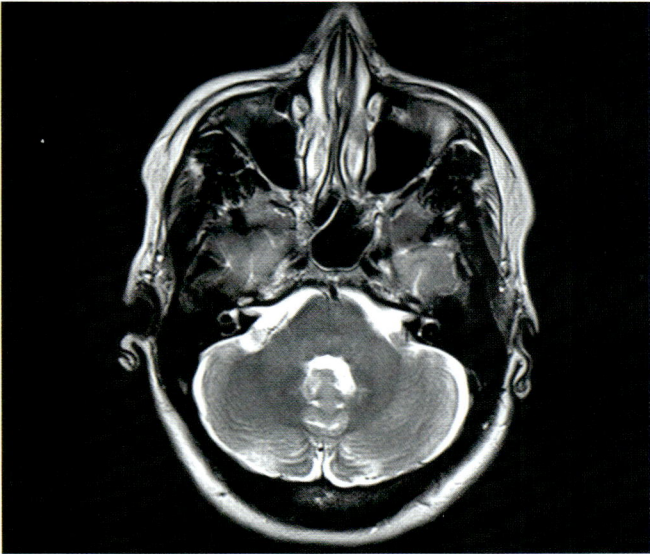

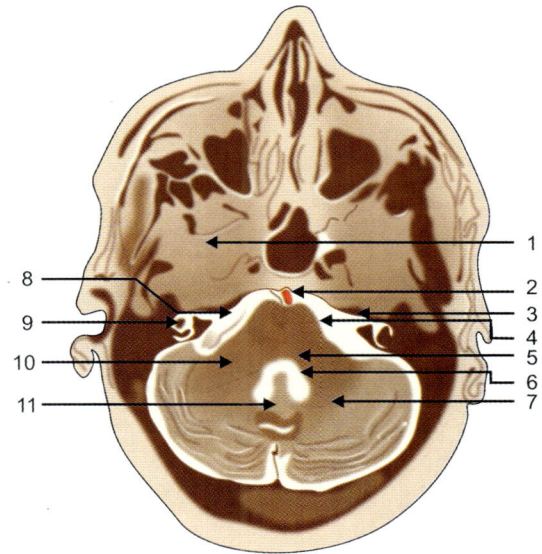

Figure 1.19

1. Temporal lobe
2. Basilar artery
3. Internal auditory canal
4. Pons
5. Medial longitudinal fasciculus
6. Fourth ventricle
7. Cerebellar white matter
8. Cerebellopontine cistern
9. Semicircular canals
10. Middle cerebellar peduncle
11. Vermis

Figure 1.20

1. Temporal pole
2. Sphenoid sinus
3. Basilar artery
4. Pons
5. Middle cerebellar peduncle
6. Superior cerebellar peduncle
7. Cerebellar vermis
8. Trigeminal nerve
9. Medial longitudinal fasciculus
10. Fourth ventricle

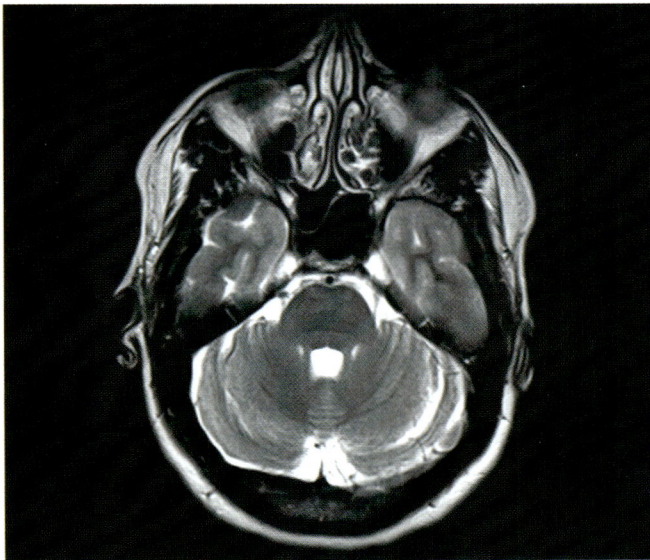

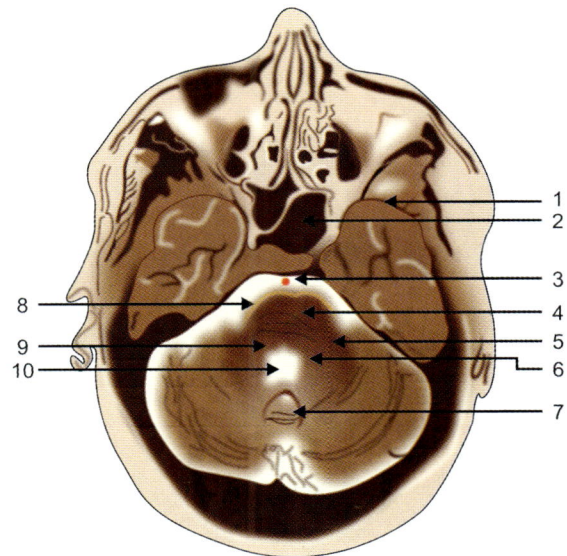

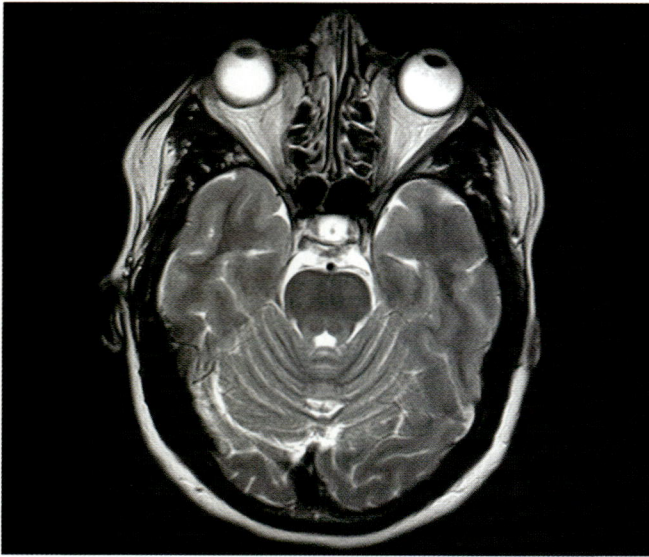

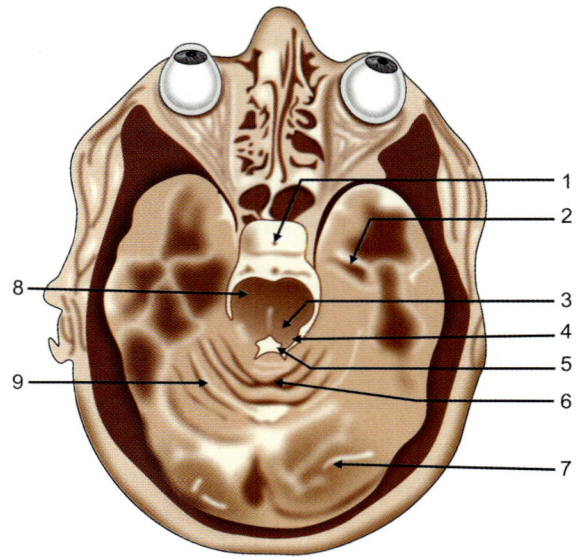

Figure 1.21

1. Pituitary stalk	4. Superior cerebellar peduncle	7. Occipital lobe
2. Temporal horn of lateral ventricle	5. Fourth ventricle	8. Pons
3. Medial longitudinal fasciculus	6. Vermis	9. Cerebellum

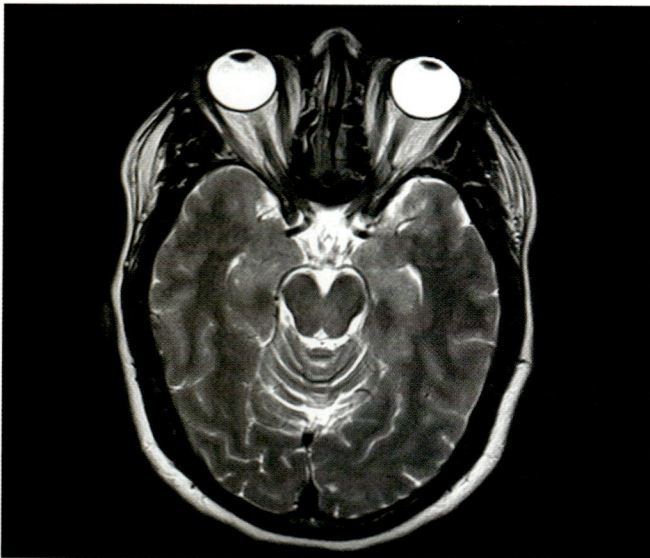

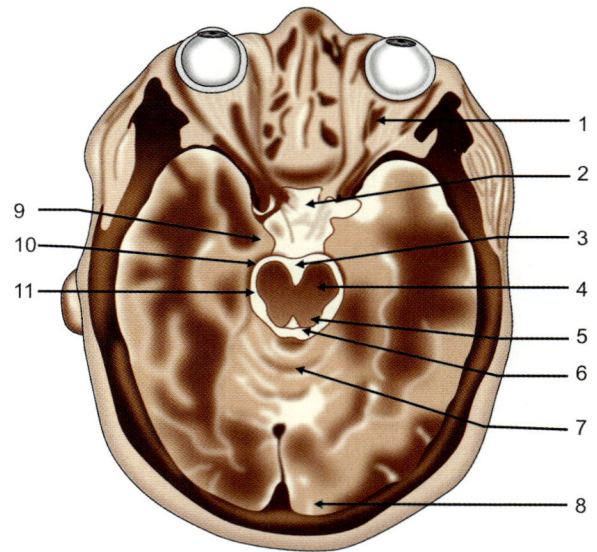

Figure 1.22

1. Optic nerve	5. Inferior colliculus	8. Occipital pole
2. Suprasellar cistern	6. Quadrigeminal plate cistern	9. Uncus
3. Interpeduncular fossa	7. Superior vermis	10. Posterior cerebellar artery
4. Cerebral peduncle		11. Ambient cistern

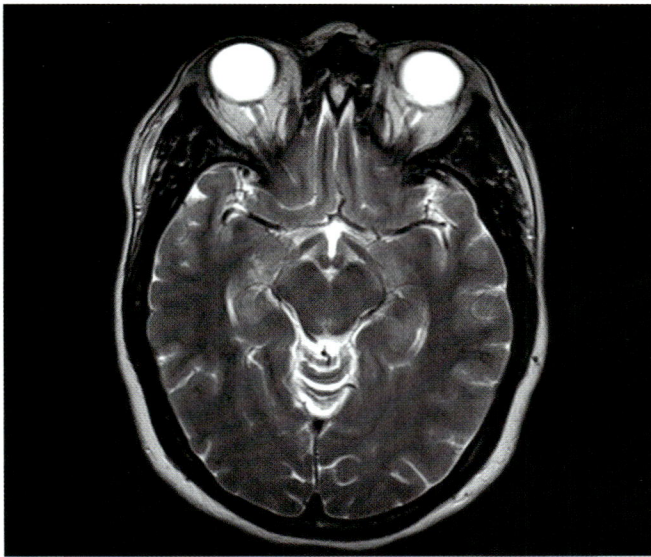

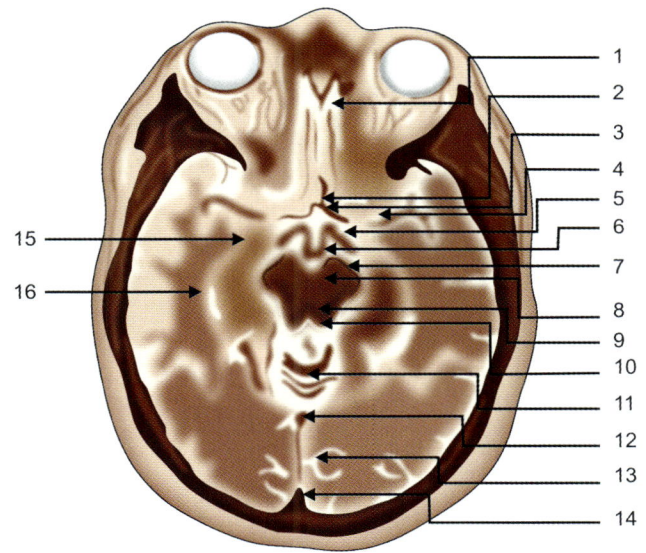

Figure 1.23

1. Gyrus rectus	7. Crus cerebri	13. Calcarine sulcus
2. Ant communicating artery	8. Red nucleus	14. Superior sagittal sinus
3. Ant cerebral artery	9. Aqueduct of sylvius	15. Uncus
4. Middle cerebral artery	10. Superior colliculus	16. Temporal horn
5. Optic tract	11. Superior vermis	
6. Mammillary body	12. Straight sinus	

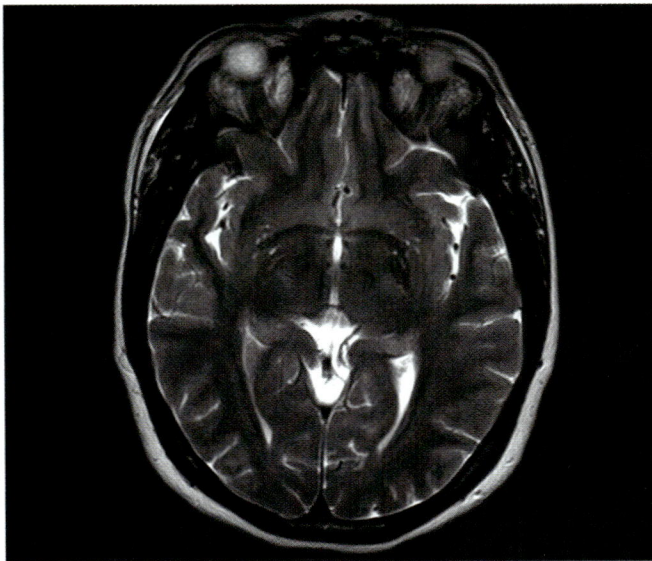

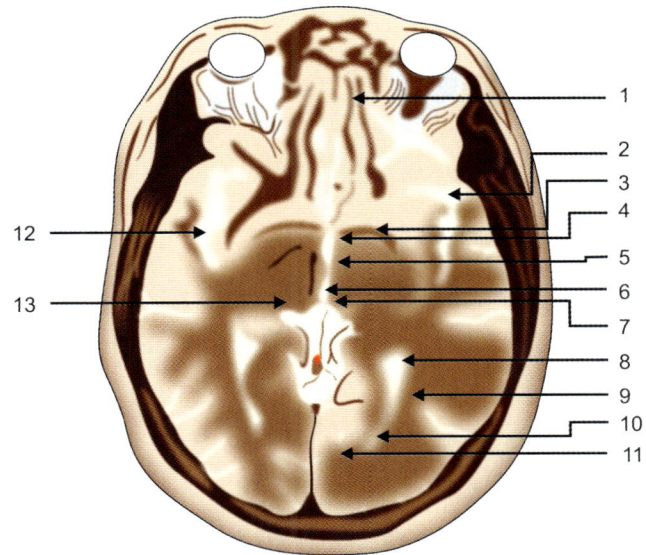

Figure 1.24

1. Gyrus rectus	6. Third ventricle	11. Calcarine fissure
2. Sylvian (lateral) fissure	7. Posterior commissure	12. Insula
3. Anterior commissure	8. Atrium of lateral ventricle	13. Pulvinar
4. Fornix	9. Optic radiation	
5. Mammillothalamic tract	10. Occipital horn	

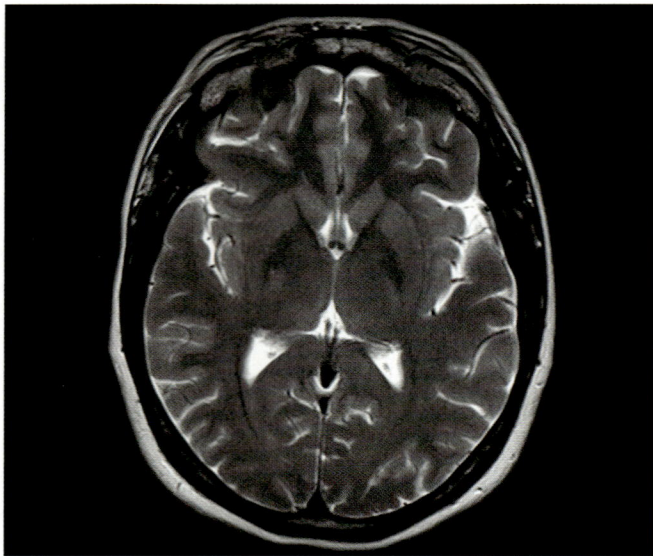

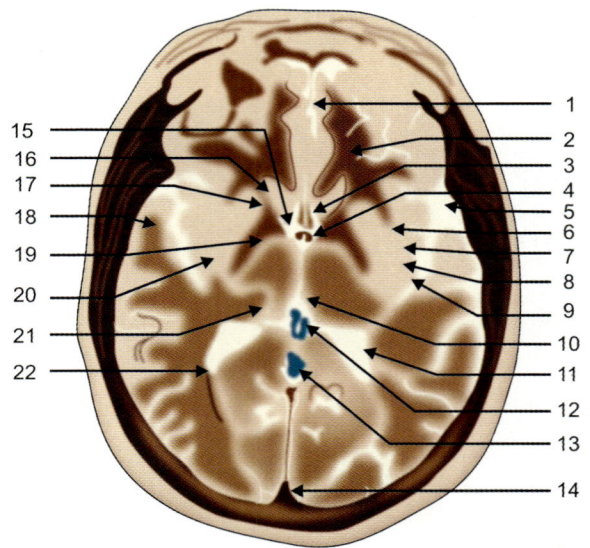

Figure 1.25

1. Anterior interhemispheric fissure	9. Insular cortex	17. Internal capsule ant.limb
2. Forceps minor	10. Stria medullaris thalami	18. Temporal operculum
3. Septum pellucidum	11. Atrium of lateral ventricle	19. Globus pallidus
4. Fornix	12. Internal cerebral veins	20. Putamen
5. Sylvian fissure	13. Vein of Galen	21. Pulvinar of thalamus
6. External capsule	14. Superior sagittal sinus	22. Optic radiation
7. Claustrum	15. Foramen of Monroe	
8. Extreme capsule	16. Caudate nucleus	

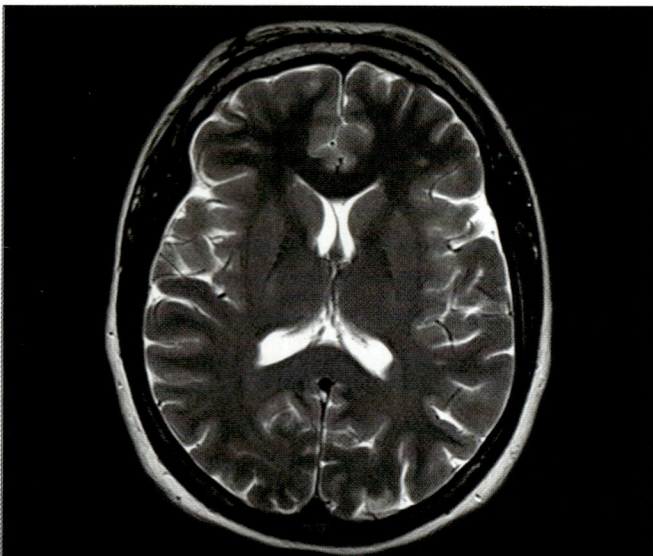

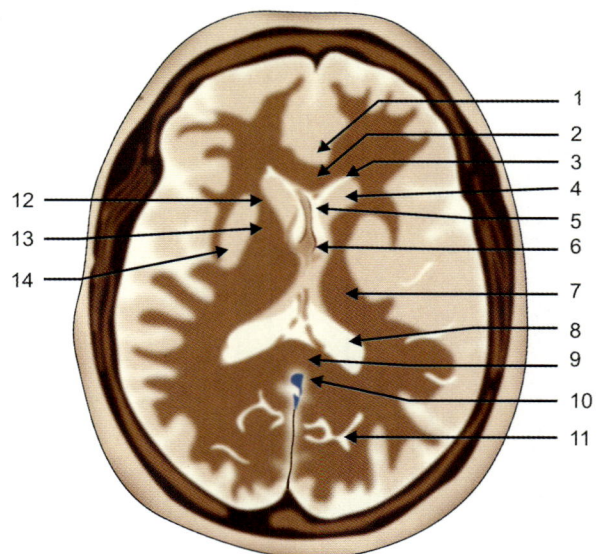

Figure 1.26

1. ACA branches	6. Fornix	11. Parieto-occipital sulcus
2. Genu of corpus callosum	7. Thalamus	12. Anterior limb of internal capsule
3. Frontal horn of lateral ventricle	8. Tail of caudate nucleus	13. Globus pallidus
4. Head of caudate nucleus	9. Splenium of corpus callosum	14. Putamen
5. Septum pellucidum	10. Vein of Galen	

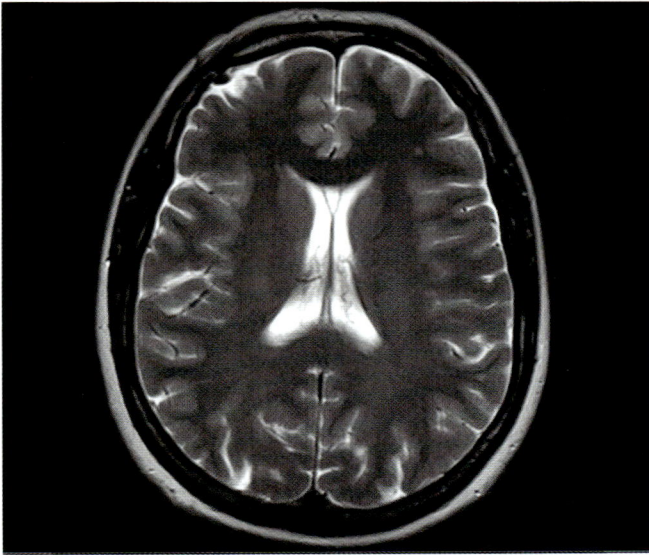

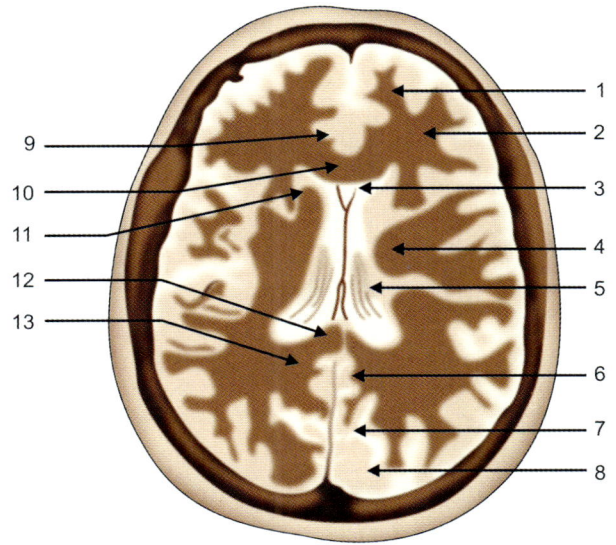

Figure 1.27

1. Superior frontal gyrus	6. Cingulate gyrus	11. Caudate nucleus head
2. Middle frontal gyrus	7. Parieto-occipital sulcus	12. Splenium corpus callosum
3. Septum pellucidum	8. Occipital lobe	13. Forceps major
4. Corona radiata	9. Cingulate gyrus	
5. Body of lateral ventricle	10. Genu of corpus callosum	

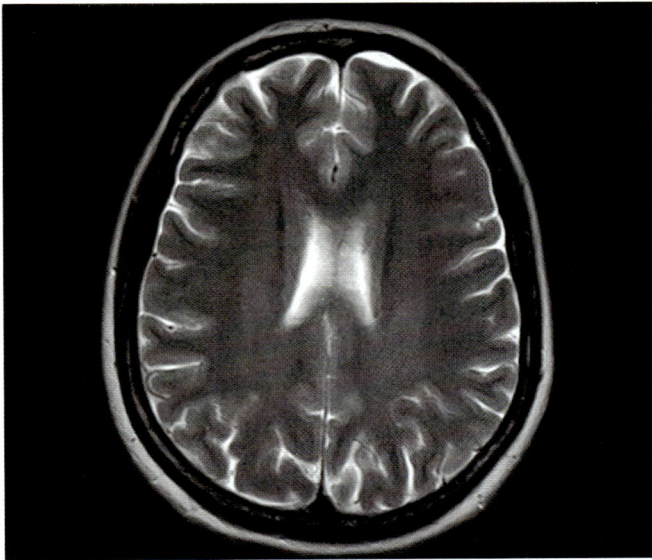

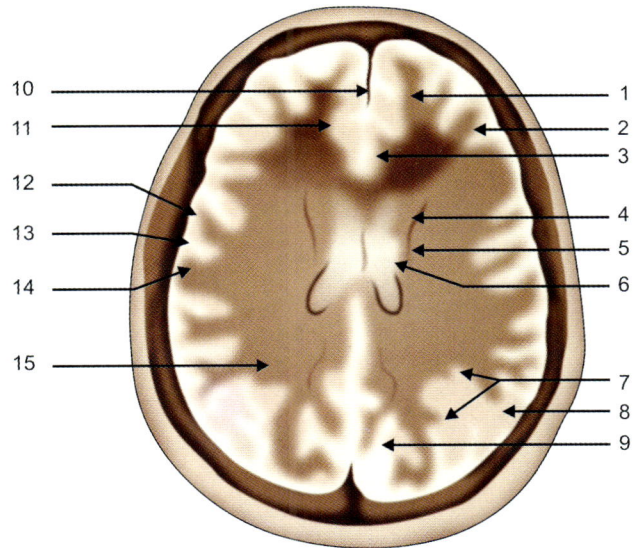

Figure 1.28

1. Superior frontal gyrus	6. Lateral ventricle	11. Cingulate sulcus
2. Middle frontal gyrus	7. Intraparietal sulcus	12. Precentral gyrus
3. Cingulate gyrus	8. Inferior parietal lobule	13. Central sulcus
4. Body of caudate nucleus	9. Parieto-occipital sulcus	14. Postcentral gyrus
5. Corona radiata	10. Interhemispheric fissure	15. Superior parietal lobule

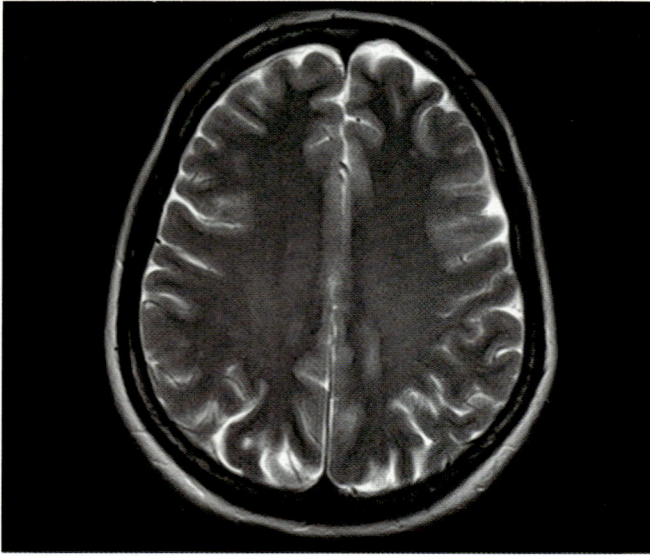

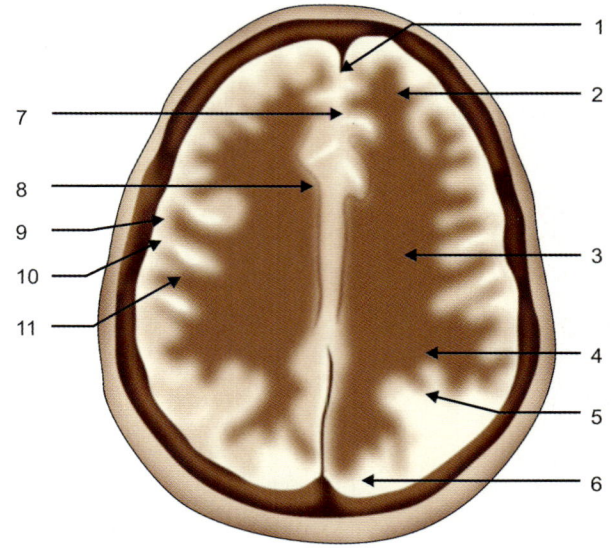

Figure 1.29

1. Interhemispheric fissure	7. Cingulate sulcus
2. Superior frontal gyrus	8. Cingulate gyrus
3. Centrum semiovale	9. Precentral gyrus
4. Superior parietal lobule	10. Central sulcus
5. Intraparietal sulcus	11. Postcentral gyrus
6. Parieto-occipital sulcus	

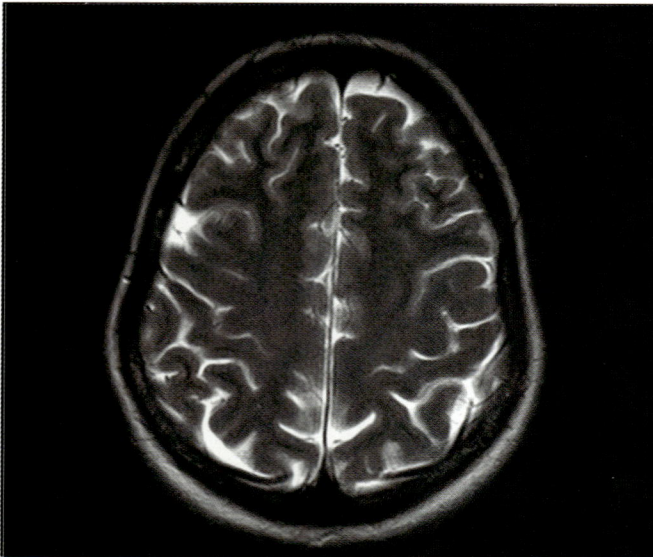

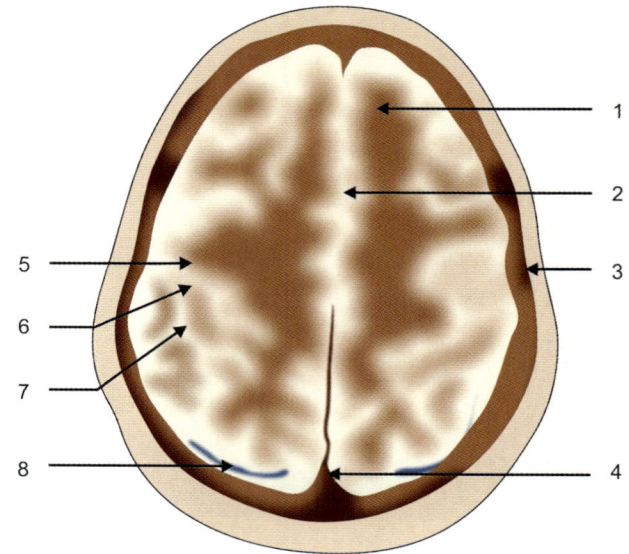

Figure 1.30

1. Superior frontal gyrus	5. Precentral gyrus
2. Interhemispheric fissure	6. Central sulcus
3. Diploic space	7. Postcentral gyrus
4. Superior sagittal sinus	8. Cortical vein

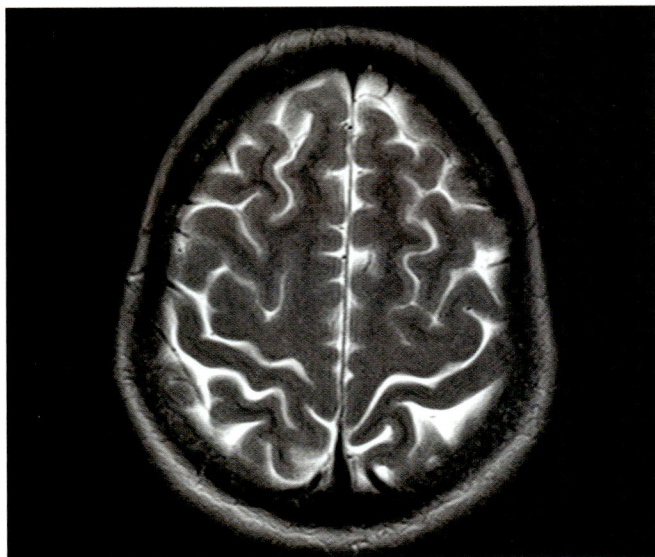

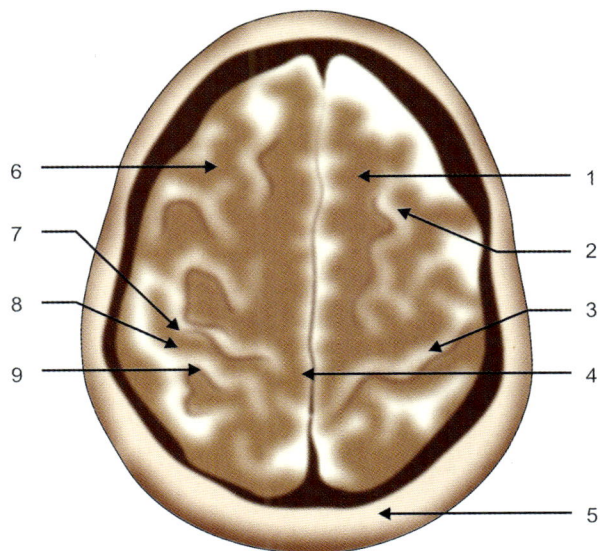

Figure 1.31

1. Superior frontal gyrus	6. Middle frontal gyrus
2. Superior frontal sulcus	7. Central sulcus
3. Central sulcus	8. Postcentral gyrus
4. Paracentral lobule	9. Postcentral sulcus
5. Scalp	

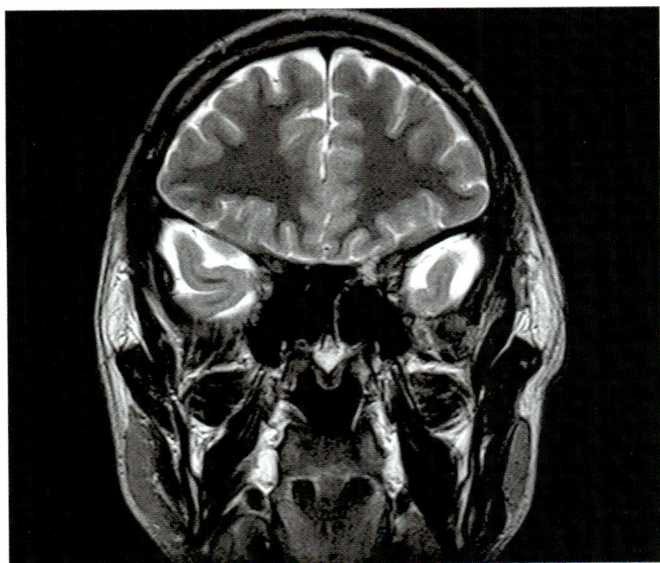

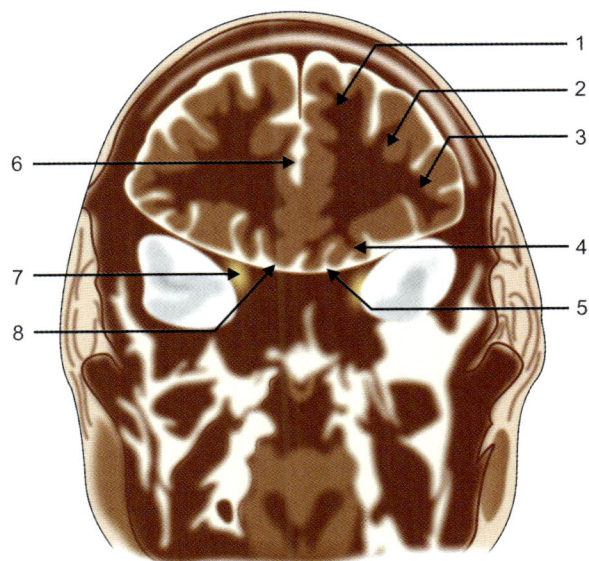

Figure 1.32

1. Superior frontal gyrus	5. Olfactory sulcus
2. Middle frontal gyrus	6. Interhemispheric fissure
3. Inferior frontal gyrus	7. Optic nerve
4. Orbital gyri	8. Gyrus rectus

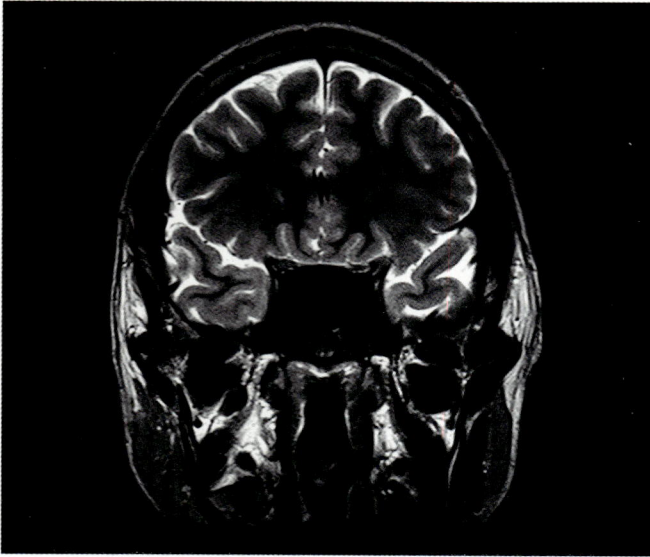

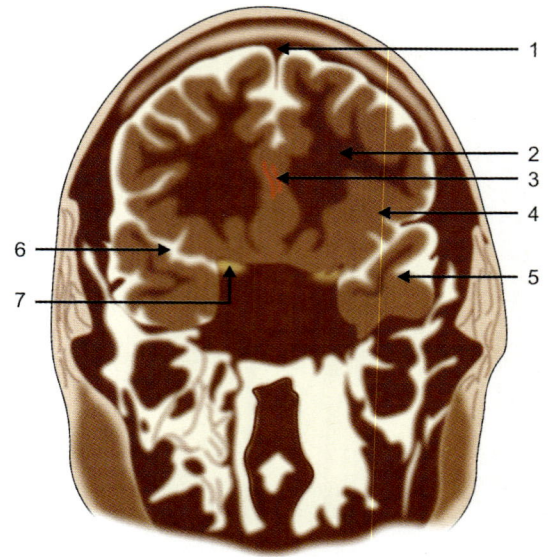

Figure 1.33

1. Superior sagittal sinus	5. Temporal lobe
2. Forceps minor	6. Sylvian fissure, stem
3. Anterior cerebral artery	7. Optic nerve
4. Frontal operculum	

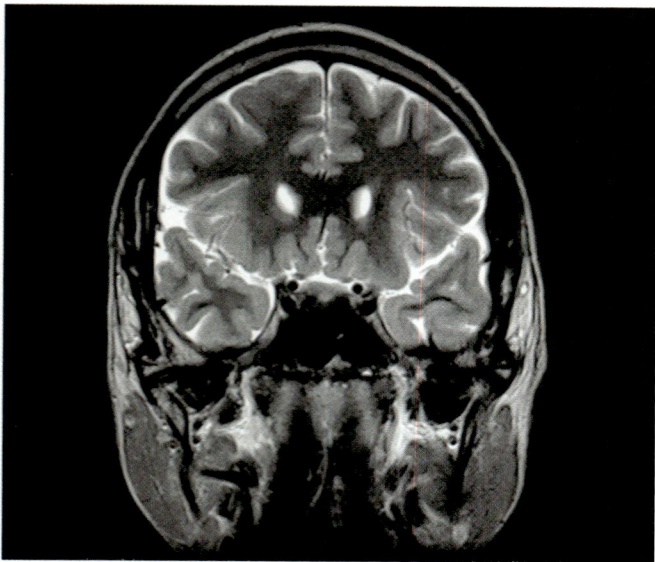

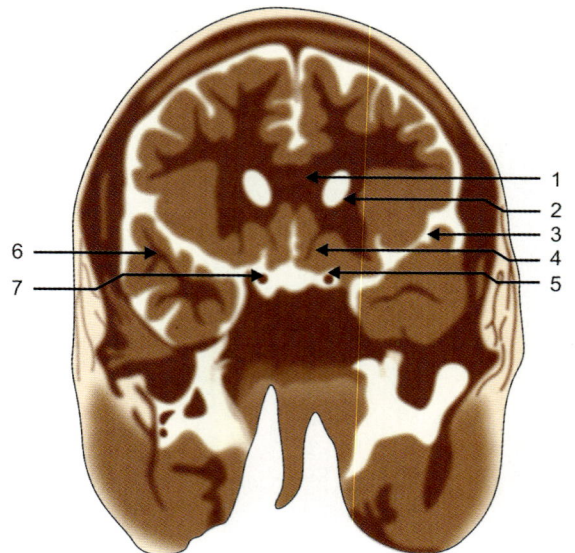

Figure 1.34

1. Genu of corpus callosum	5. Optic nerve
2. Frontal horn of lateral ventricle	6. Temporal operculum
3. Sylvian fissure	7. ICA
4. Gyrus rectus	

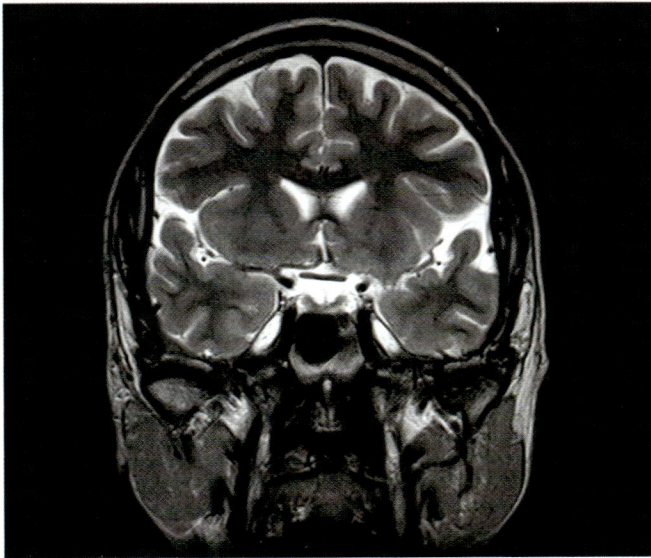

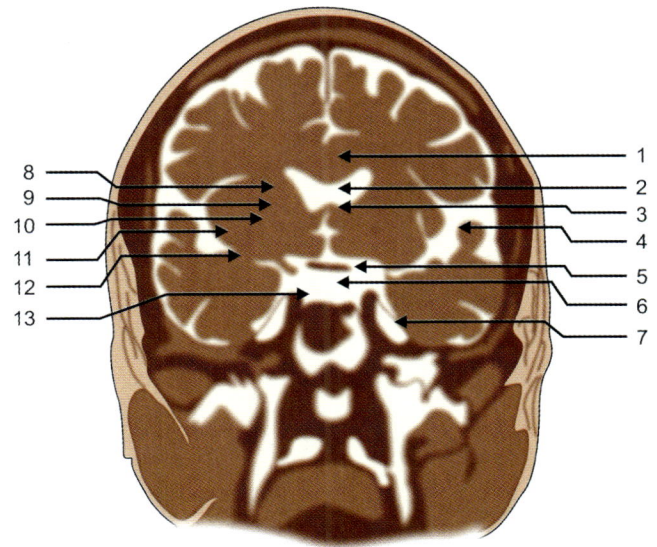

Figure 1.35

1. Pericallosal artery	8. Caudate nucleus head
2. Septum pellucidum	9. Internal capsule
3. Rostrum of corpus callosum	10. Putamen
4. Sylvian fissure	11. Insula
5. Optic chiasm	12. MCA
6. Suprasellar cistern	13. Pituitary gland
7. Meckel's cave	

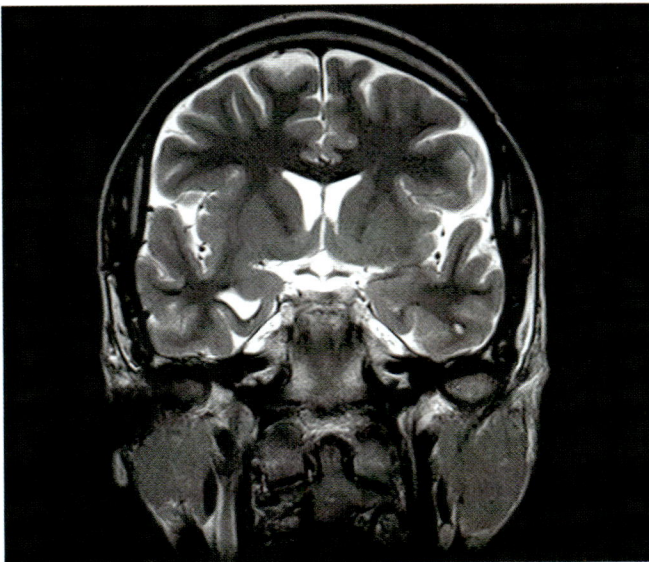

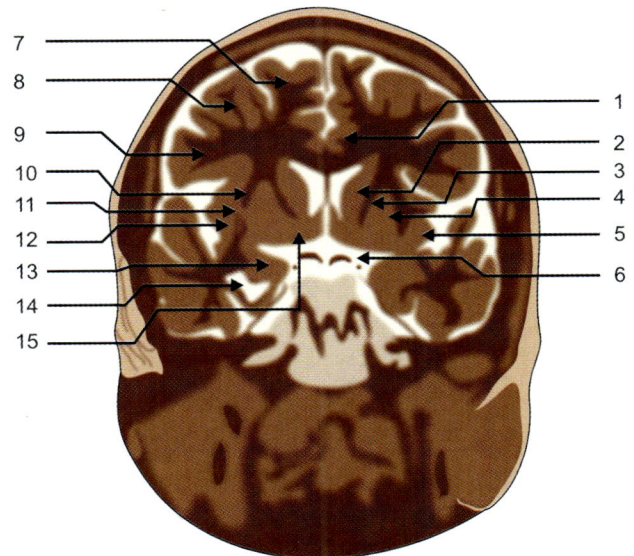

Figure 1.36

1. Cingulate gyrus	6. Optic tract	11. Claustrum
2. Caudate nucleus	7. Superior frontal gyrus	12. External capsule
3. Internal capsule	8. Middle frontal gyrus	13. Uncus
4. Putamen	9. Inferior frontal gyrus	14. Temporal horn
5. Insula	10. External capsule	15. Fundus striati

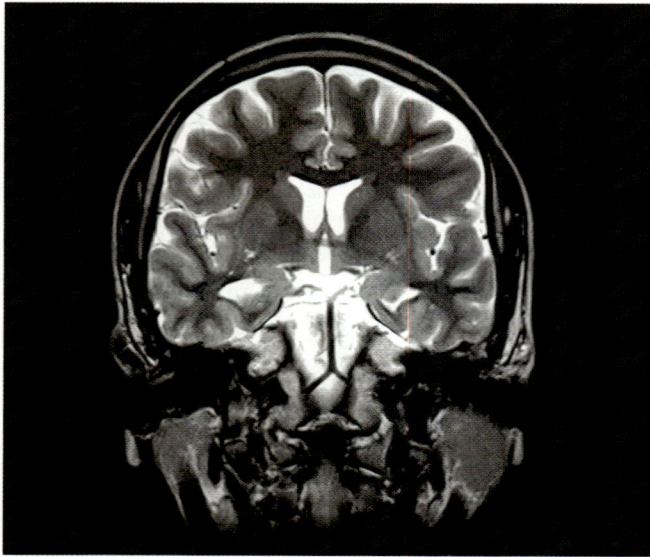

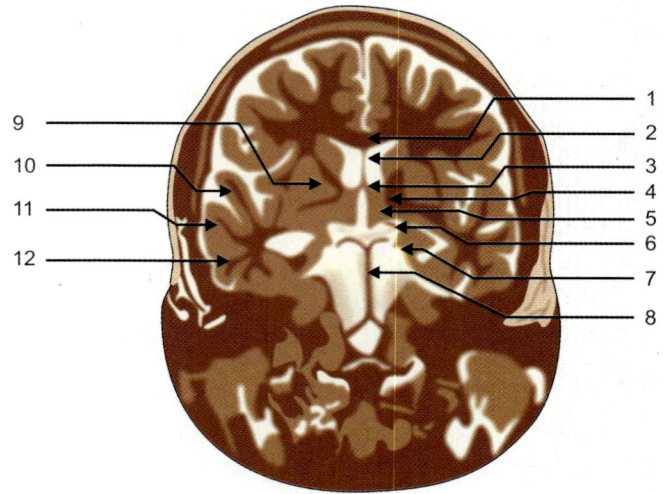

Figure 1.37

1.	Corpus callosum body	7.	Oculomotor nerve
2.	Septum pellucidum	8.	Basilar artery
3.	Fornix	9.	Globus pallidus
4.	Anterior commissure	10.	Superior temporal gyrus
5.	Innominate substance	11.	Middle temporal gyrus
6.	Optic tract	12.	Inferior temporal gyrus

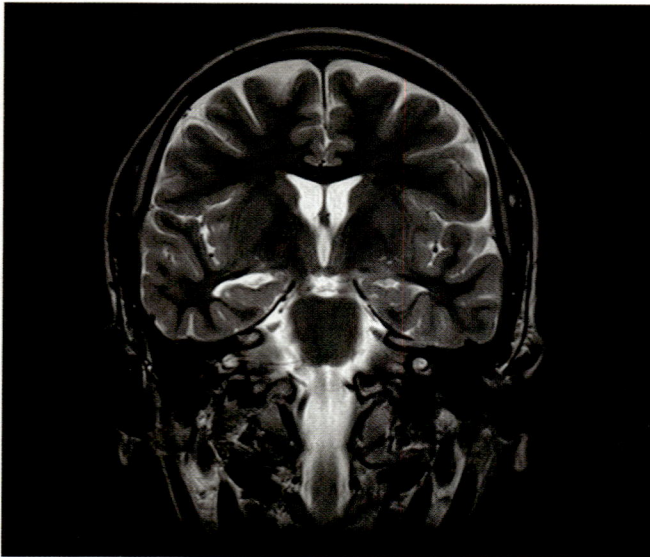

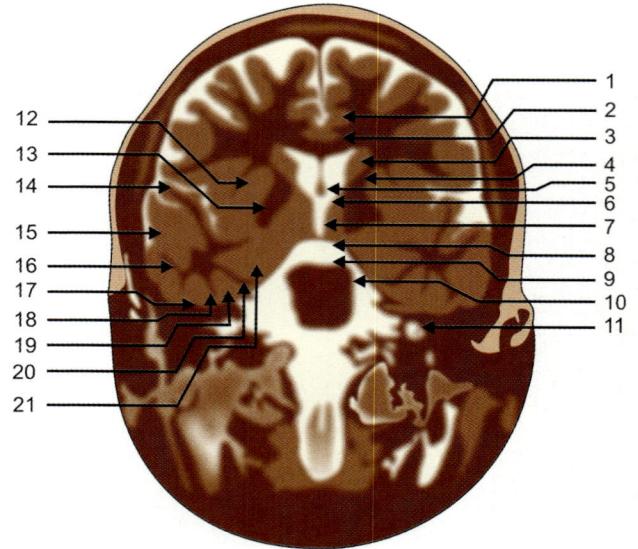

Figure 1.38

1.	Cingulate sulcus	8.	Mammillary body	15.	Middle temporal gyrus
2.	Pericallosal sulcus	9.	Interpeduncular cistern	16.	Inferior temporal gyrus
3.	Caudate nucleus	10.	Pons	17.	Occipitotemporal sulcus
4.	Internal capsule	11.	Cochlea	18.	Occipitotemporal gyrus
5.	Fornix	12.	Putamen	19.	Collateral sulcus
6.	Foramen of Monro	13.	Globus pallidus	20.	Parahippocampal
7.	Third ventricle	14.	Superior temporal gyrus	21.	Hippocampus

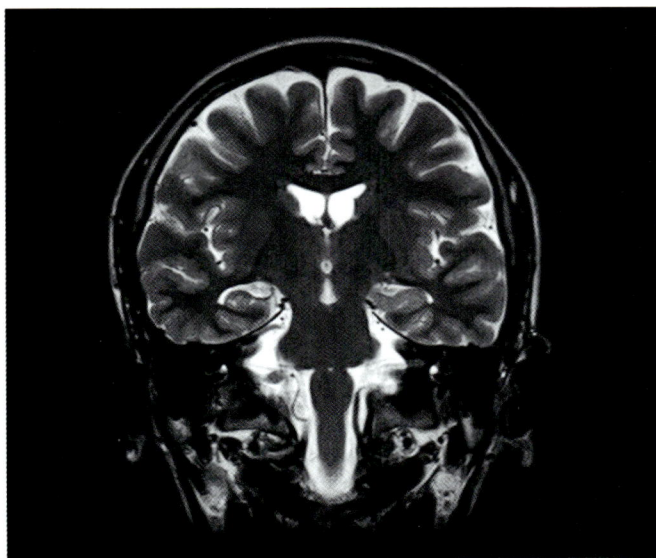

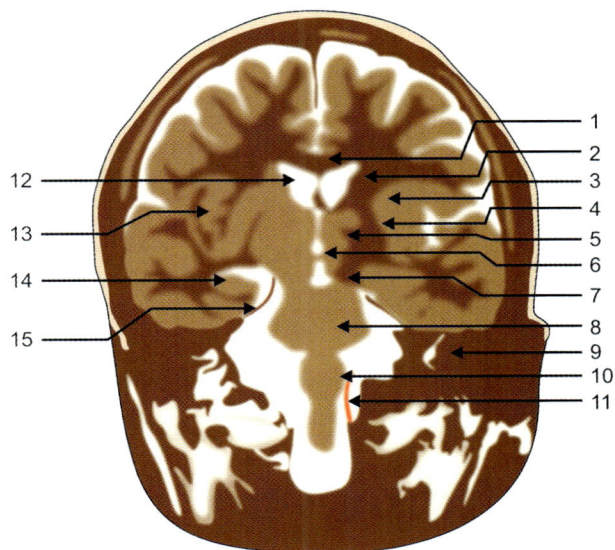

Figure 1.39

1. Corpus callosum	6. Third ventricle	11. Vertebral artery
2. Caudate nucleus	7. Cerebral peduncle	12. Lateral ventricle
3. Putamen	8. Pons	13. Insula
4. Internal capsule	9. Vestibule	14. Hippocampus
5. Thalamus	10. Medulla	15. Tentorium

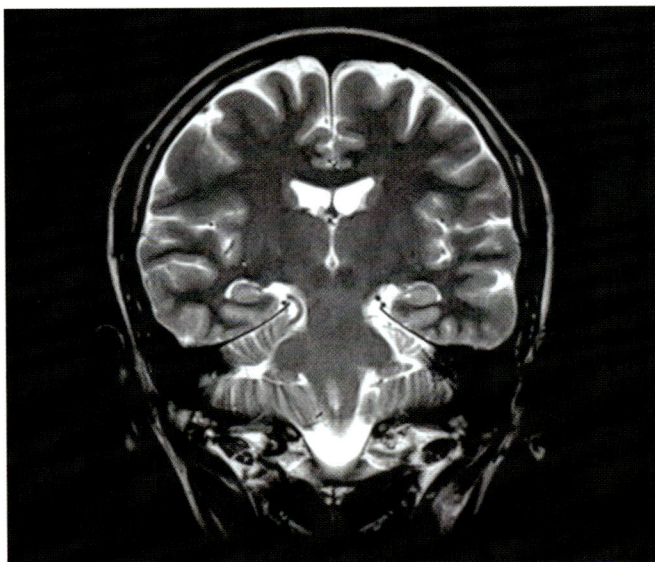

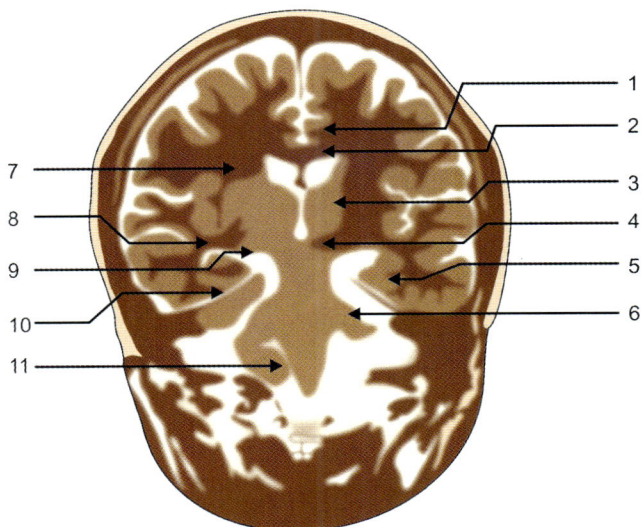

Figure 1.40

1. Cingulate gyrus	7. Corona radiata
2. Corpus callosum	8. Lateral geniculate body
3. Thalamus	9. Medial geniculate body
4. Red nucleus	10. Tentorium cerebelli
5. Parahippocampal gyrus	11. Inferior cerebellar peduncle
6. Middle cerebellar peduncle	

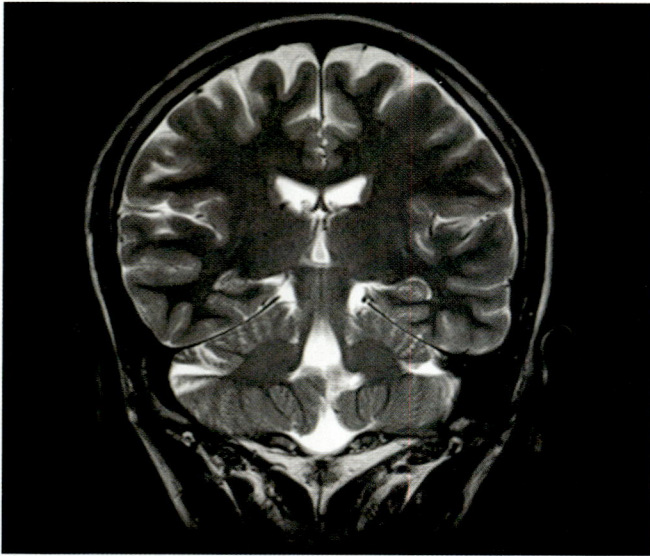

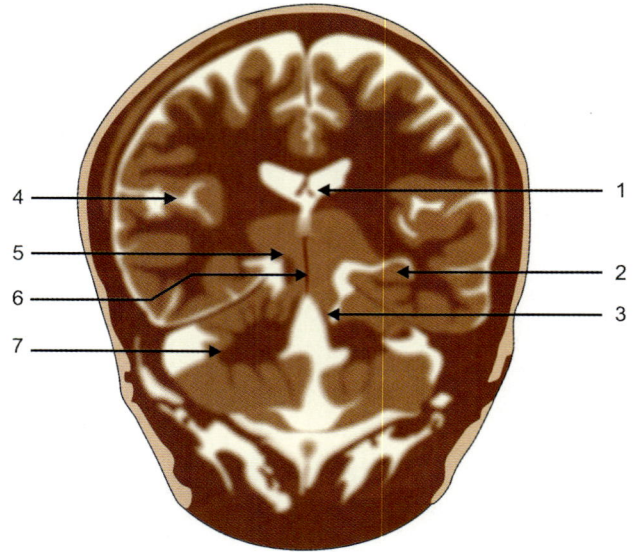

Figure 1.41

1. Fornix	5. Superior colliculus
2. Hippocampus body	6. Aqueduct of sylvius
3. Superior cerebellar peduncle	7. Cerebellum
4. Sylvian fissure	

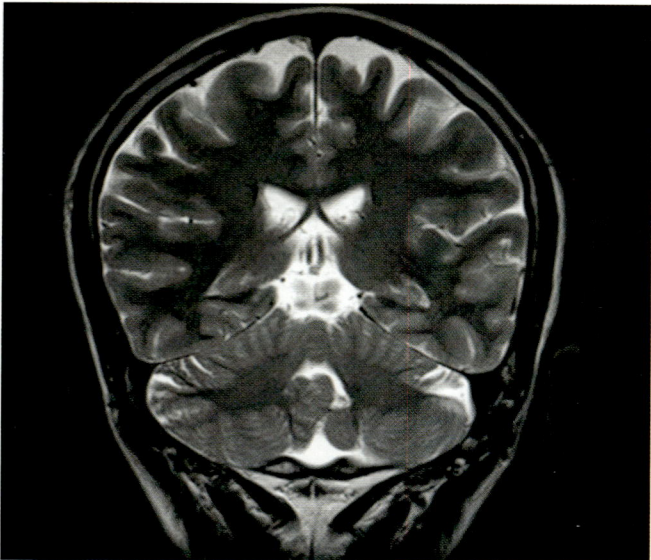

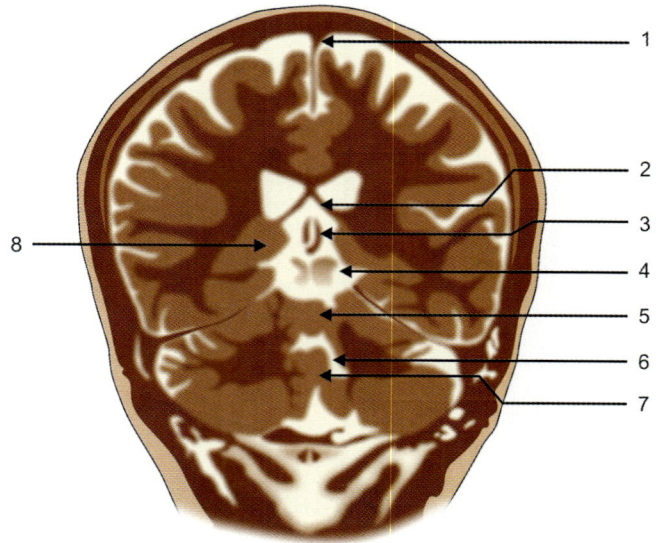

Figure 1.42

1. Superior sagittal sinus	5. Vermis
2. Fornix	6. Fourth ventricle
3. Internal cerebral vein	7. Nodule of cerebellum
4. Quadrigeminal plate cistern	8. Pulvinar of thalamus

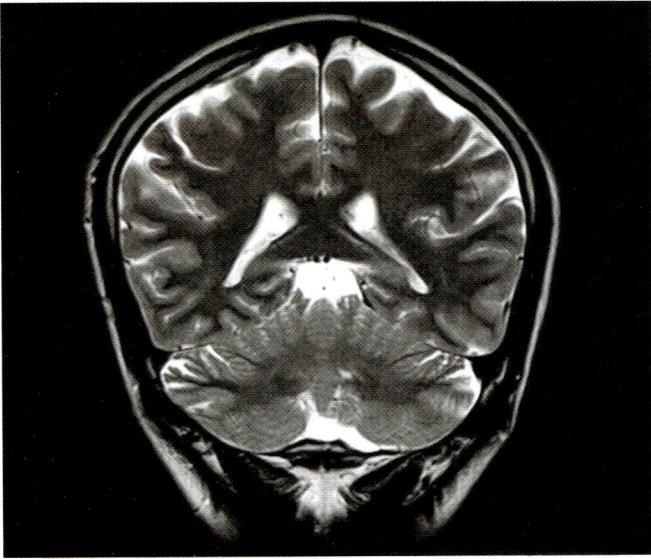

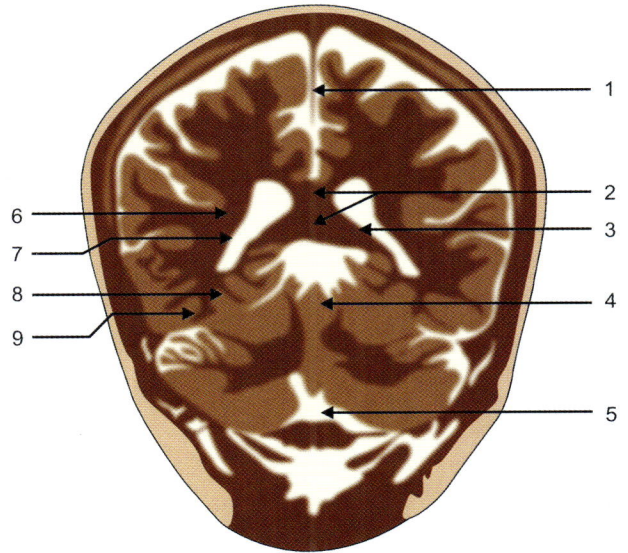

Figure 1.43

1. Interhemispheric fissure	6. Optic radiation
2. Splenium of corpus callosum	7. Atrium of lateral ventricle
3. Fornix	8. Lingular gyrus
4. Vermis	9. Fusiform gyrus
5. Cisterna magna	

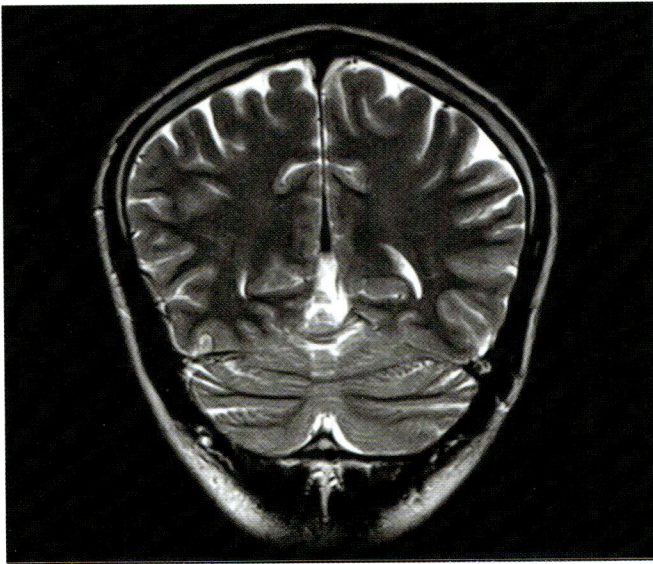

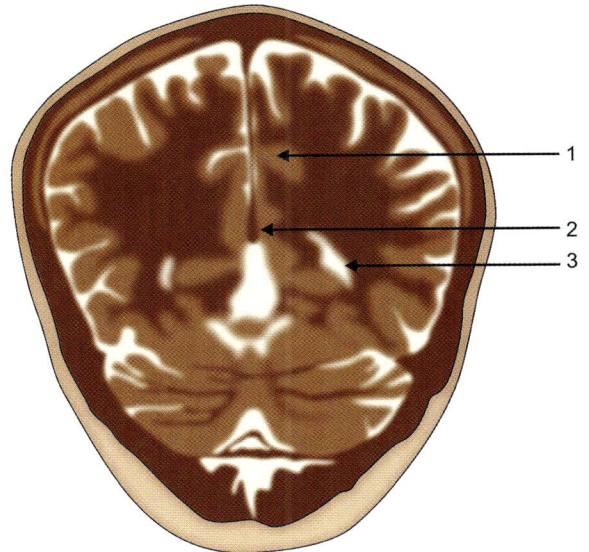

Figure 1.44

1. Cingulate sulcus, marginal branch
2. Straight sinus
3. Occipital horn

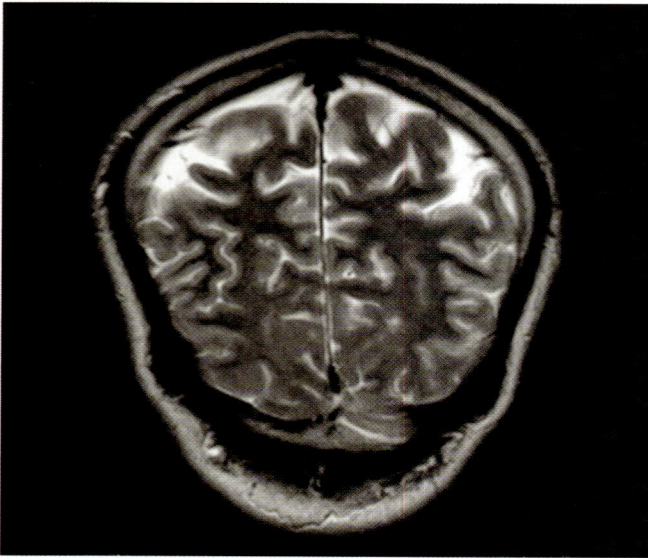

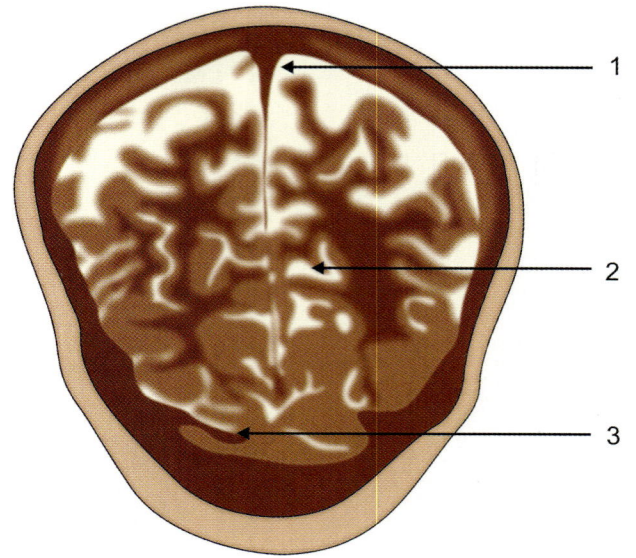

Figure 1.45

1. Superior sagittal sinus
2. Calcarine sulcus
3. Transverse sinus

CHAPTER 2

Orbit

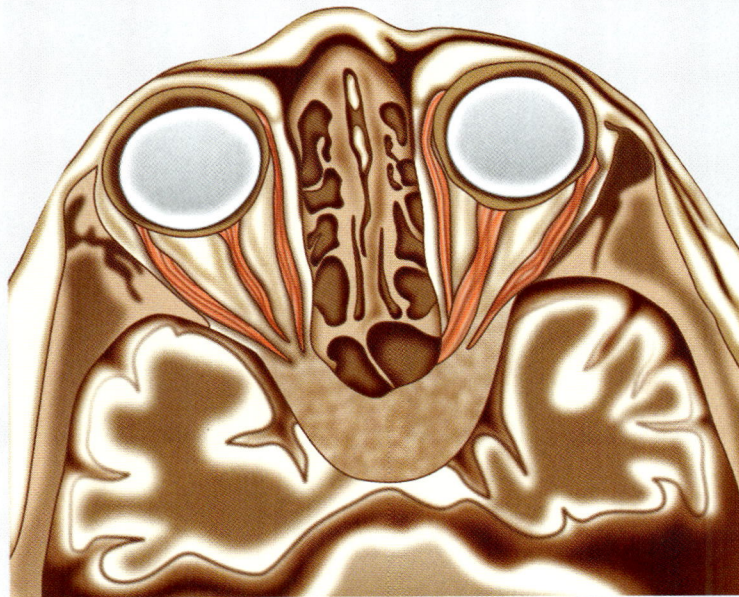

AXIAL IMAGES: INFERIOR TO SUPERIOR

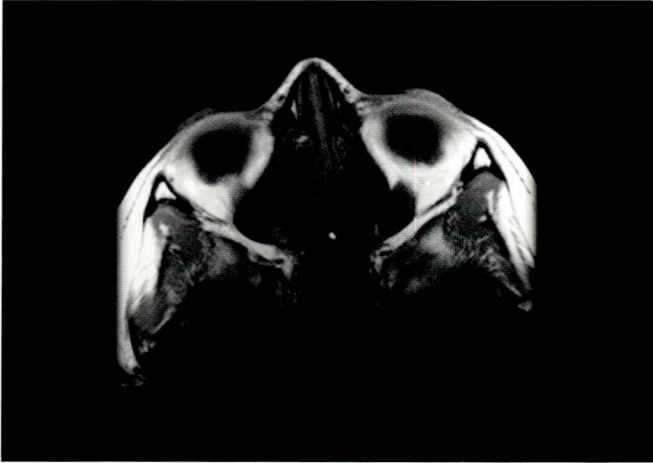
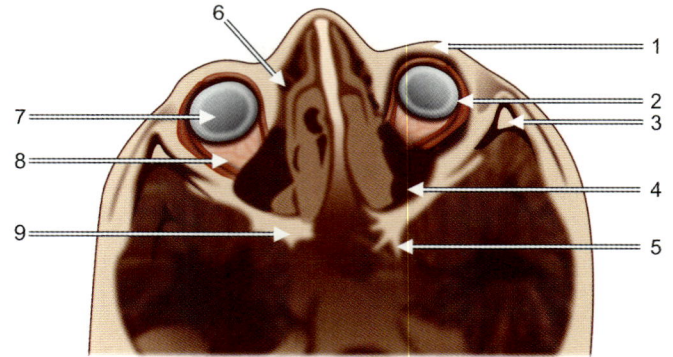

Figure 2.1

1. Lower eyelid
2. Insertion of inferior oblique
3. Zygoma
4. Maxillary sinus
5. Vidian canal
6. Nasolacrimal duct
7. Eyeball
8. Inferior rectus
9. Pterygopalatine fossa

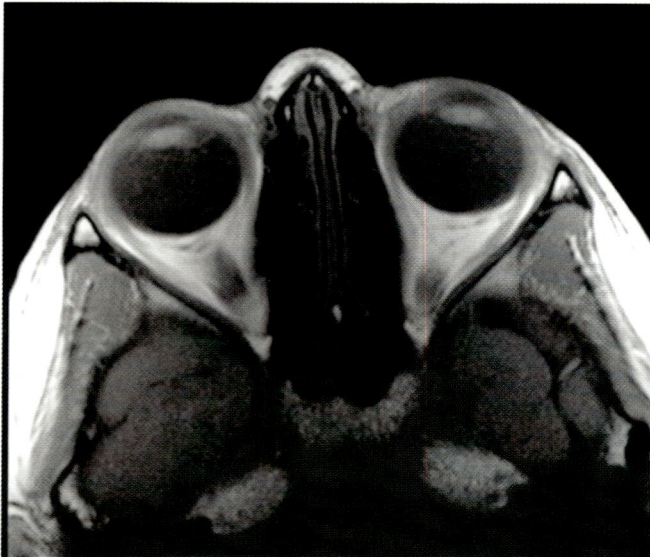
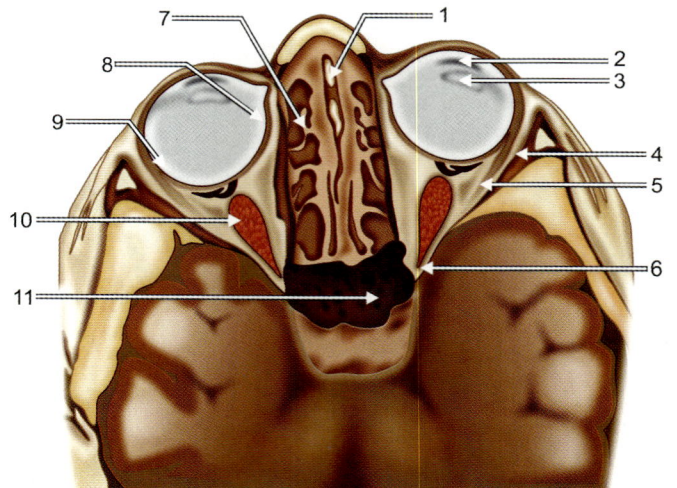

Figure 2.2

1. Nasal septum
2. Anterior chamber
3. Lens
4. Extraconal fat
5. Lateral rectus
6. Superior orbital fissure
7. Ethmoid air cells
8. Medial rectus
9. Sclera
10. Inferior rectus
11. Sphenoid sinus

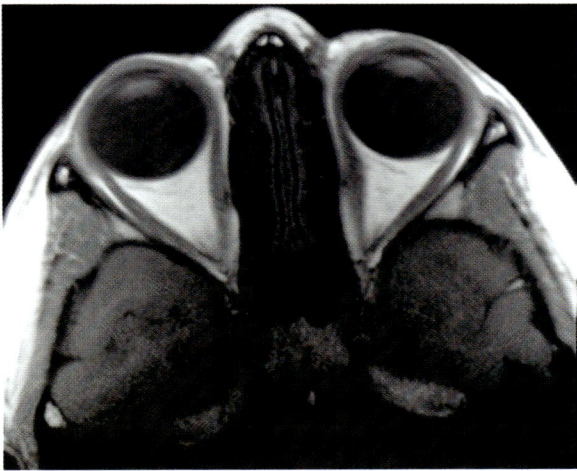

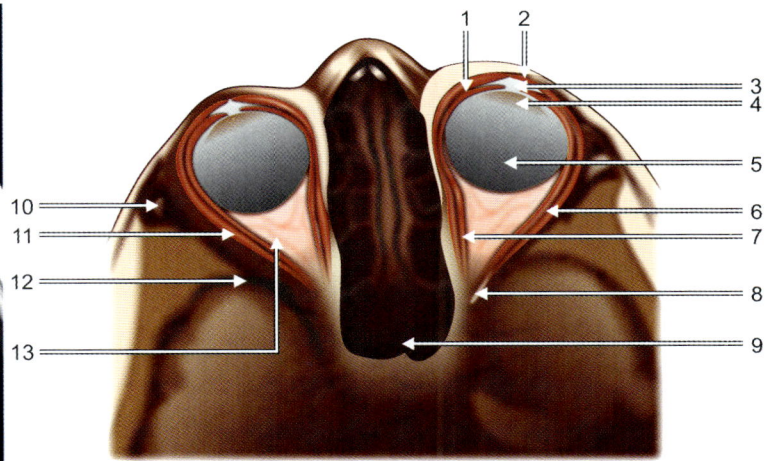

Figure 2.3

1. Ciliary body	8. Superior orbit fissure
2. Cornea	9. Sphenoid sinus
3. Anterior chamber	10. Zygoma
4. Lens	11. Extraconal fat
5. Vitreous	12. Greater wing of sphenoid
6. Lateral rectus	13. Intraconal fat
7. Medial rectus	

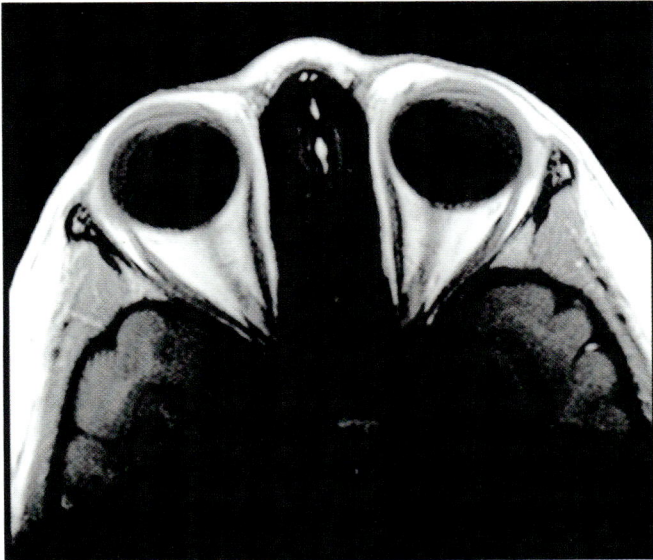

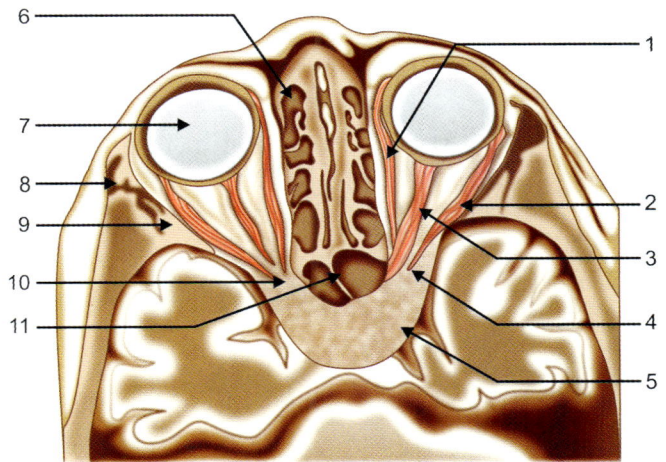

Figure 2.4

1. Medial rectus	7. Vitreous
2. Lateral rectus	8. Zygomatic bone
3. Optic nerve	9. Lateral wall, orbit
4. Superior orbit fissure	10. Optic canal
5. Internal carotid artery	11. Sphenoid sinus
6. Ethmoid air cells	

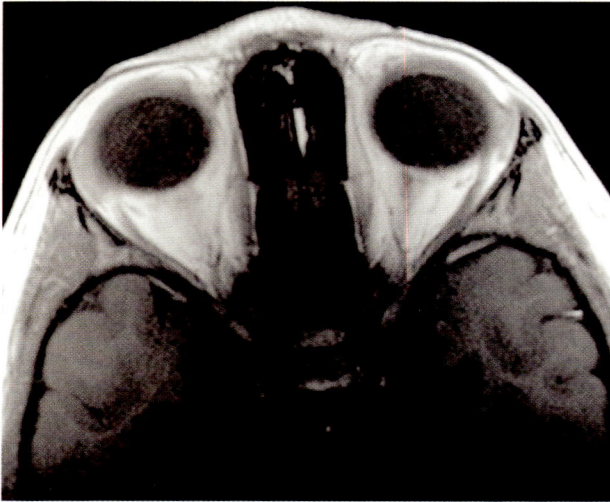

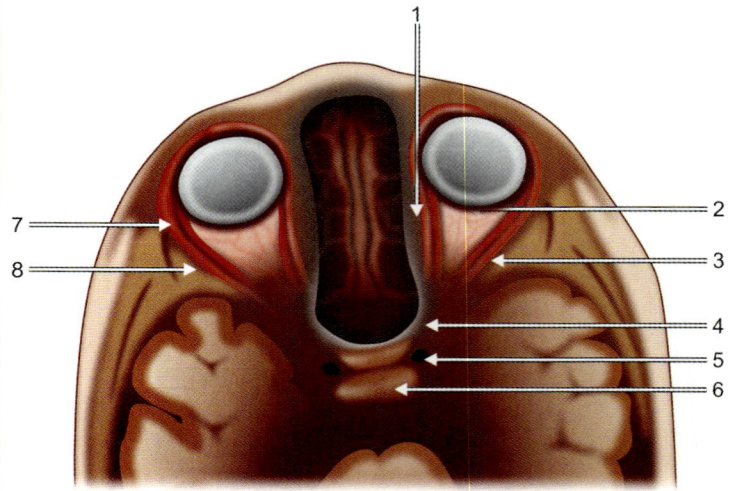

Figure 2.5

1. Superior rectus	5. ICA
2. Optic disk	6. Sella
3. Lateral rectus	7. Lacrimal gland
4. Optic nerve	8. Lateral wall, orbit

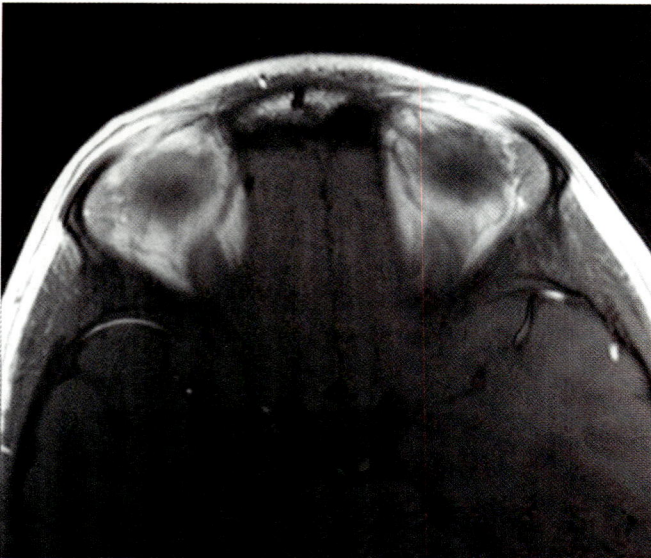

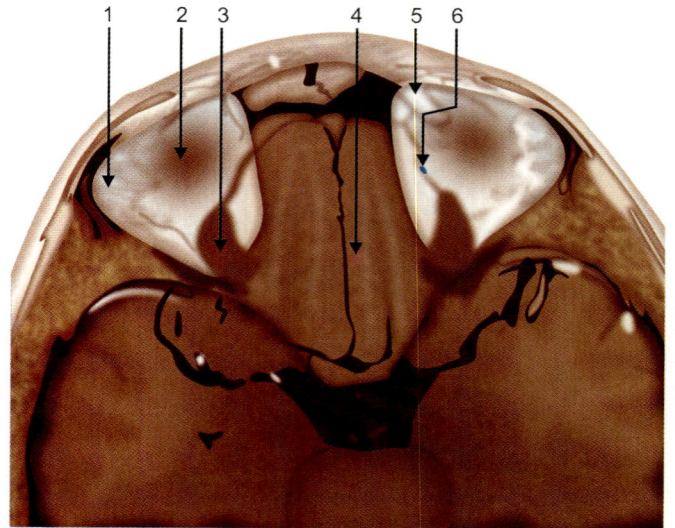

Figure 2.6

1. Lacrimal gland	4. Gyrus rectus
2. Globe, superior part	5. Reflected tendon of superior oblique
3. Superior rectus	6. Superior ophthalmic vein

CORONAL IMAGES: POSTERIOR TO ANTERIOR

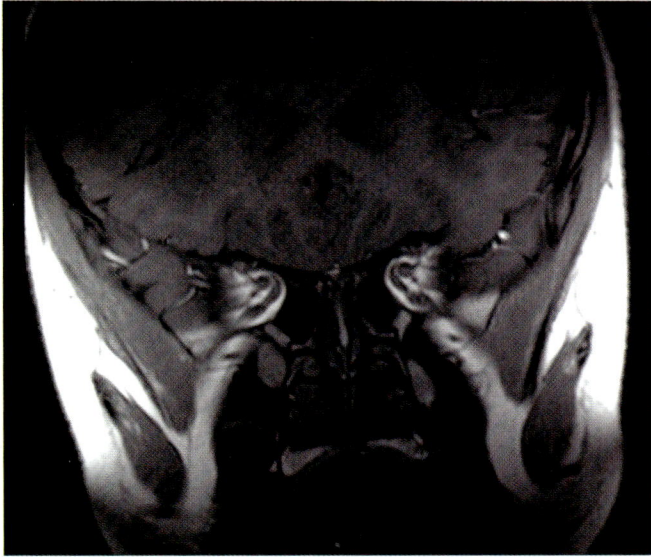

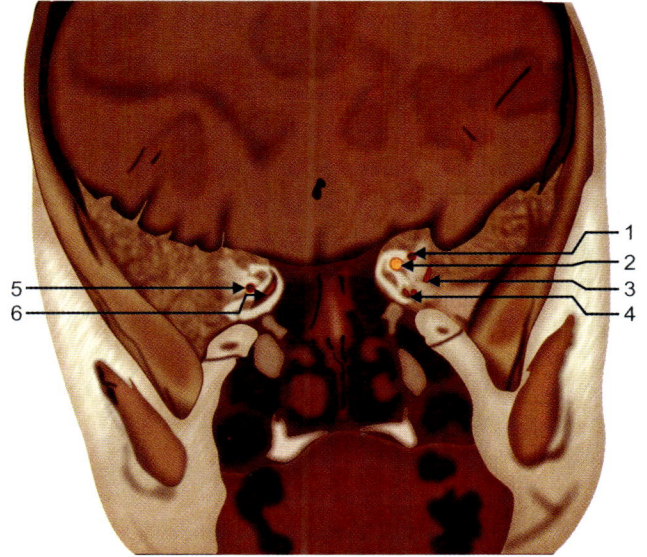

Figure 2.7

1. Long posterior ciliary artery	4. Inferior rectus
2. Optic nerve	5. Ophthalmic artery
3. Lateral rectus	6. Medial rectus

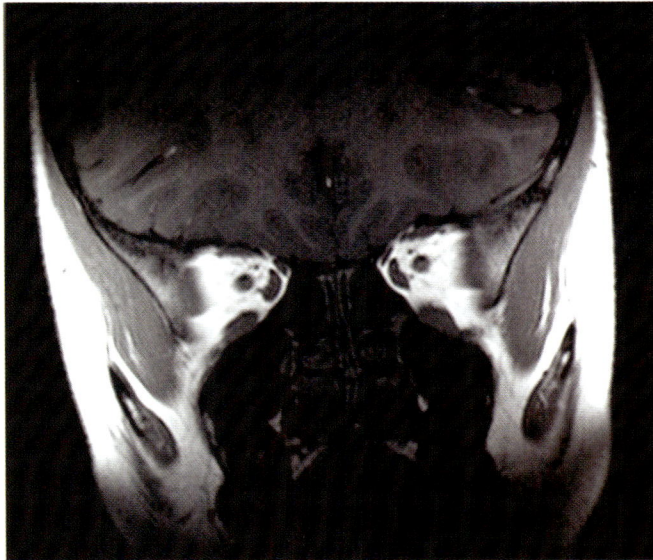

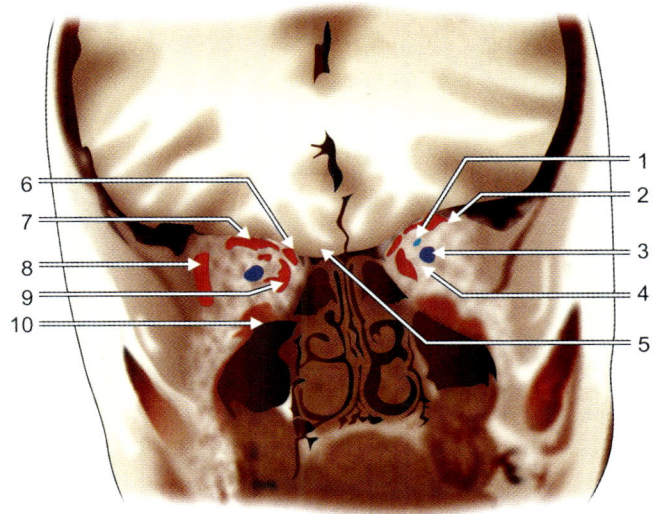

Figure 2.8

1. Long posterior ciliary artery	6. Superior oblique
2. Superior Ophthalmic vein	7. Superior rectus
3. Optic nerve	8. Lateral rectus
4. Ophthalmic artery	9. Medial rectus
5. Gyrus rectus	10. Inferior rectus

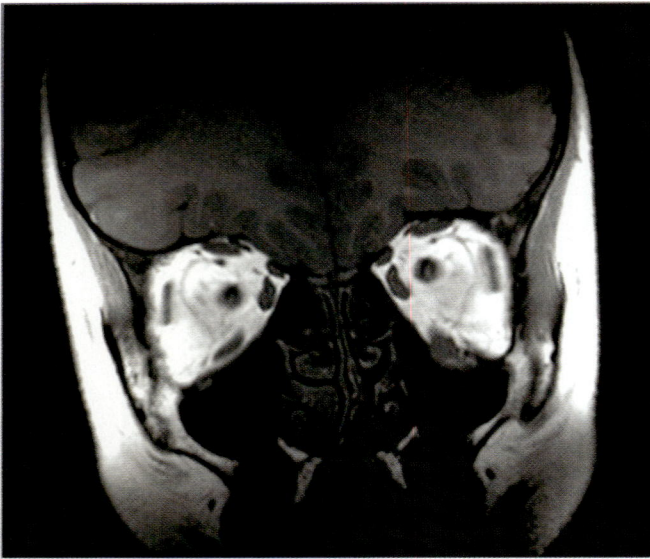

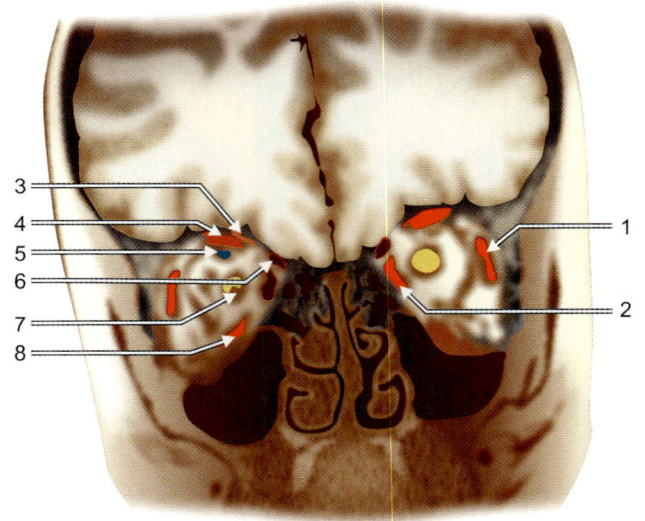

Figure 2.9

1. Lateral rectus	5. Superior ophthalmic vein
2. Medial rectus	6. Superior oblique
3. Levator palpebrae superioris muscle	7. Optic nerve
4. Superior rectus	8. Inferior rectus

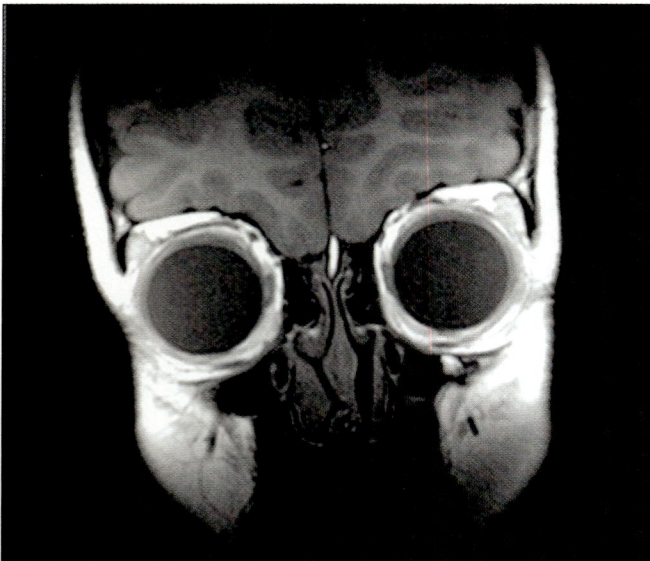

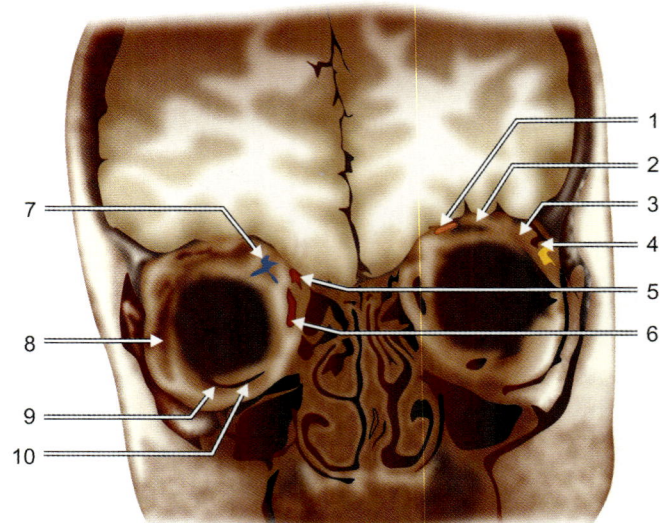

Figure 2.10

1. Levator palpebrae superioris muscle	6. Medial rectus
2. Superior rectus	7. Superior ophthalmic vein
3. Intermuscular septum	8. Lateral rectus
4. Lacrimal gland	9. Inferior oblique
5. Superior oblique	10. Inferior rectus

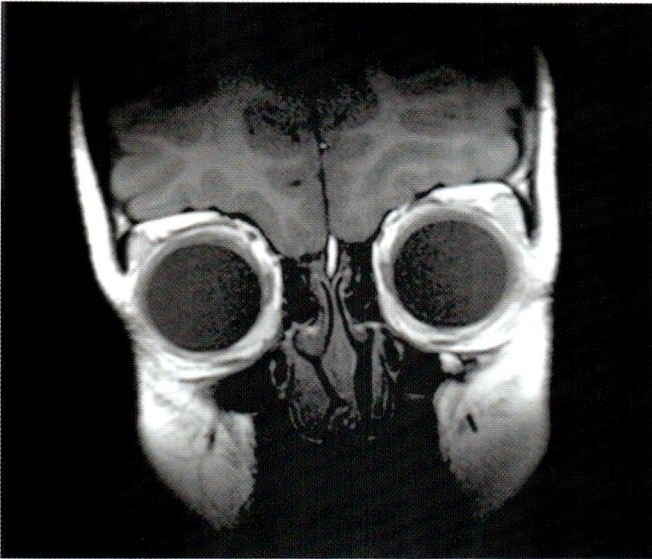

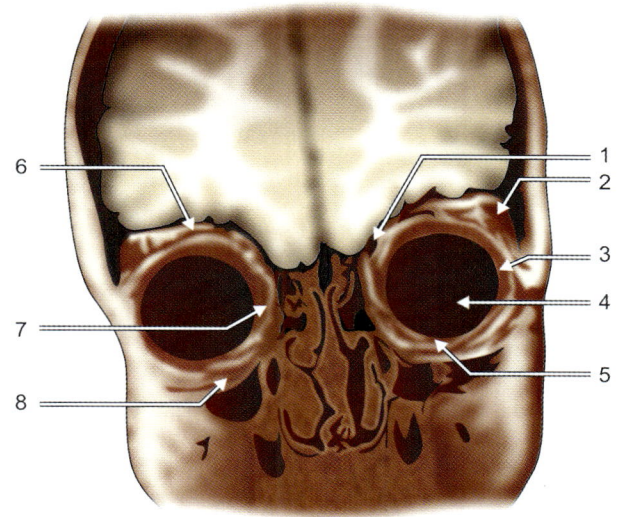

Figure 2.11

1. Superior oblique	5. Inferior rectus
2. Lacrimal gland	6. Superior rectus and levator palpebrae muscles
3. Sclera	7. Medial rectus
4. Vitreous	8. Inferior oblique

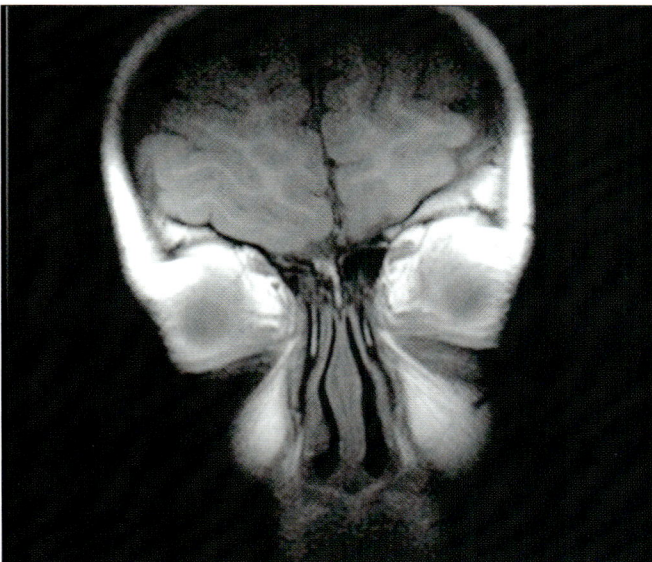

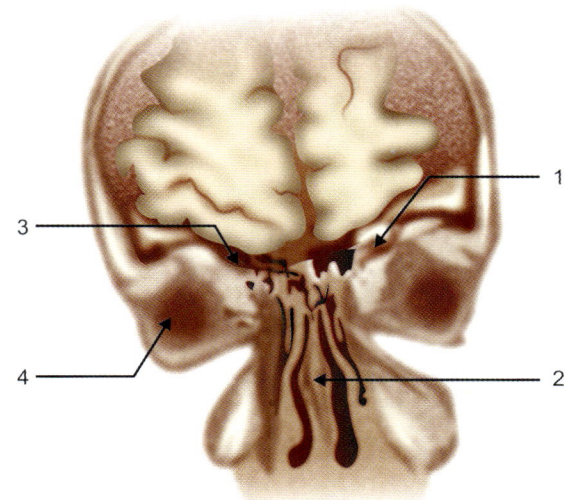

Figure 2.12

1. Reflected tendon of superior oblique	3. Trochlea
2. Nasal septum	4. Globe

CHAPTER 3

PNS and Skull Base

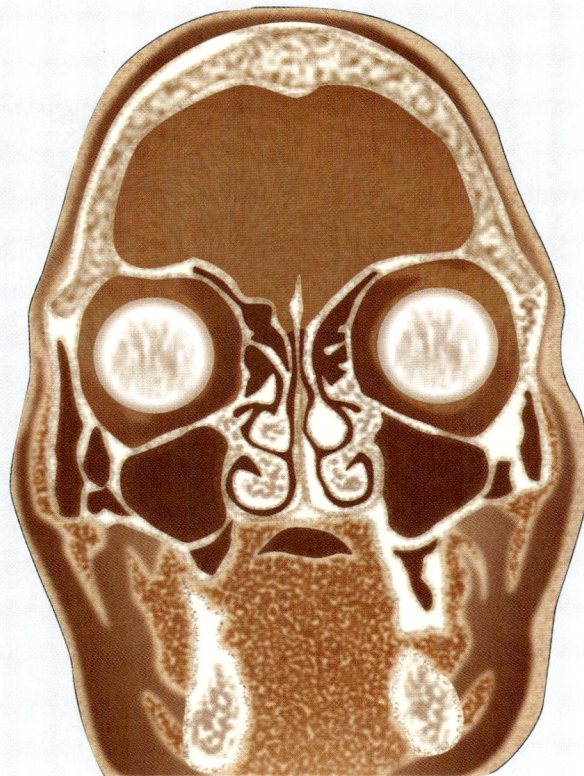

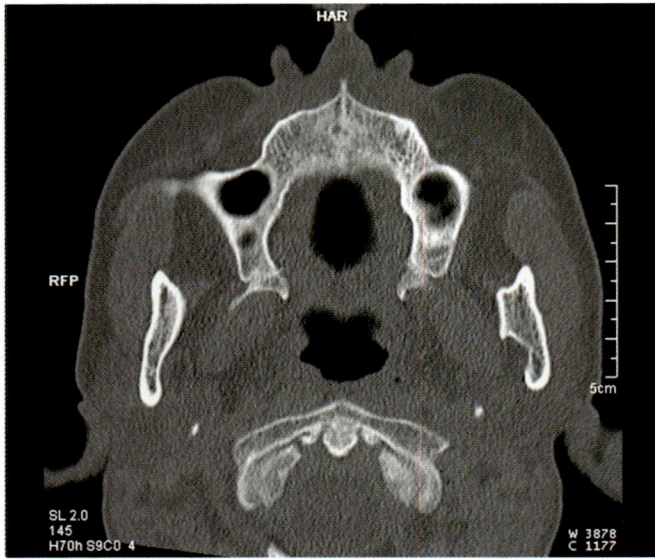

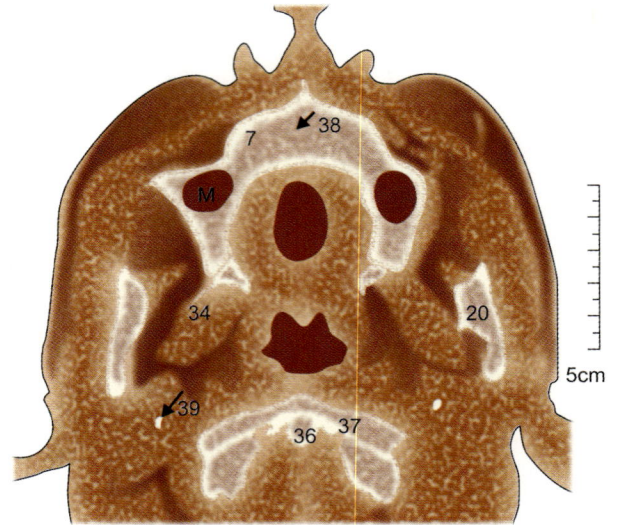

Figure 3.1: 38; Incisive canal, 7; Alveolar margin of maxilla, M; Maxillary sinus, 34; Lateral pterygoid plate, 39; Styloid process, 36; Dens of axis, 37; Anterior arch of atlas, 20; Mandible

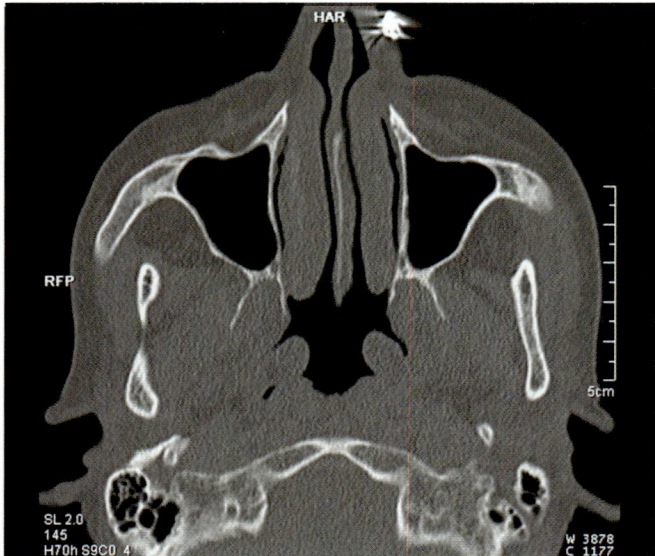

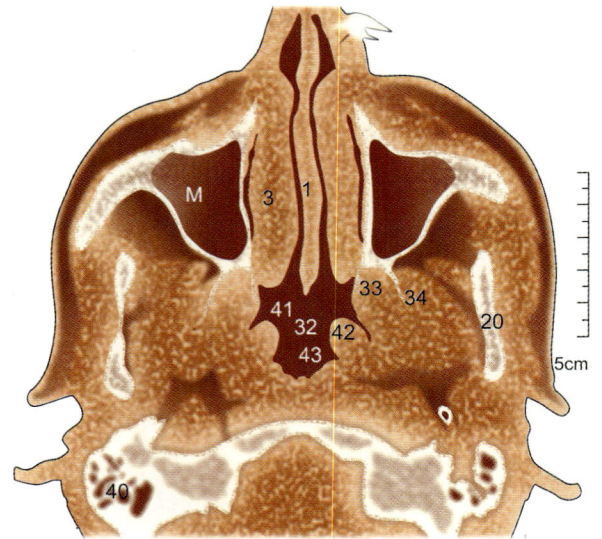

Figure 3.2: 1; Nasal septum, 3; Inferior turbinate, M; Maxillary sinus, 20; Mandible 32; Nasopharynx 33; Medial pterygoid plate 34; Lateral pterygoid plate, 41; Eustachian tube opening 42; Torus tubrius 43; Fossa of Rosenmuller

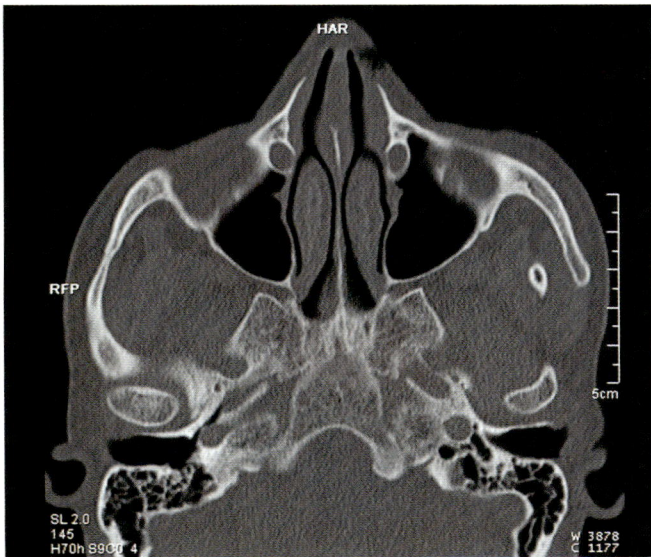

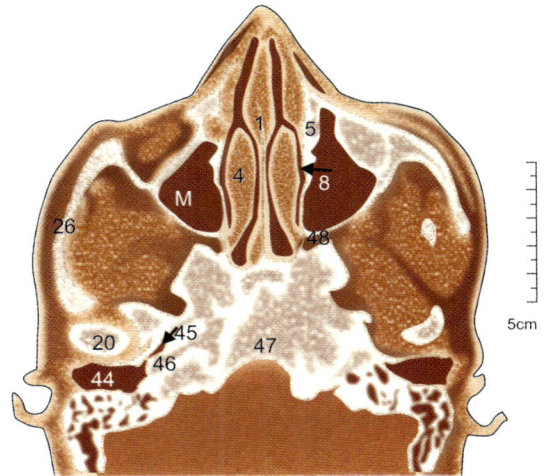

Figure 3.3: 1; Nasal septum, 4; Middle turbinate, 8; Middle meatus, M; Maxillary sinus, 48; Pterygopalatine fossa, 45; Eustachian tube 46; Internal carotid artery, 47; Basi-occiput 44; External auditory canal, 20; Mandible, 26; Zygomatic arch

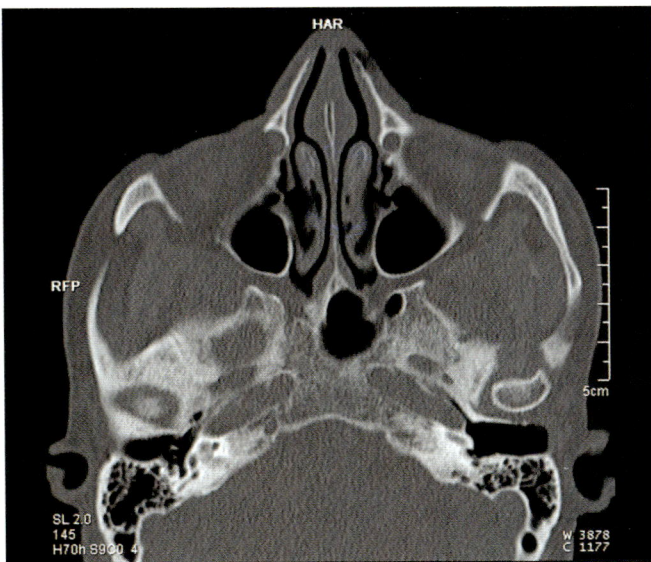

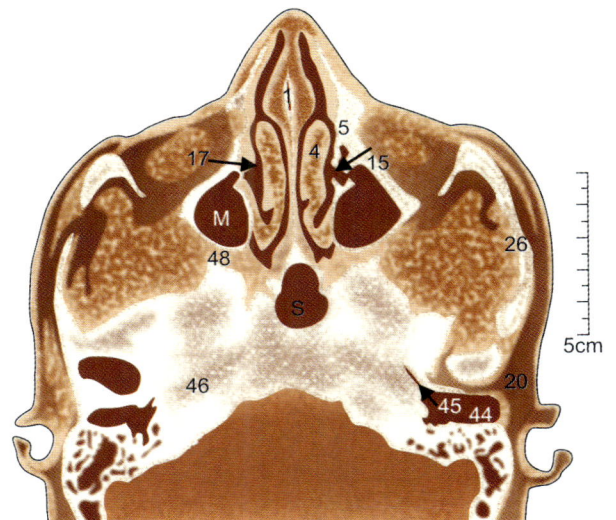

Figure 3.4: 1; Nasal septum, 4; Middle turbinate, 5; Nasolacrimal duct 15; Hiatus semilunaris, M; maxillary sinus; S; sphenoid sinus 48; Pterygopalatine fossa, 20; Mandible, 44; External auditory meatus 45; Eustachian tube 46; Internal carotid artery, 26; Zygomatic arch

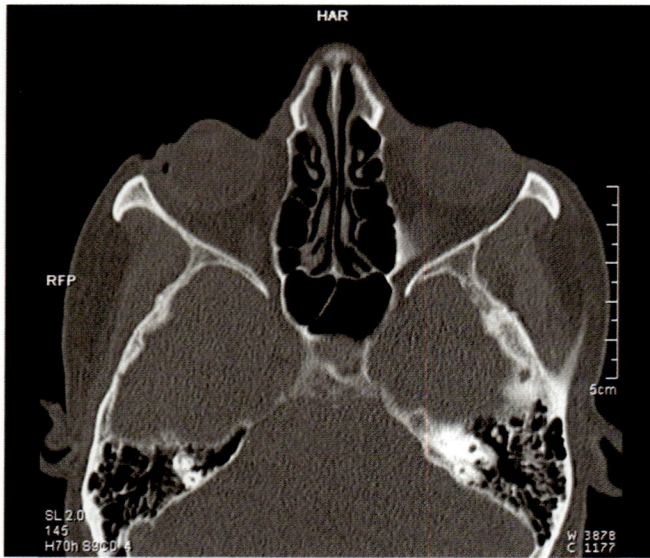

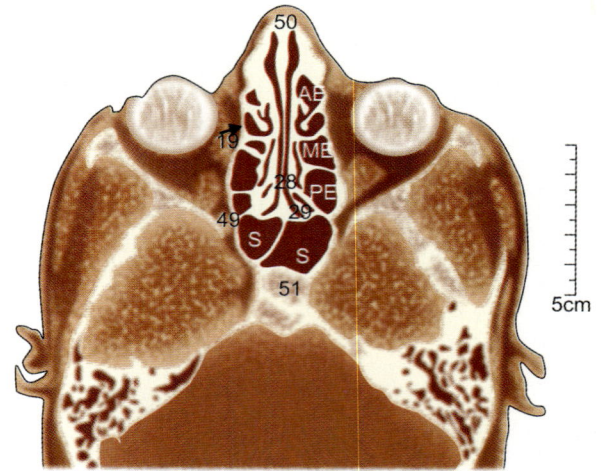

Figure 3.5: 50; Nasal bone; S; Sphenoid sinus, AE; Anterior ethmoid cells, ME; Middle ethmoid cells, PE; Posterior ethmoid cells, 28; Perpendicular plate of ethmoid, 29; Spheno-ethmoidal recess, 49; Superior orbital fissure, 51; Pituitary fossa

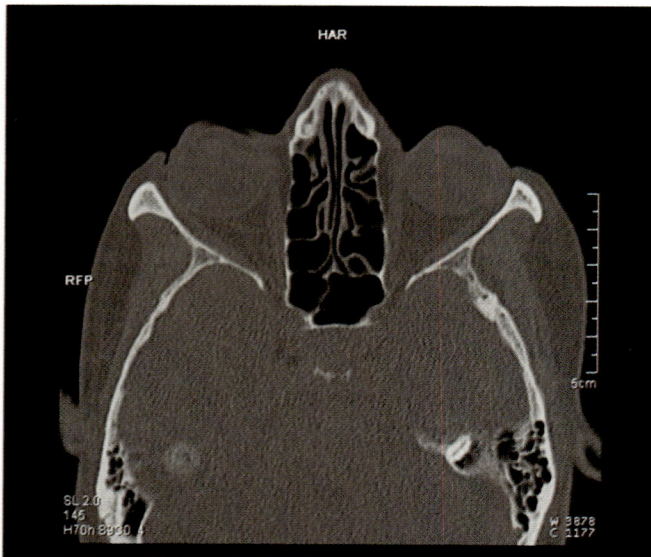

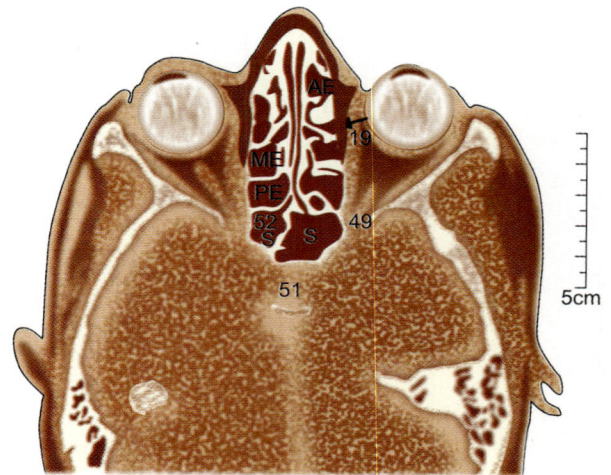

Figure 3.6: AE; Anterior ethmoid cells, ME; Middle ethmoid cells, PE; Posterior ethmoid cells, 49; Superior orbital fissure 51; Pituitary fossa, 52; Sphenoid ostium

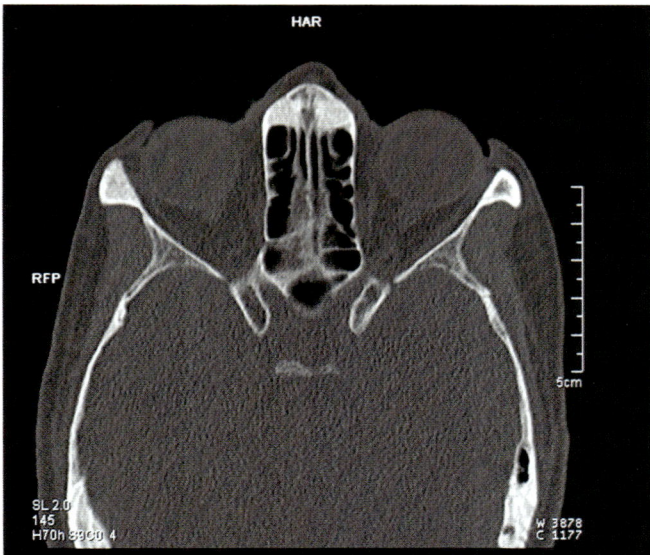

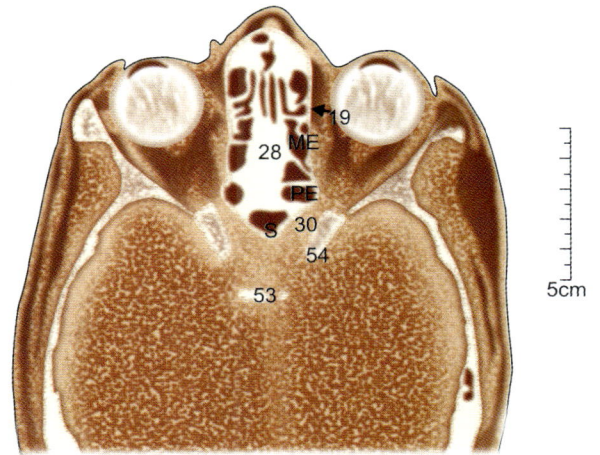

Figure 3.7: ME; Middle ethmoid cells, PE; Posterior ethmoid cells, S; Sphenoid sinus, 19; Lamina papyracea 28; Perpendicular plate of ethmoid, 30; Optic canal, 54; Anterior clinoid, 53; Dorsum sella

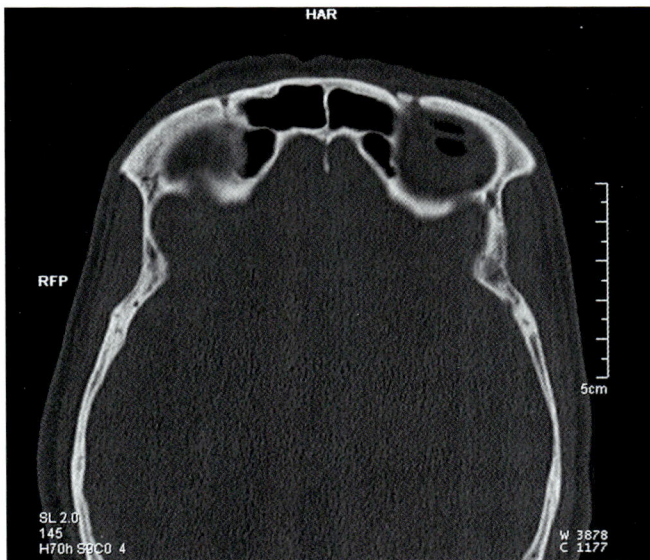

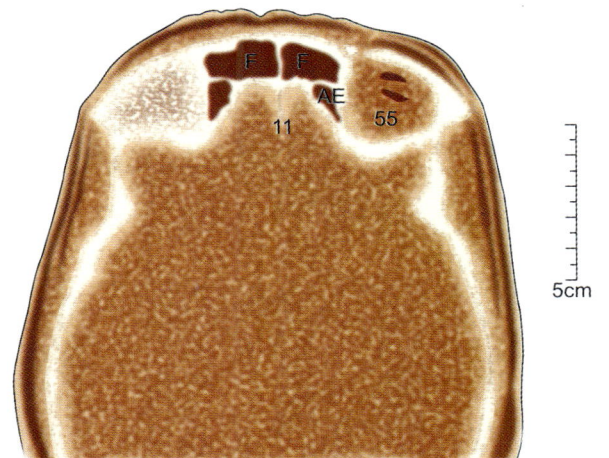

Figure 3.8: F; Frontal sinus, AE; Anterior ethmoid cells 11; Crista galli, 55; Orbit

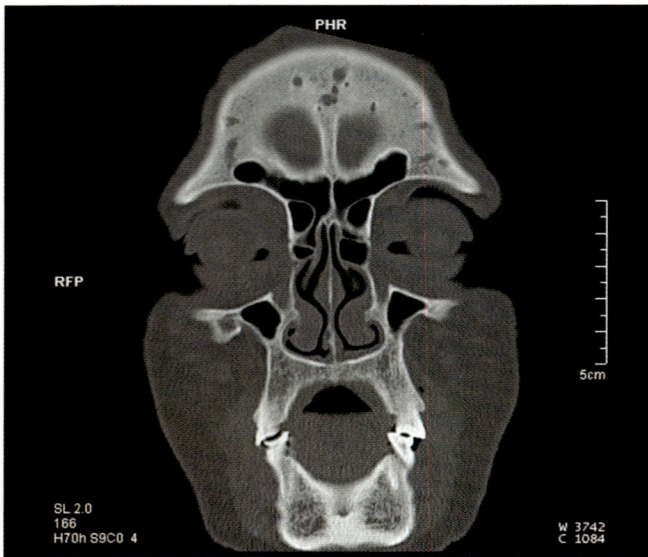

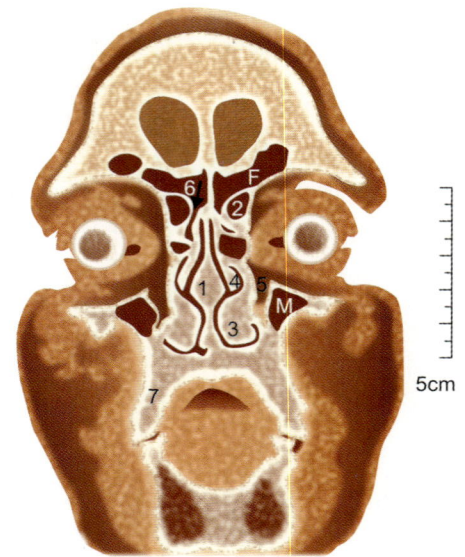

Figure 3.9: F; Frontal sinus, M; Maxillary sinus, 1; Nasal septum 2; Agger nasi cells, 3; Inferior turbinate, 4; Middle turbinate 5; Nasolacrimal duct, 6; Frontal recess, 7; Alveolar margin of maxilla

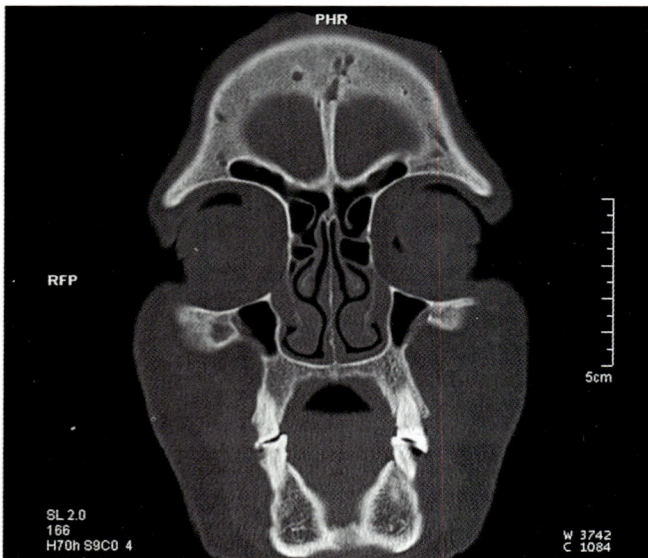

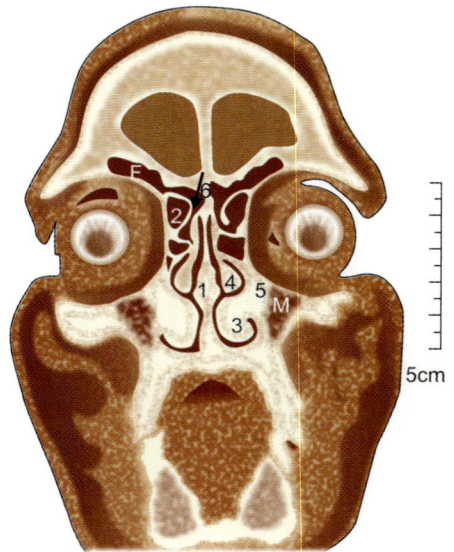

Figure 3.10: F; Frontal sinus, M; maxillary sinus, 1; Nasal septum 2; Agger nasi cells 3; Inferior turbinate 4; Middle turbinate 5; Nasolacrimal duct 6; Frontal recess

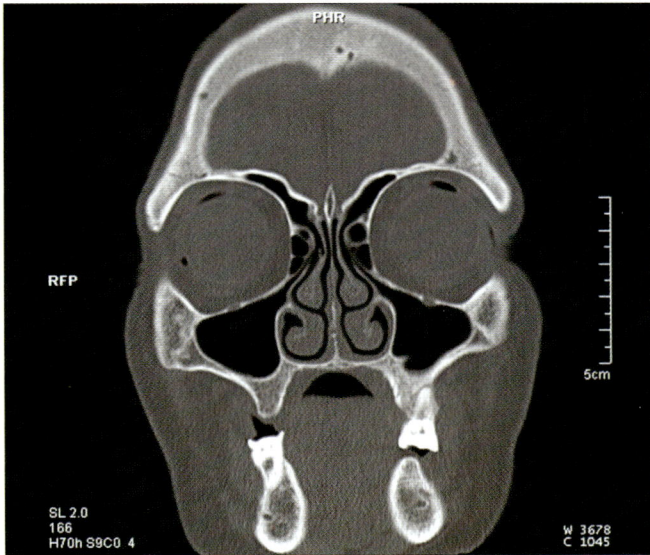

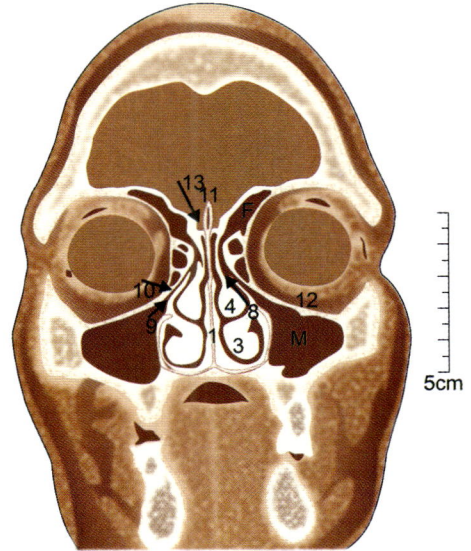

Figure 3.11. F; Frontal sinus, M; Maxillary sinus, 1; Nasal septum, 3; Inferior turbinate 4; Middle turbinate, 8; Middle meatus, 9; Primary ostium of maxillary antrum 10. Infundibulum 11. Crista galli, 12; Infraorbital foramen, 13; Cribriform plate

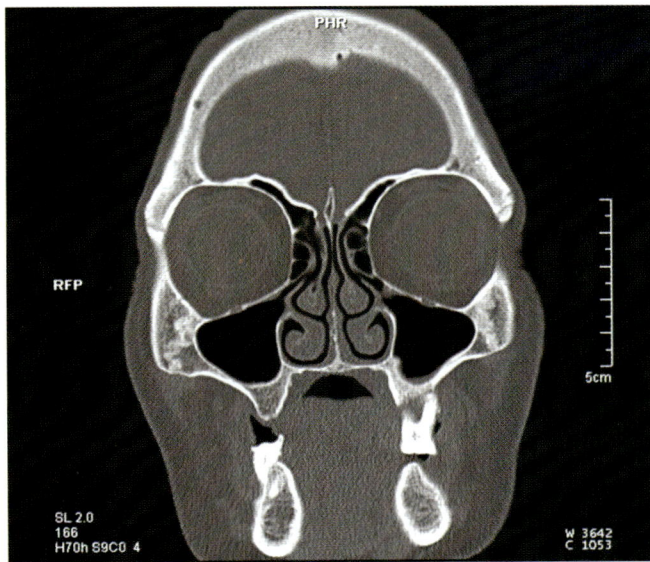

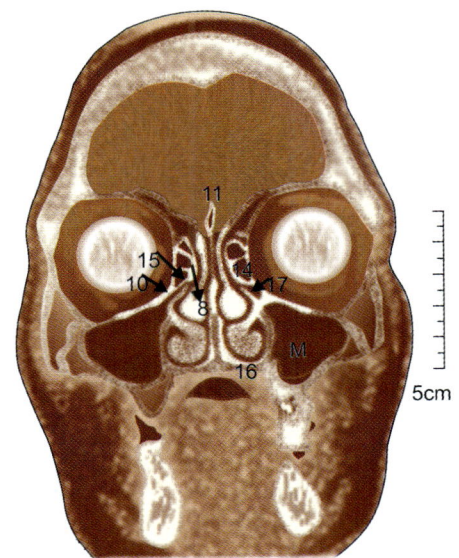

Figure 3.12: M; maxillary sinus, 8; Middle meatus, 11; Crista galli 10; Infundibulum 14; Bulla ethmoidalis, 15; Hiatus semilunaris 16; Hard palate, 17; Uncinate process

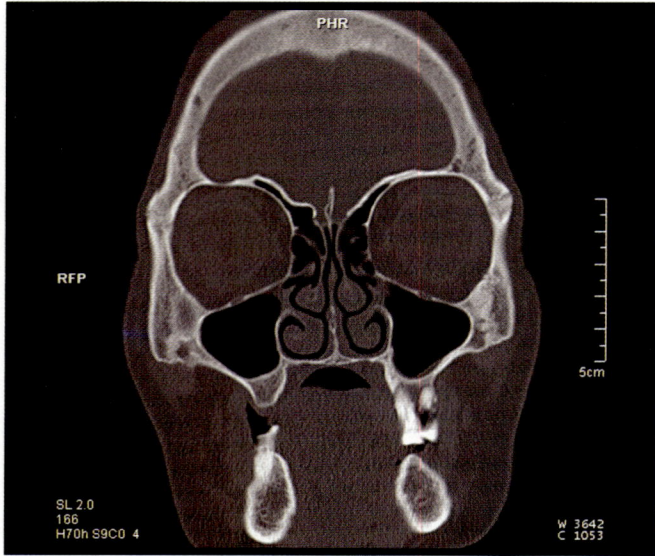

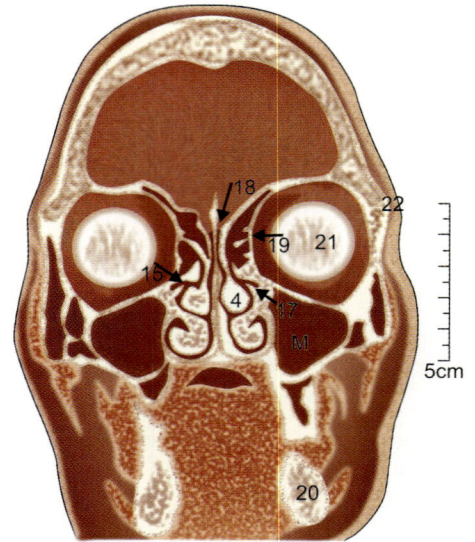

Figure 3.13: M; Maxillary sinus, 4; Middle turbinate 15; Hiatus semilunaris 17; Uncinate process 18; Fovea ethmoidalis 19; Lamina papyracea, 20; Mandible, 21; Globe

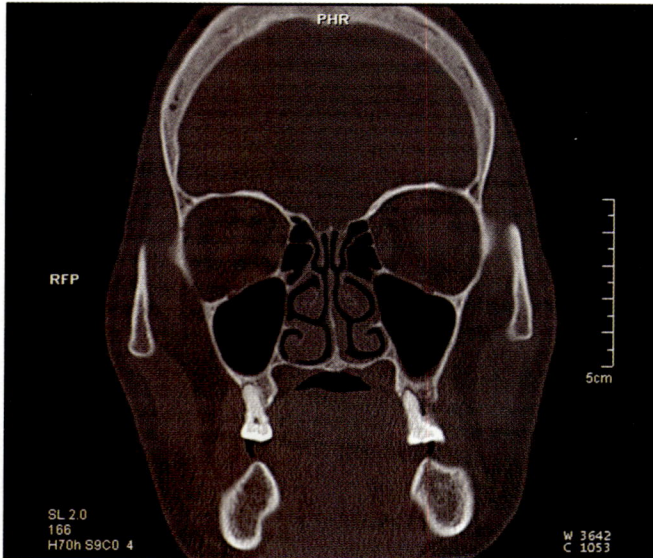

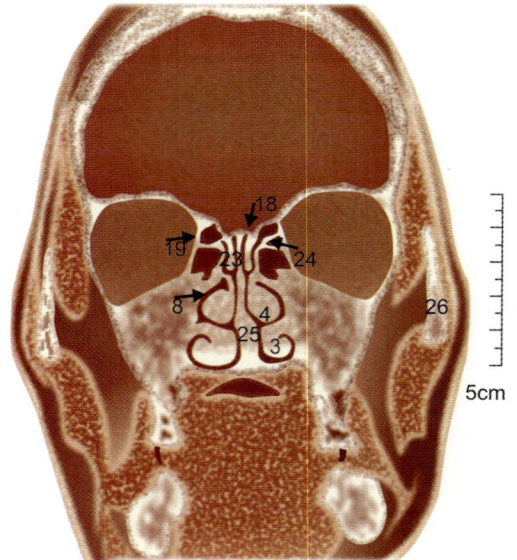

Figure 3.14: 3; Inferior turbinate, 4; Middle turbinate, 8; Middle meatus 18; Fovea ethmoidalis, 19; Lamina papyracea, 23; superior turbinate 24; Basal lamina, 25; Vomer bone, 26; Zygomatic arch

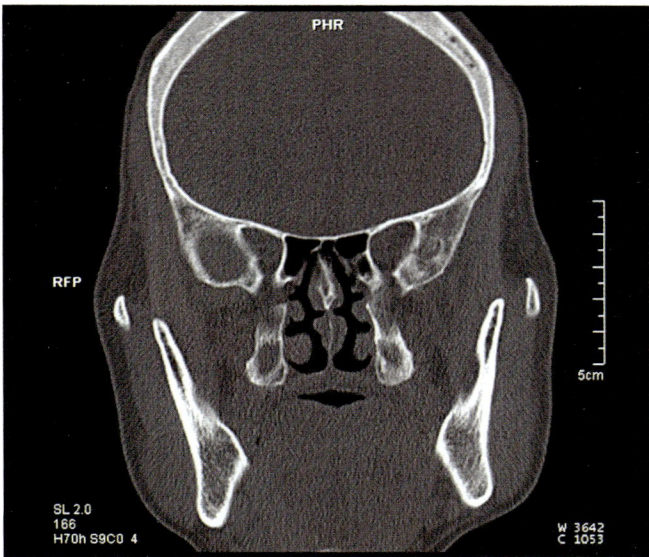

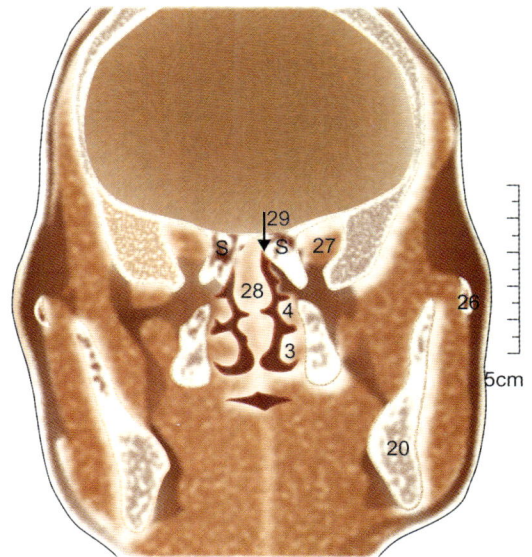

Figure 3.15: S; Sphenoid sinus, 3; Inferior turbinate, 4; Middle turbinate, 20; Mandible, 26; Zygomatic arch, 27; Orbital apex 28; Perpendicular plate of ethmoid, 29; Spheno-ethmoidal recess

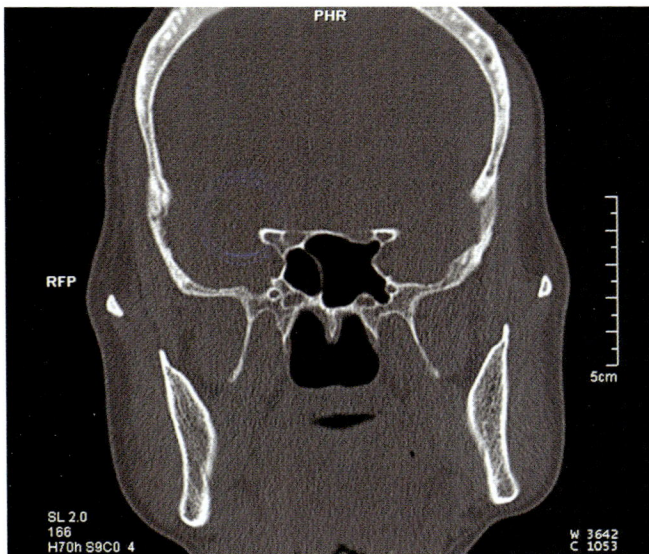

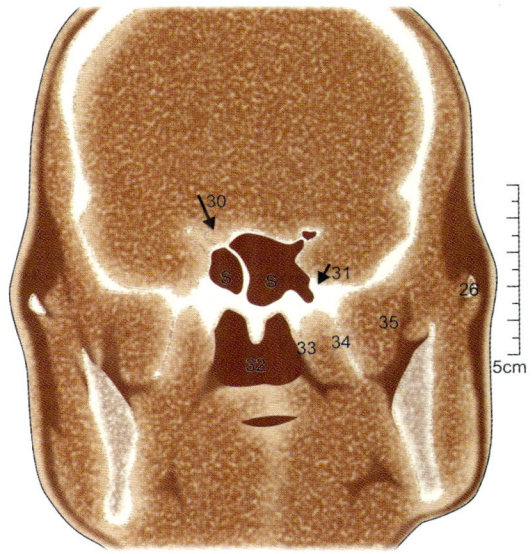

Figure 3.16: S; Sphenoid sinus, 28; Perpendicular plate of ethmoid, 30; Optic canal, 31; Foramen rotundum, 32; Nasopharynx, 33; Medial pterygoid plate, 34; Lateral pterygoid plate, 35; Infratemporal fossa

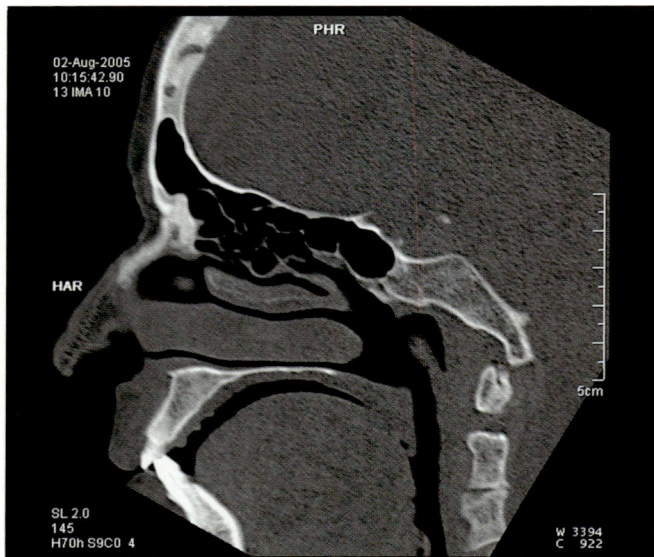

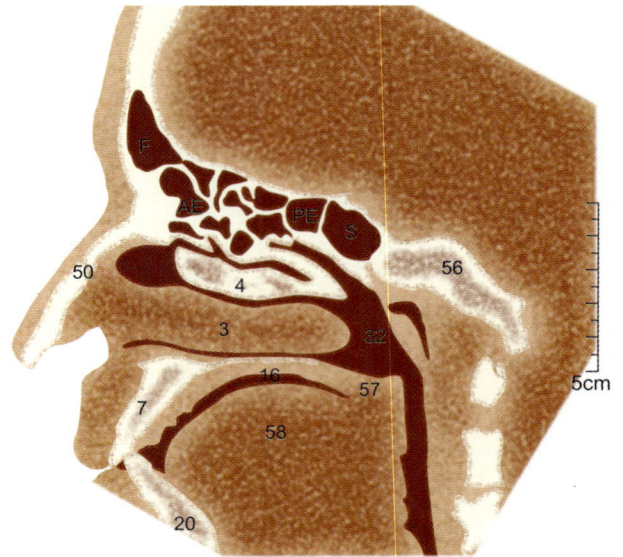

Figure 3.17: AE; Anterior ethmoid cells, PE; Posterior ethmoidal cells 3; Inferior turbinate, 4; Middle turbinate, 32; nasopharynx, 50; Nasal bone 56; Clivus, 57; Soft palate, 58; Tongue, 20; Mandible, F; Frontal sinus, S; Sphenoid sinus

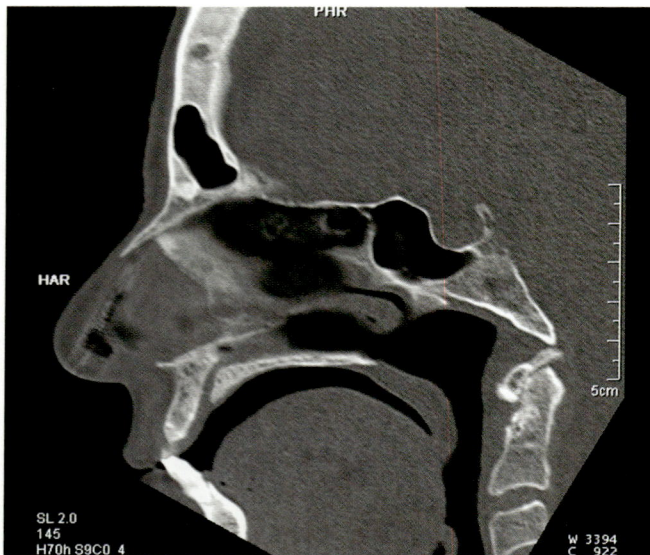

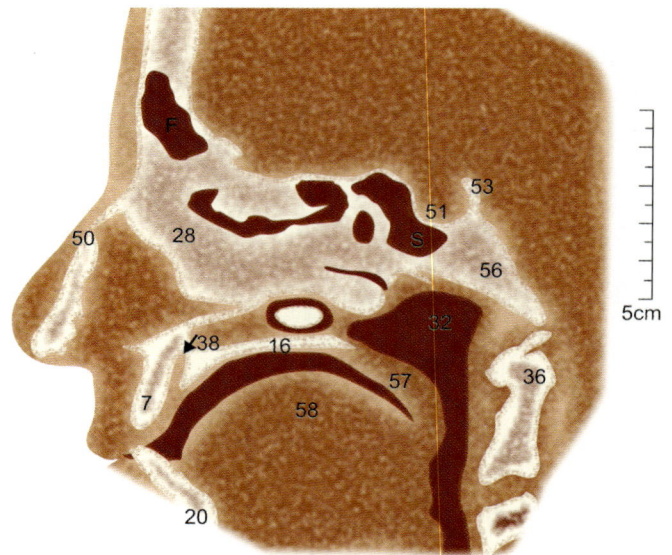

Figure 3.18: F; Frontal sinus, S; Sphenoid sinus, 7; Alveolar margin of Maxilla 16; Hard palate, 28; Perpendicular plate of ethmoid, 32; Nasopharynx, 36; Dens of axis, 38; Incisive canal, 51; Pituitary fossa, 53; Dorsum sella, 56; Clivus, 57; Soft palate, 58; Tongue, 50; Nasal bone, 20; Mandible

KEYS: PNS

1. Nasal septum
2. Agger nasi cells
3. Inferior turbinate
4. Middle turbinate
5. Nasolacrimal duct
6. Frontal recess
7. Alveolar margin of maxilla
8. Middle meatus
9. Primary ostium of maxillary antrum
10. Infundibulum
11. Crista galli
12. Infraorbital foramen
13. Cribriform plate
14. Bulla ethmoidalis
15. Hiatus semilunaris
16. Hard palate
17. Uncinate process
18. Fovea ethmoidalis
19. Lamina papyracea
20. Mandible
21. Globe
22. Zygomatico-frontal suture
23. Superior turbinate
24. Basal lamina
25. Vomer
26. Zygomatic arch
27. Orbital apex
28. Perpendicular plate of ethmoid
29. Spheno-ethmoidal recess
30. Optic canal
31. Foramen rotundum
32. Nasopharynx
33. Medial pterygoid plate
34. Lateral pterygoid plate
35. Infratemporal fossa
36. Dens of axis
37. Anterior arch of atlas
38. Incisive canal
39. Styloid process
40. Mastoid sinus
41. Eustachian tube opening
42. Torus tubarius
43. Fossa of Rosenmuller
44. External auditory meatus
45. Eustachian tube
46. Internal carotid artery
47. Basi-occiput
48. Pterygopalatine fossa
49. Superior orbital fissure
50. Nasal bone
51. Pituitary fossa
52. Sphenoid ostium
53. Dorsum sella
54. Anterior clinoid
55. Orbit
56. Clivus
57. Soft palate
58. Tongue

M= Maxillary sinus

S= Sphenoid sinus

F= Frontal sinus

AE= Anterior Ethmoid cells

ME= Middle Ethmoid cells

PE= Posterior Ethmoid cells

CHAPTER 4

Temporal Bones and TM Joint

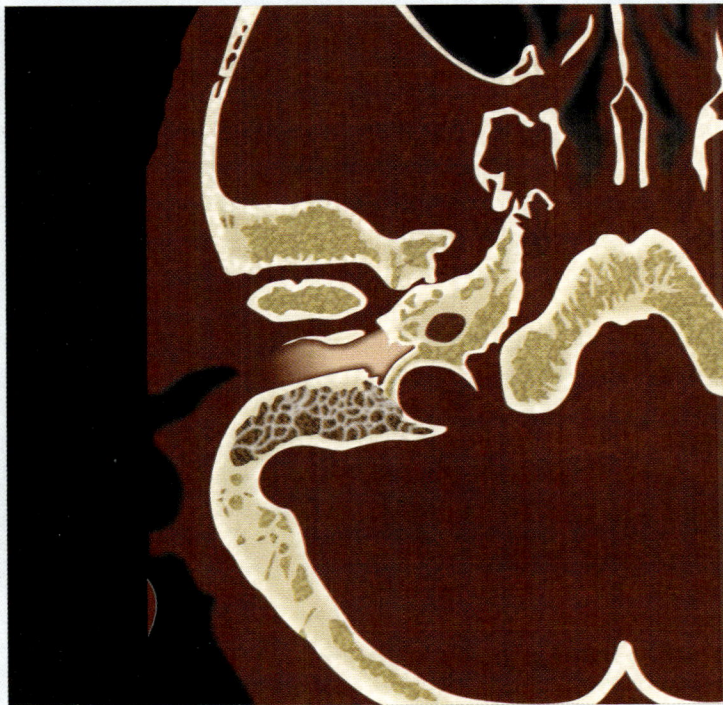

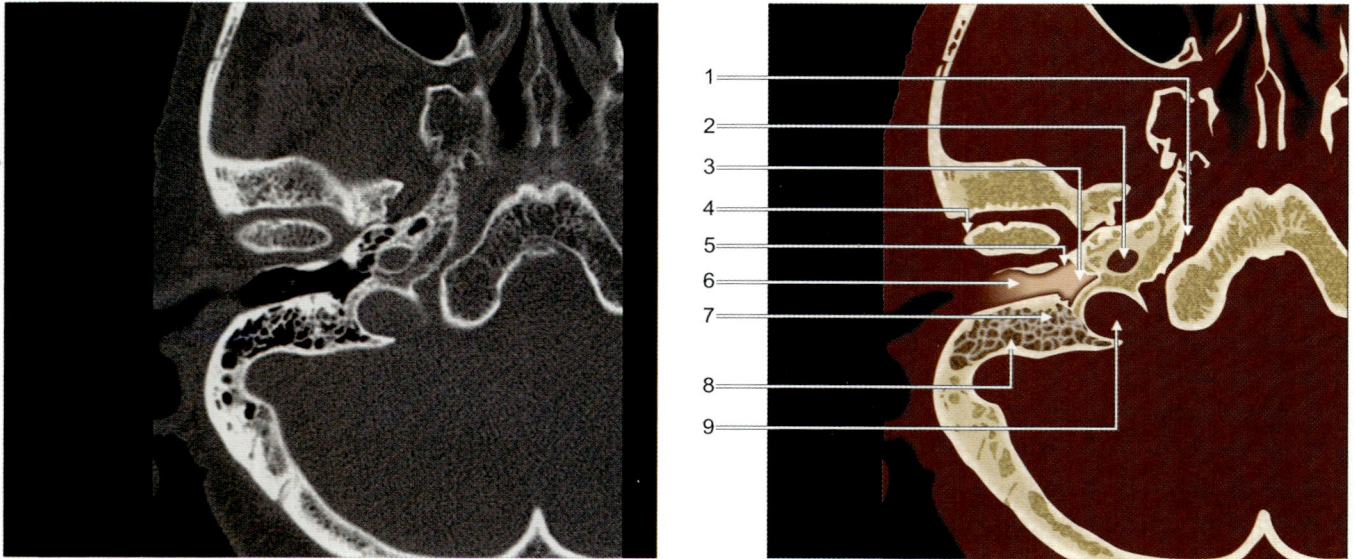

Figure 4.1

1. Petro-occipital fissure
2. Carotid canal
3. Hypotympanum
4. TM joint
5. Limbus
6. External auditory canal
7. Facial nerve canal
8. Mastoid sinus
9. Jugular fossa

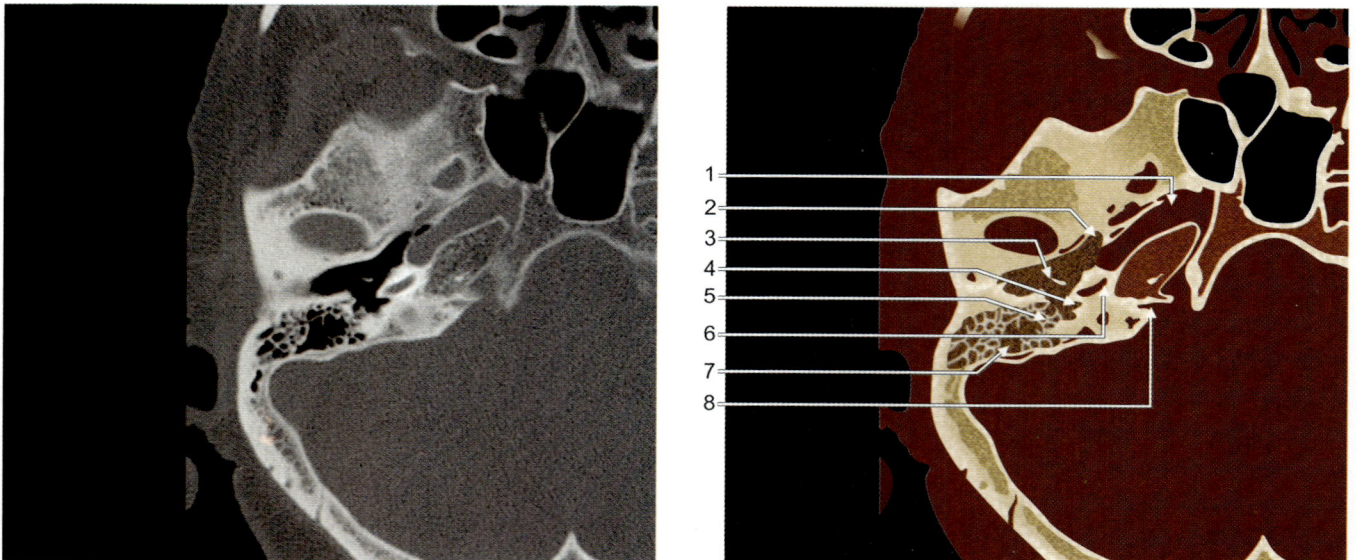

Figure 4.2

1. Carotid canal
2. Eustachian tube
3. Malleous, long process
4. Round window
5. Facial nerve
6. Basal turn of cochlea
7. Mastoid sinus
8. Cochlear aqueduct

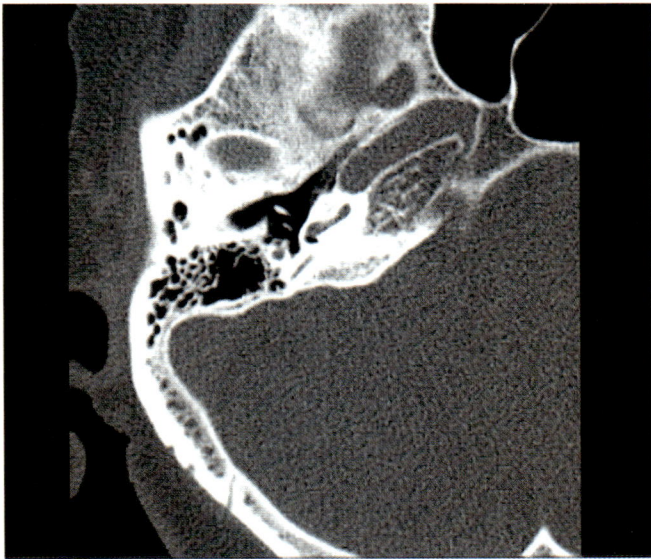
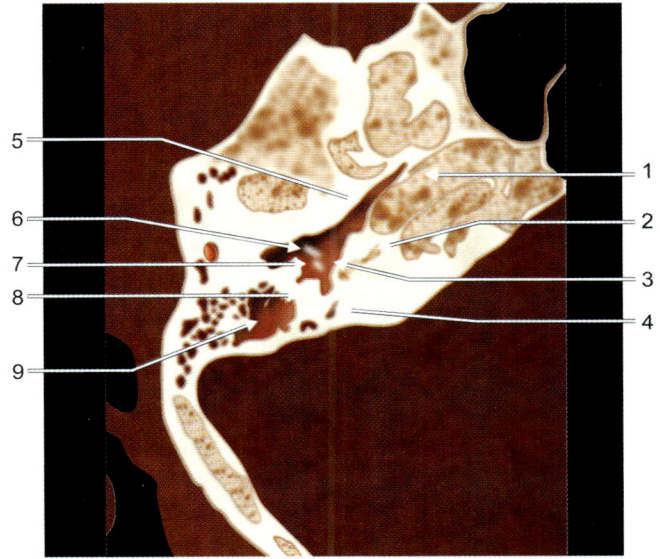

Figure 4.3

1. Carotid canal
2. Basal turn of cochlea
3. Middle ear
4. Posterior semicircular canal
5. Tensor tympani
6. Malleus, manubrium
7. Incus, long process
8. Facial nerve
9. Mastoid

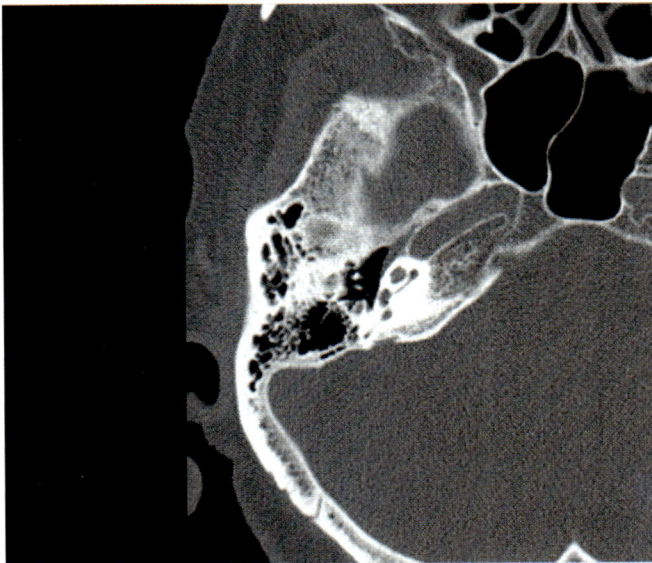
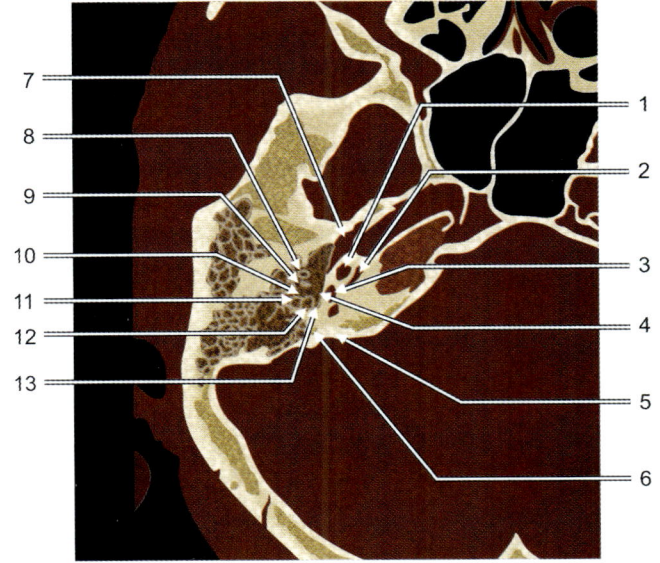

Figure 4.4

1. Apical turn, cochlea
2. Basal turn of cochlea
3. Vestibule
4. Stapes bone
5. Vestibular aqueduct
6. Posterior semicircular canal
7. Tensor tympani muscle
8. Malleus
9. Incus
10. Pyramidal eminence
11. Facial recess
12. Facial nerve
13. Sinus tympani

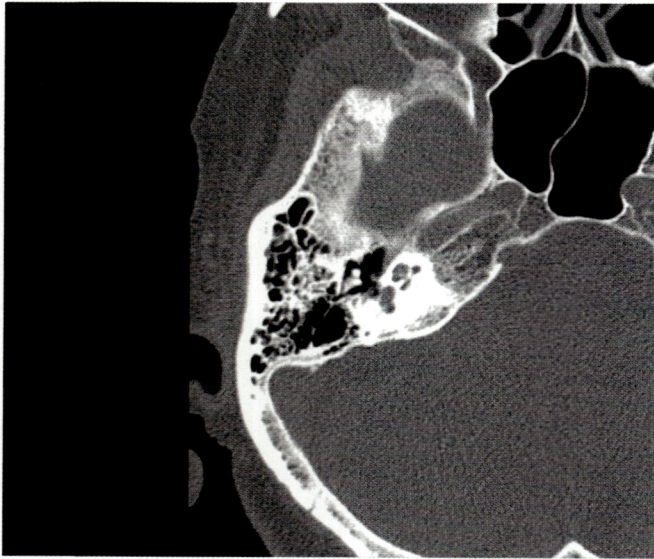
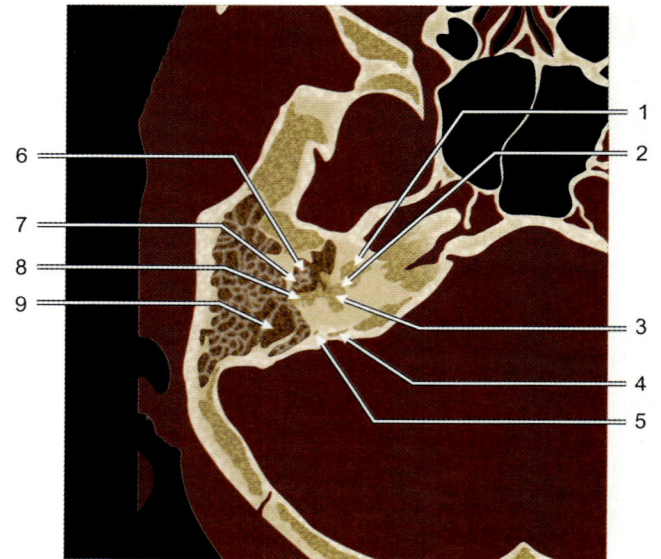

Figure 4.5

1. Cochlea
2. Vestibule
3. Oval window
4. Vestibular aqueduct
5. Posterior semicircular canal
6. Malleus
7. Incus
8. Facial nerve
9. Mastoid

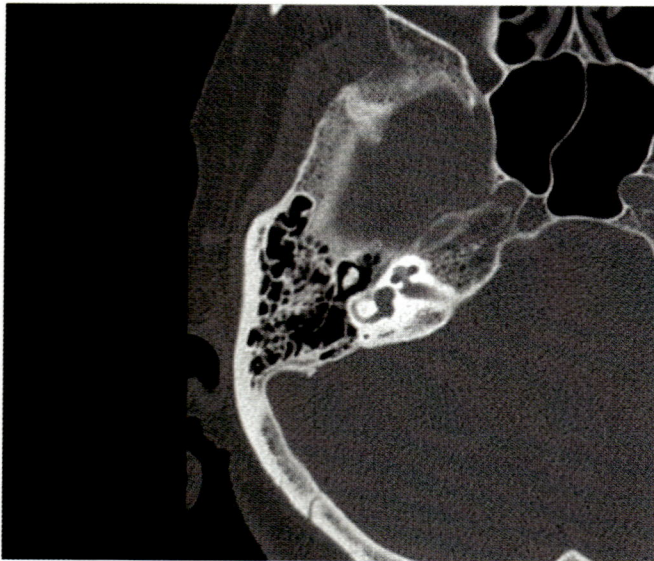
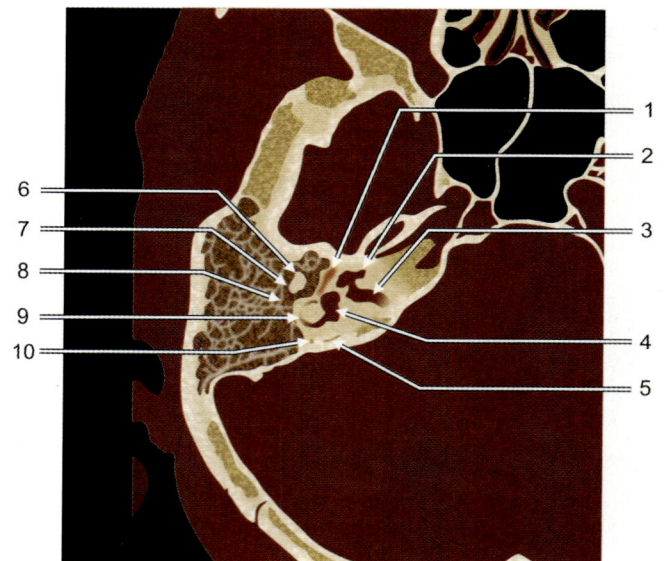

Figure 4.6

1. Facial nerve
2. Cochlea
3. Internal auditory canal
4. Vestibule
5. Vestibular aqueduct
6. Malleus
7. Incus
8. Aditus ad antrum
9. Lateral semicircular canal
10. Posterior semicircular canal

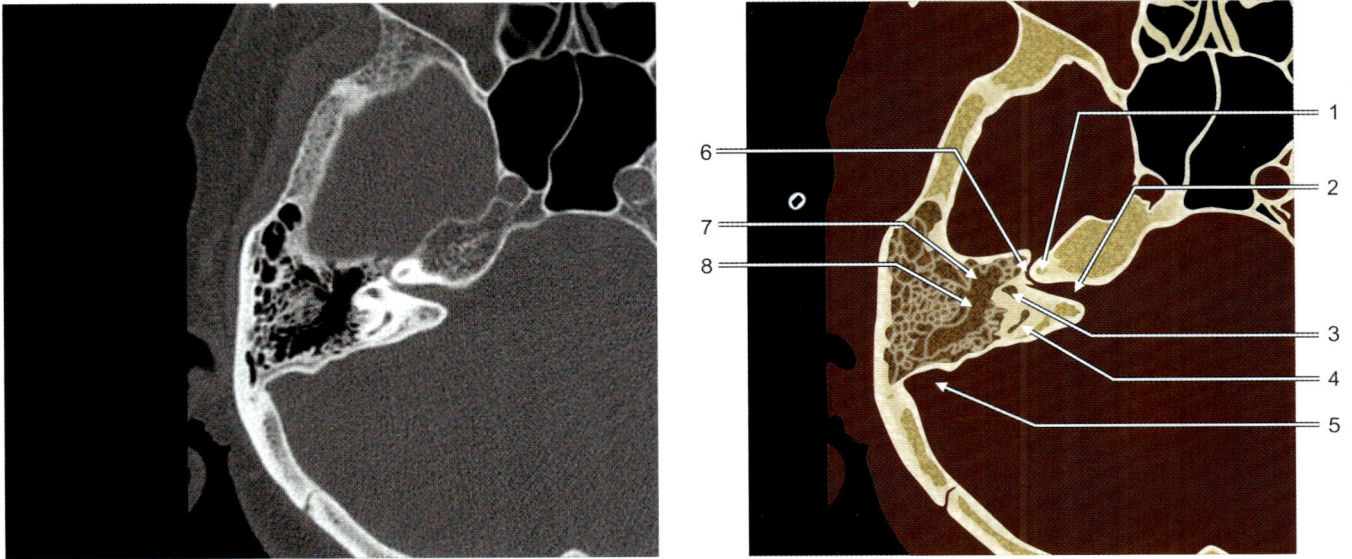

Figure 4.7

1. Cochlea
2. Internal auditory canal
3. Vestibule
4. Posterior semicircular canal
5. Sigmoid groove
6. Facial nerve
7. Epitympanum
8. Aditus ad antrum

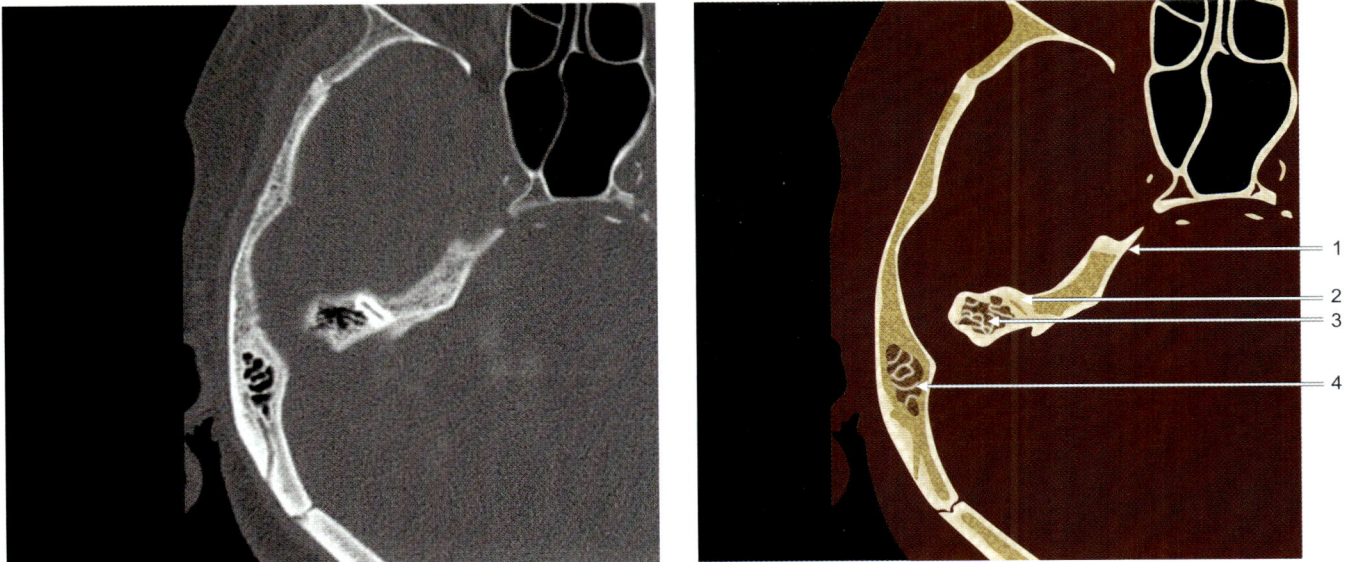

Figure 4.8

1. Petrous apex
2. Superior semicircular canal
3. Epitympanum
4. Mastoid

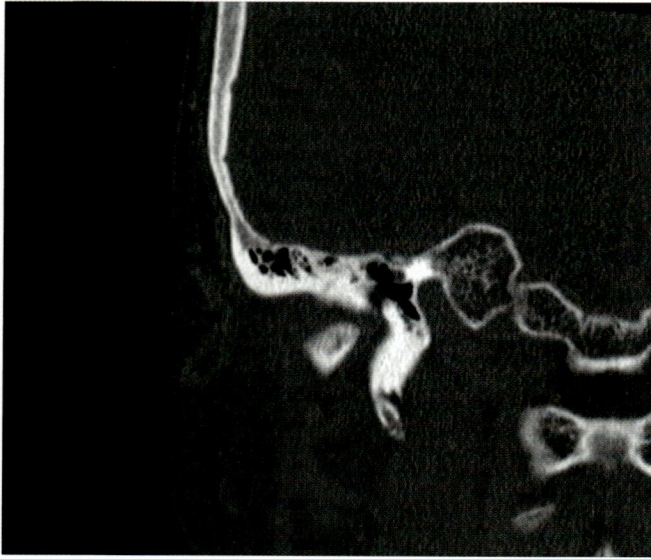

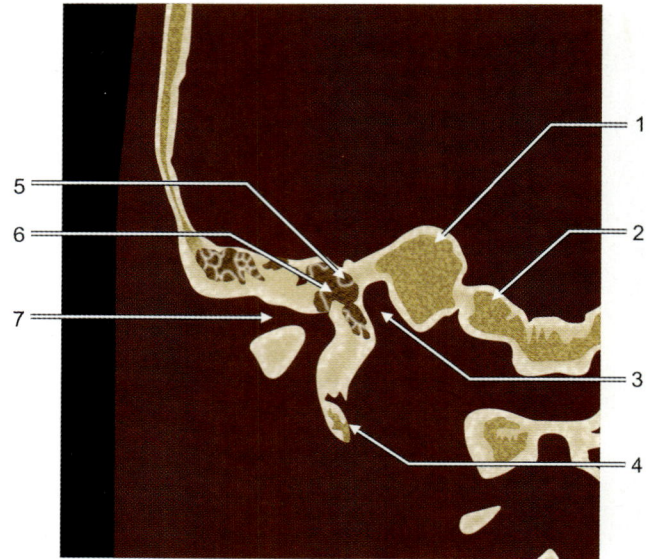

Figure 4.9

1. Petrous bone	5. Tensor tympani muscle
2. Basi-occiput	6. Eustachian tube
3. Carotid canal	7. TM joint
4. Styloid process	

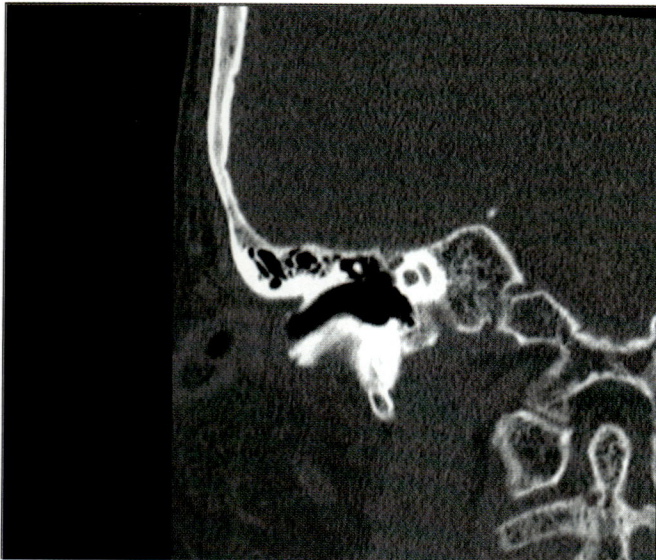

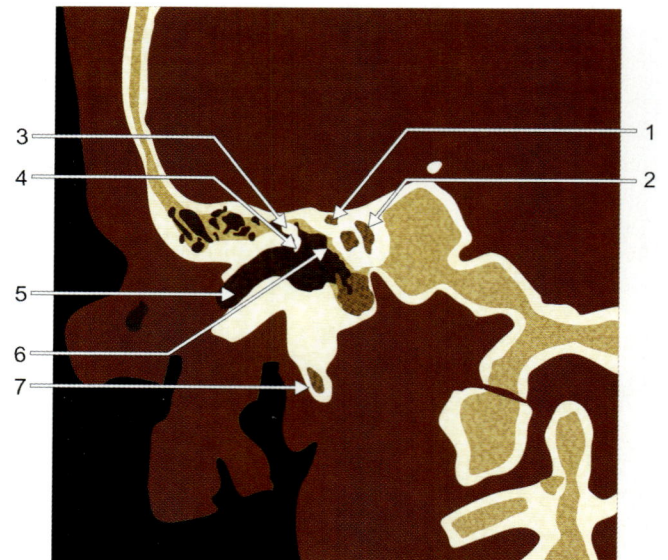

Figure 4.10

1. Facial nerve, anterior genu	5. External auditory canal
2. Cochlea	6. Tensor tympani
3. Malleus	7. Styloid process
4. Incus	

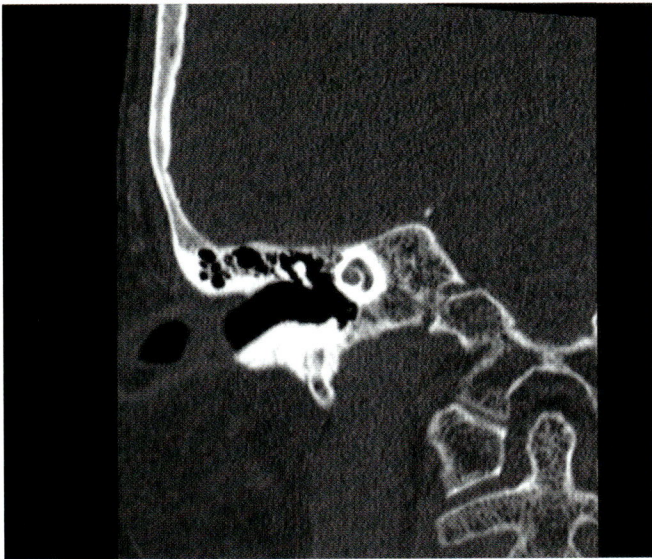
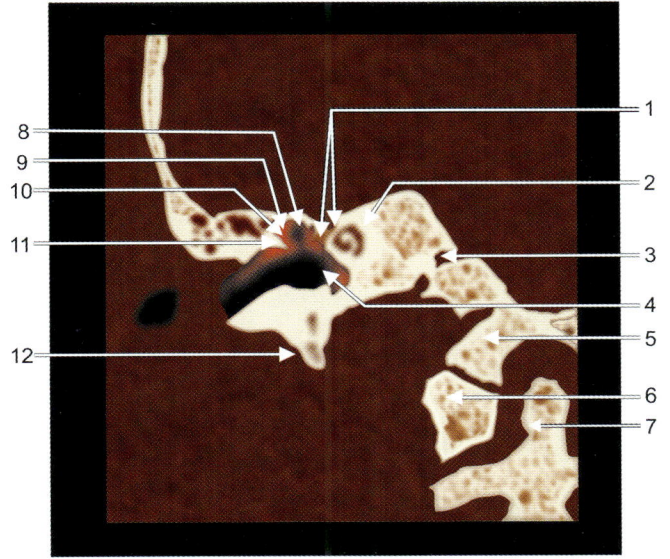

Figure 4.11

1. Facial nerve	7. Dens
2. Cochlea	8. Epitympanum
3. Petro-occipital fissure	9. Malleus
4. Middle ear	10. Prussak's space
5. Occipital condyle	11. Scutum
6. Lateral mass, atlas	12. Styloid process

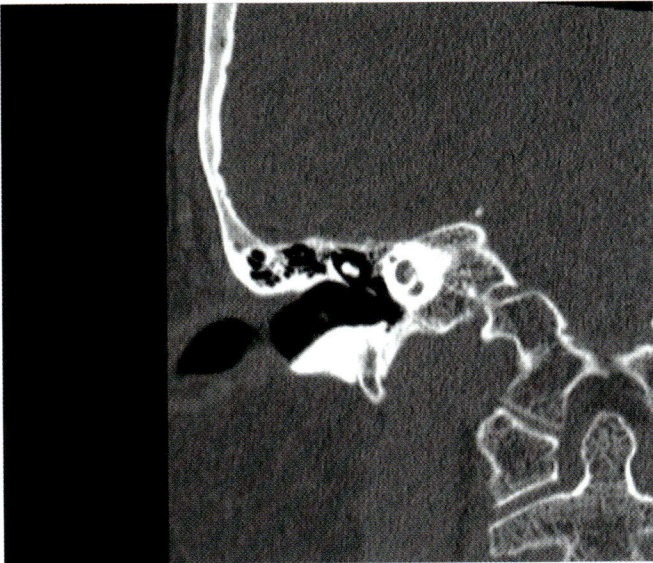
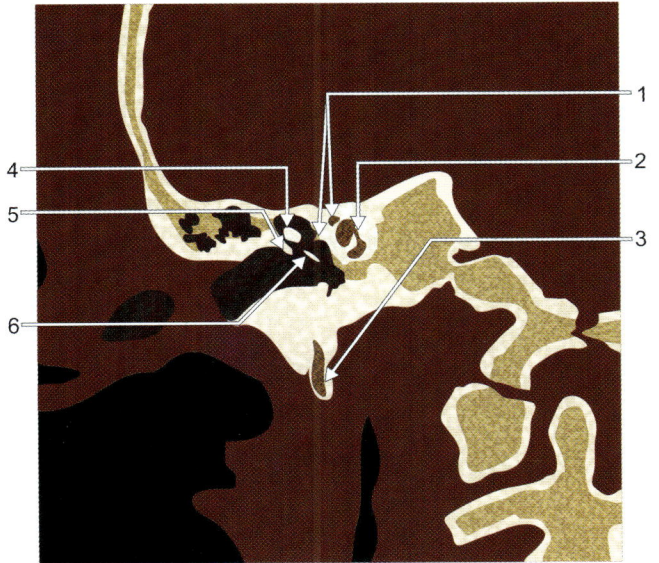

Figure 4.12

1. Facial nerve	4. Malleus
2. Cochlea	5. Scutum
3. Styloid process	6. Incus

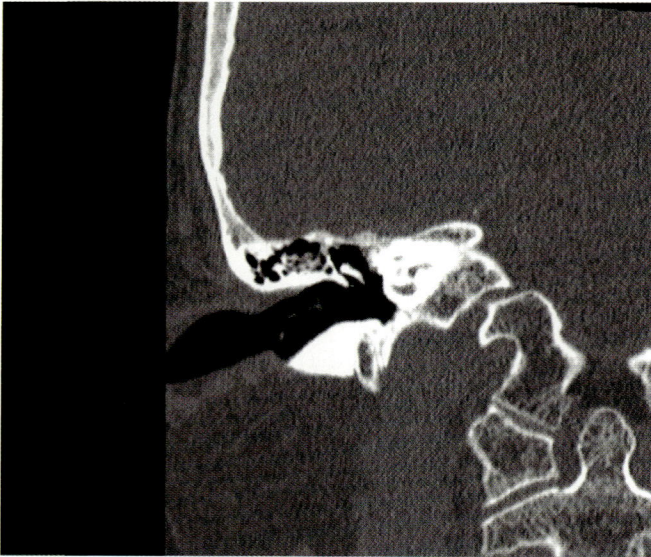

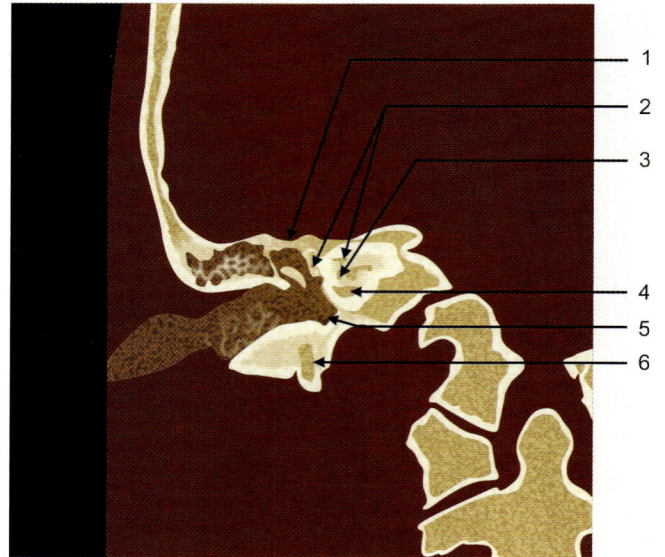

Figure 4.13

1. Tegmen tympanum	4. Cochlea, basal turn
2. Facial nerve	5. Hypotympanum
3. Cochlea, middle turn	6. Styloid process

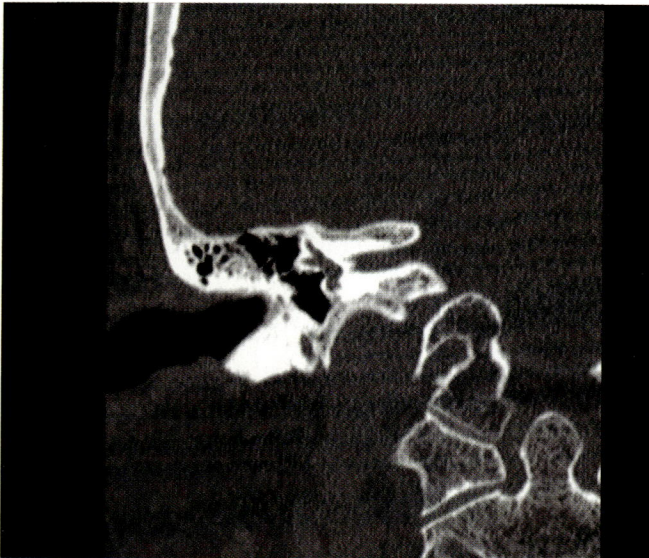

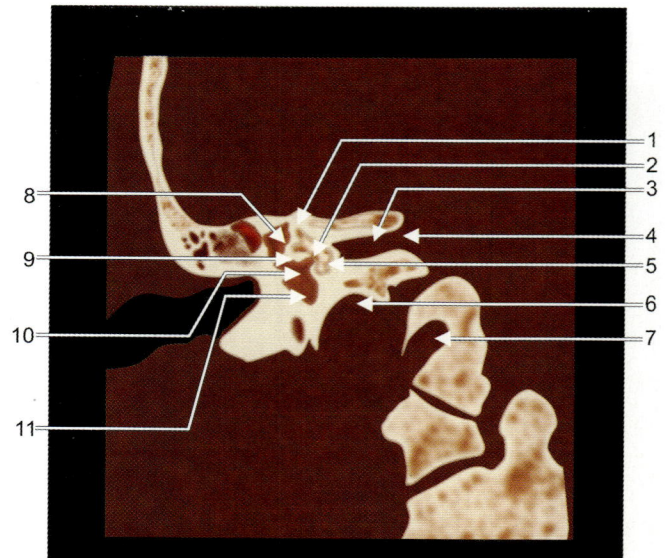

Figure 4.14

1. Superior semicircular canal	7. Hypoglossal cana
2. Oval window	8. Lateral semicircular canal
3. Internal auditory canal	9. Facial nerve
4. Porus acusticus	10. Stapes
5. Vestibule	11. Hypotympanum
6. Jugular fossa	

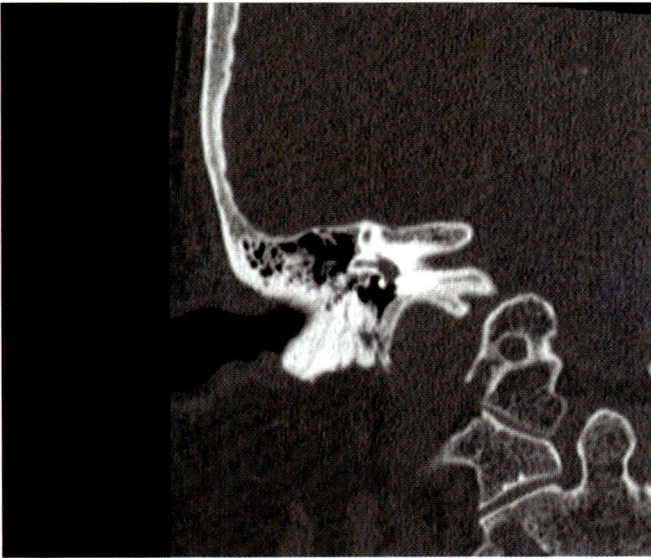

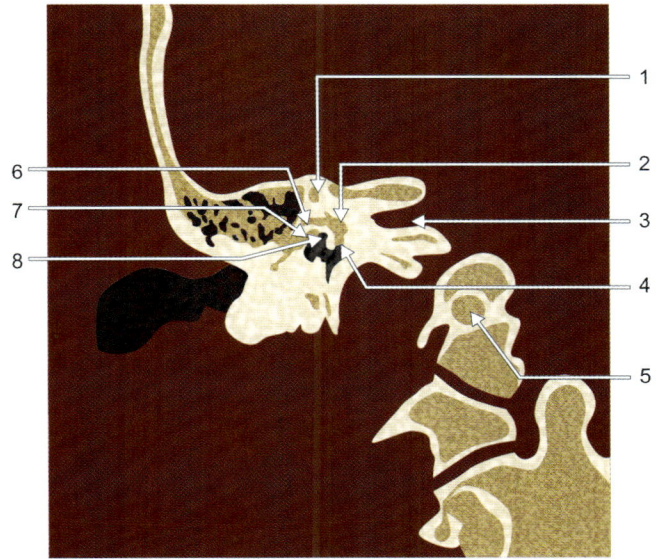

Figure 4.15

1. Superior semicircular canal	5. Hypoglossal canal
2. Vestibule	6. Lateral semicircular canal
3. Internal auditory canal	7. Facial nerve
4. Round window	8. Sinus tympani

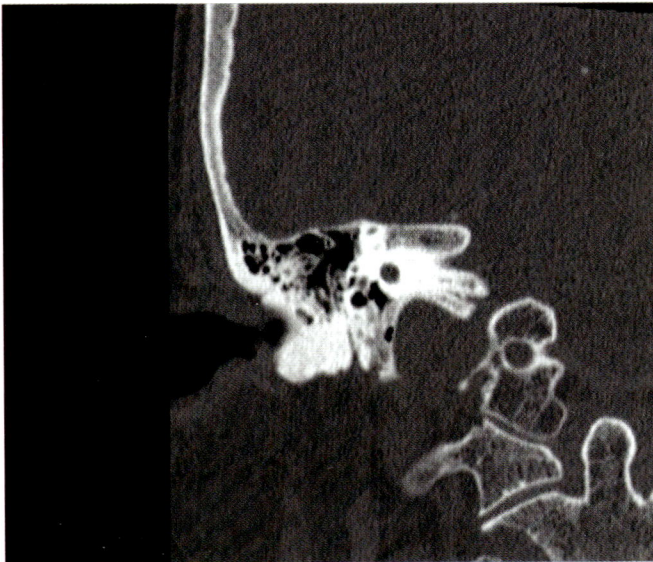

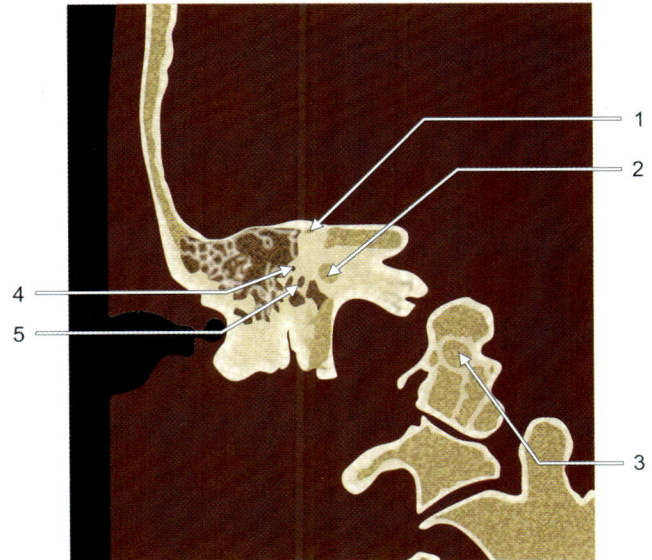

Figure 4.16

1. Superior semicircular canal
2. Vestibule
3. Hypoglossal canal
4. Lateral semicircular canal
5. Facial nerve

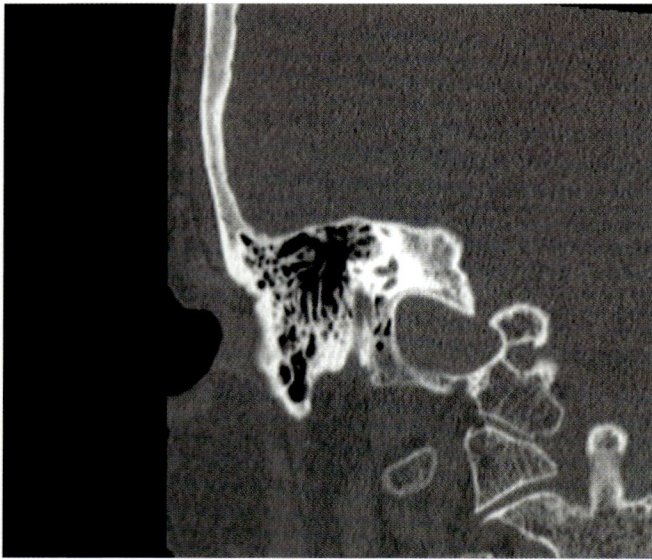

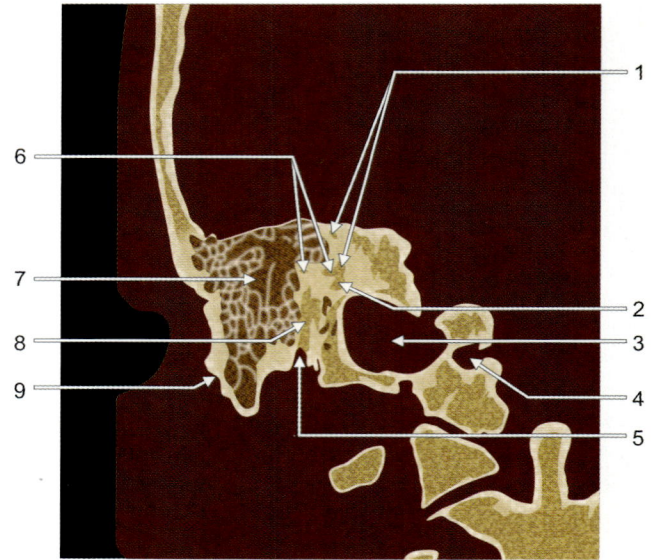

Figure 4.17

1. Superior semicircular canal	6. Lateral semicircular canal
2. Posterior semicircular canal	7. Mastoid sinus
3. Jugular fossa	8. Facial nerve
4. Hypoglossal canal	9. Mastoid process
5. Stylomastoid foramen	

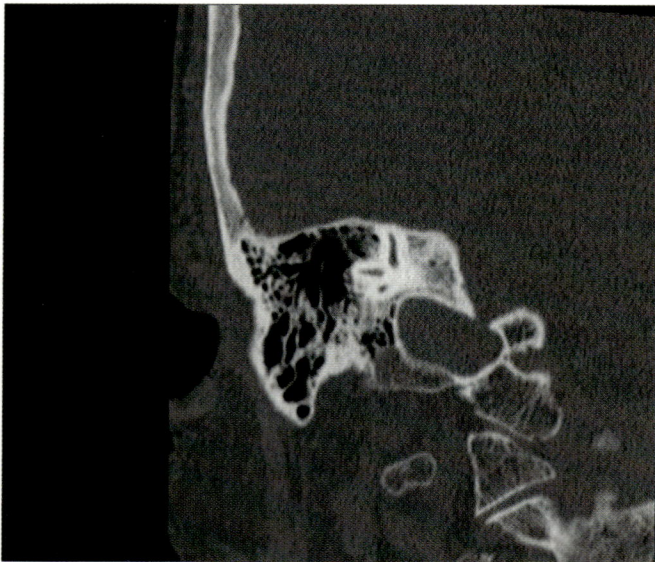

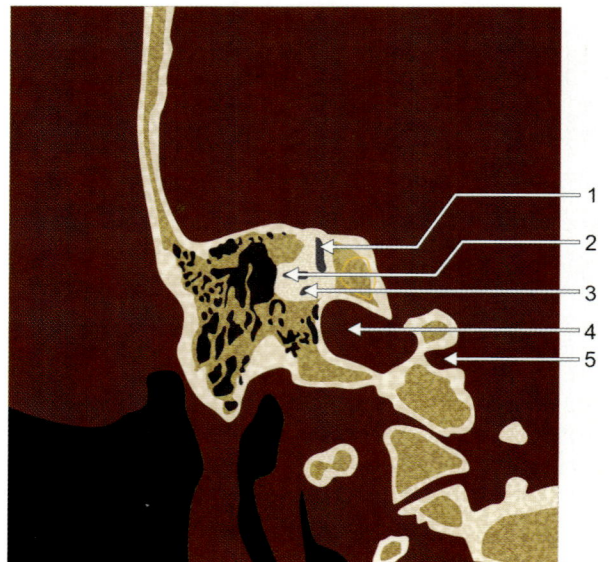

Figure 4.18

1. Superior semicircular canal	4. Jugular fossa
2. Lateral semicircular canal	5. Hypoglossal canal
3. Posterior semicircular canal	

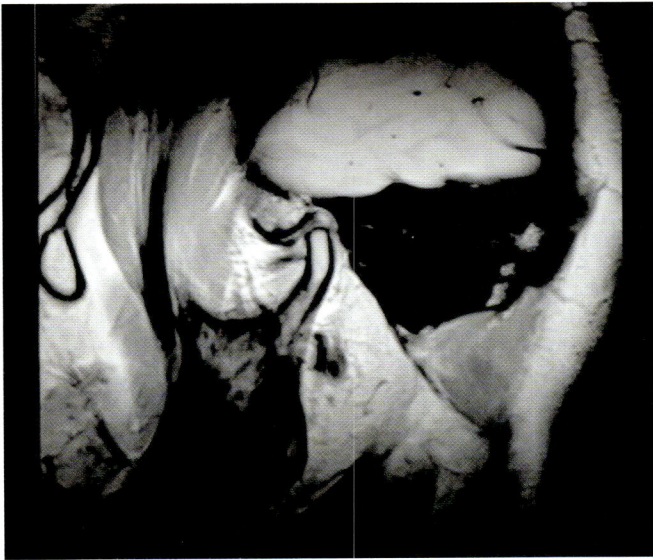
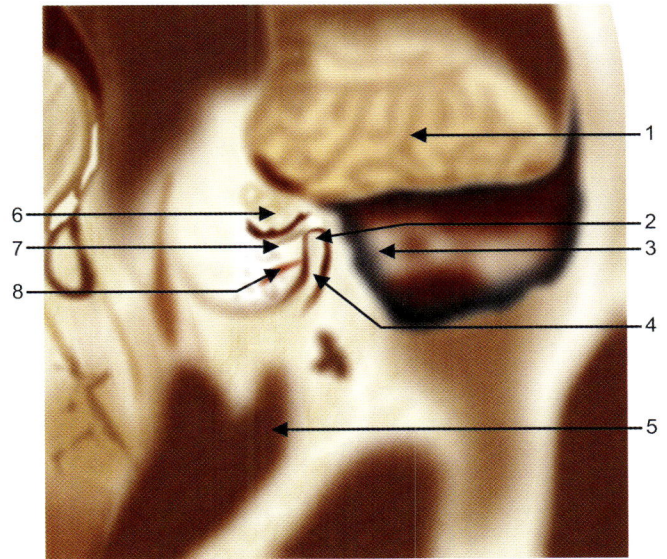

Figure 4.19

1. Temporal lobe, brain
2. Head of the mandible
3. External auditory canal
4. Neck of the mandible
5. Ramus of the mandible
6. Articular tubercle of temporal bone
7. Articular disk
8. Lateral pterygoid muscle

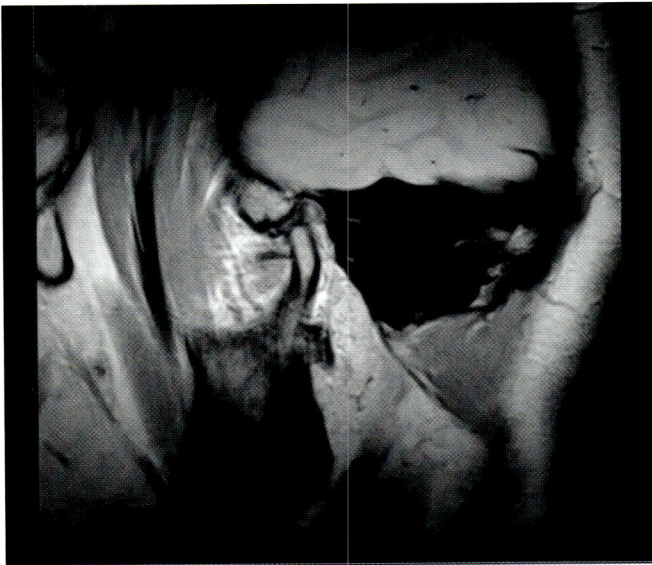
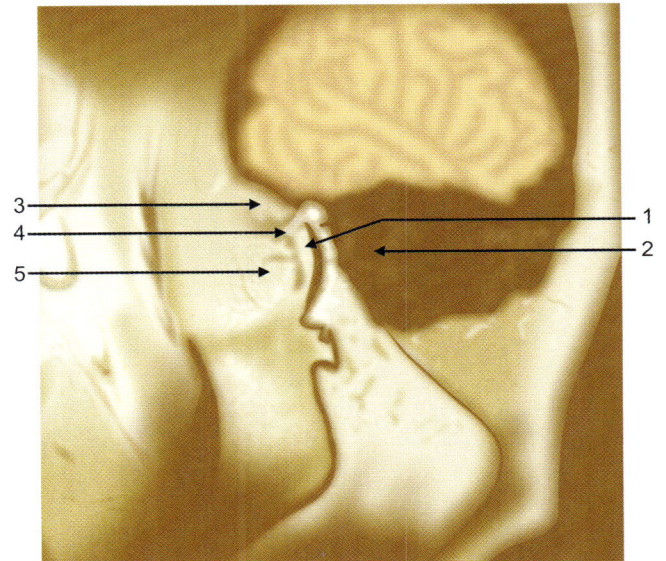

Figure 4.20

1. Head, mandible
2. External auditory canal
3. Articular tubercle
4. Articular disk
5. Lateral pterygoid muscle

CHAPTER 5

Neck

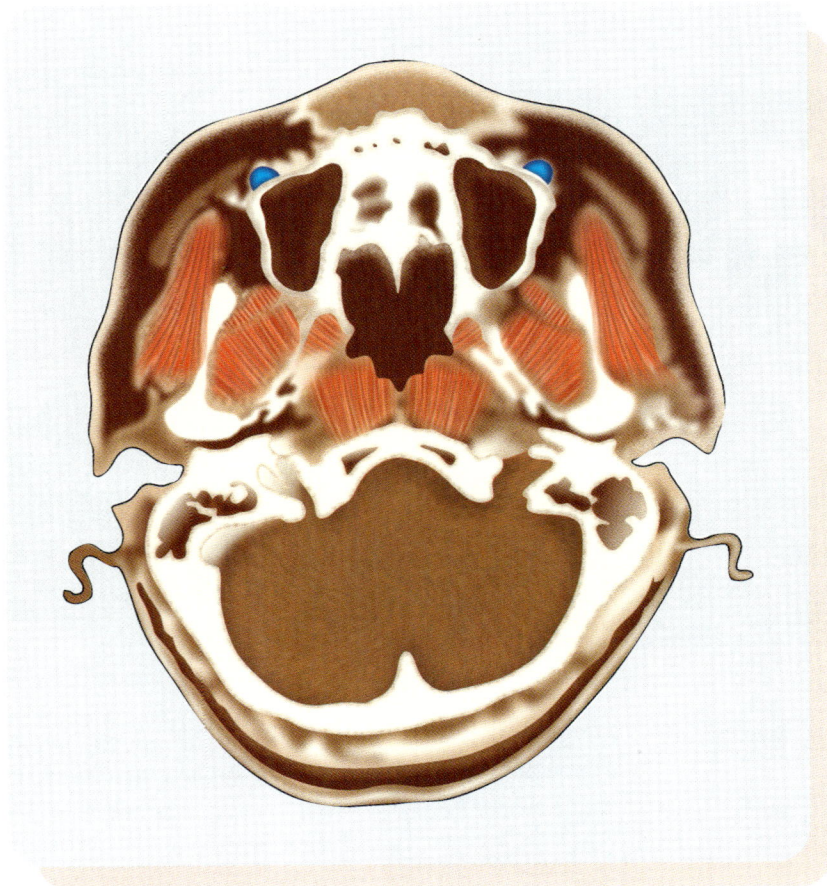

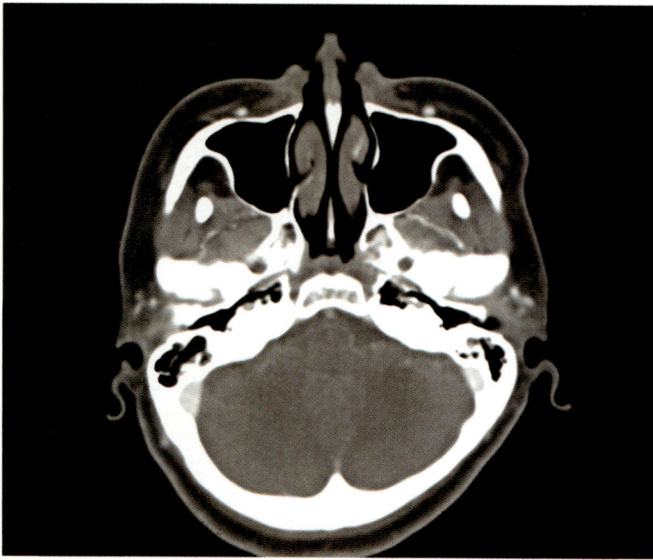
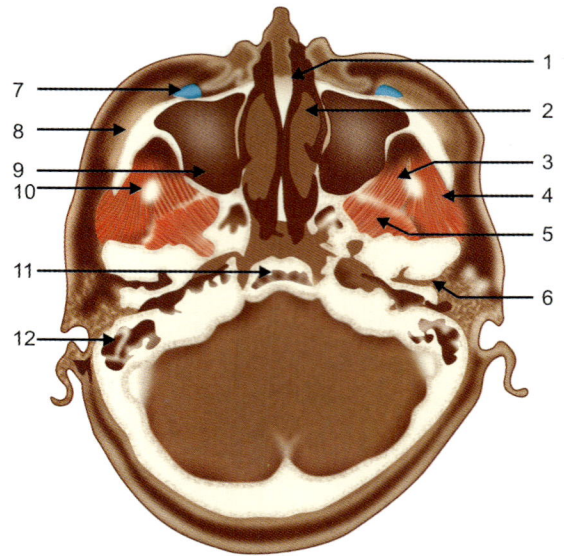

Figure 5.1

1. Nasal septum	5. Lateral pterygoid muscle	9. Maxillary antrum
2. Inferior turbinate	6. TM joint	10. Coronoid process, mandible
3. Temporalis muscle	7. Facial vein	11. Clivus
4. Masseter muscle	8. Zygoma	12. Mastoid sinus

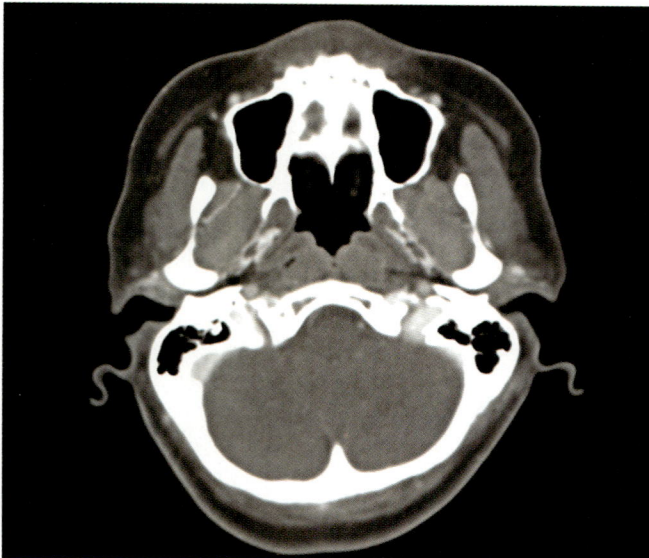
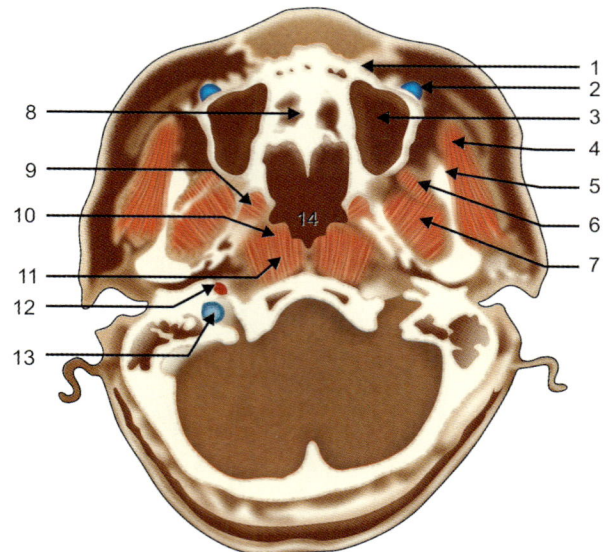

Figure 5.2

1. Alveolar margin, maxilla	6. Temporalis muscle	11. Longus capitis/collis muscle
2. Facial vein	7. Lateral pterygoid muscle	12. Internal carotid artery
3. Maxillary antrum	8. Hard palate	13. Jugular fossa
4. Masseter muscle	9. Medial pterygoid muscle	
5. Mandible	10. Torus tubarius	

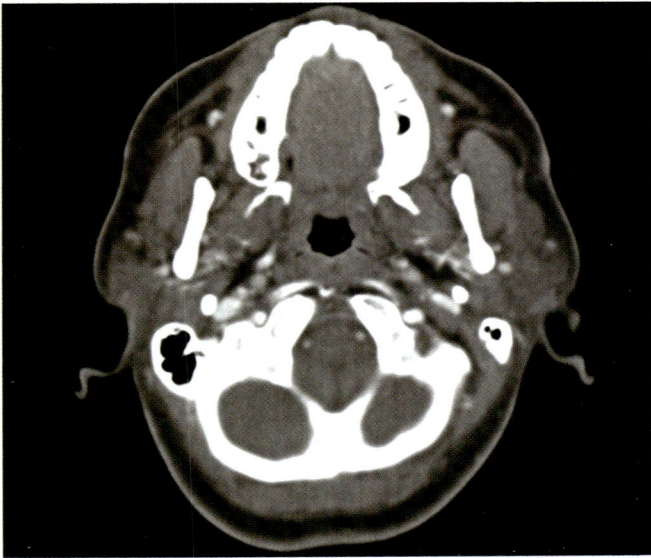

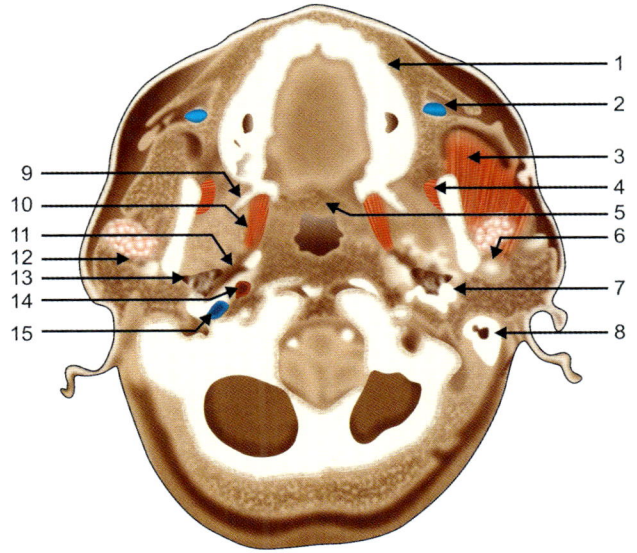

Figure 5.3

1. Maxilla, alveolar margin	6. Retromandibular vein	11. Parapharyngeal space
2. Facial vein	7. Styloid process	12. Parotid gland, superficial
3. Masseter	8. Mastoid	13. Parotid gland, deep lobe
4. Temporalis muscle	9. Lateral pterygoid plate	14. ICA
5. Soft palate	10. Medial pterygoid muscle	15. IJV

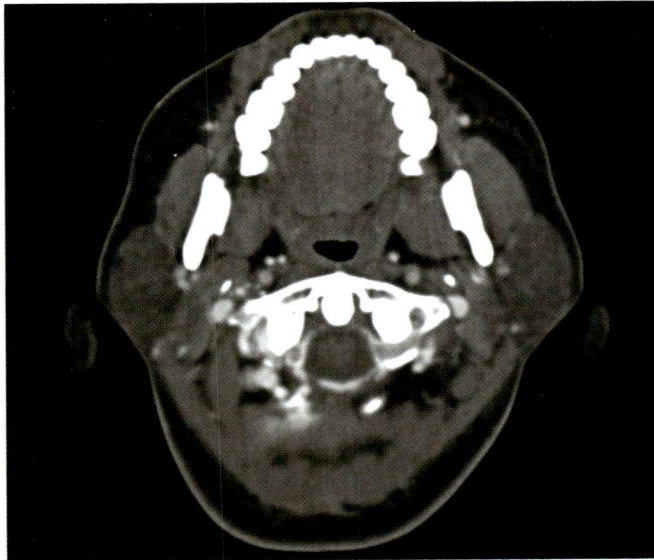

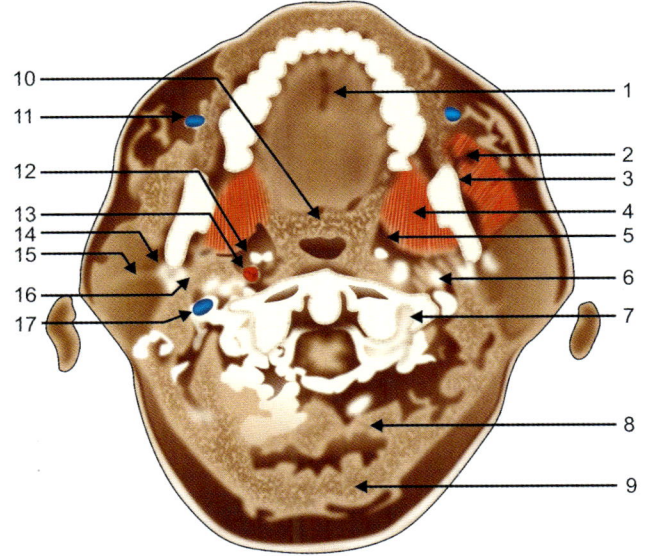

Figure 5.4

1. Tongue	7. Transverse foramen	13. ICA
2. Masseter	8. Paraspinal muscles	14. Retromandibular vein
3. Mandible	9. Trapezius muscle	15. Parotid gland
4. Medial pterygoid muscle	10. Soft palate	16. Parotid, deep lobe
5. Parapharyngeal space	11. Facial vein	17. IJV
6. Styloid process	12. Ascending pharyngeal vessels	

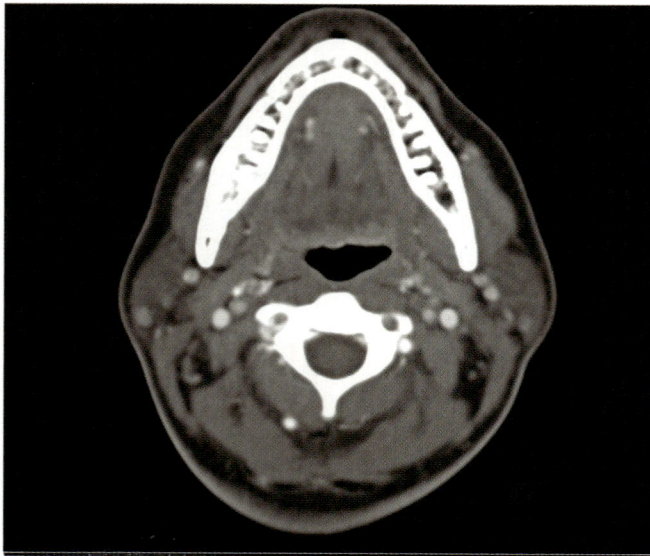

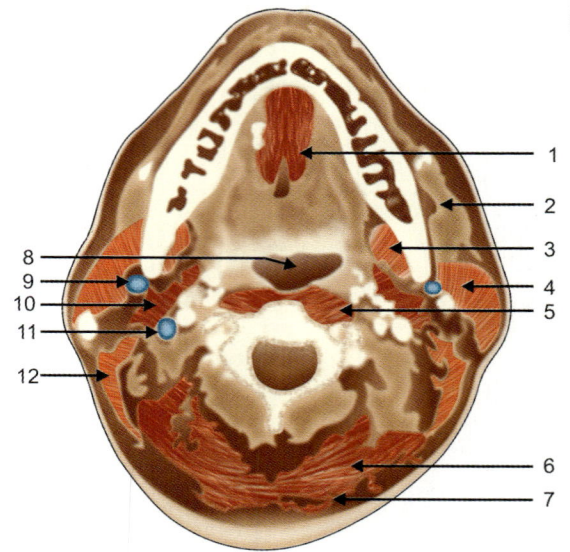

Figure 5.5

1. Genioglossus muscle	5. Longus collis muscle	9. Retromandibular vein
2. Masseter muscle	6. Splenius muscle	10. Digastric muscle, post belly
3. Medial pterygoid muscle	7. Trapezius muscle	11. IJV
4. Parotid gland	8. Oropharynx	12. Sternocleidomastoid muscle

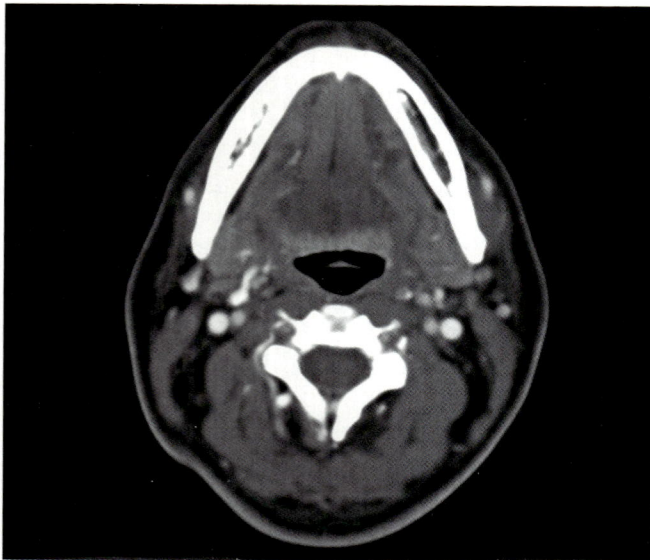

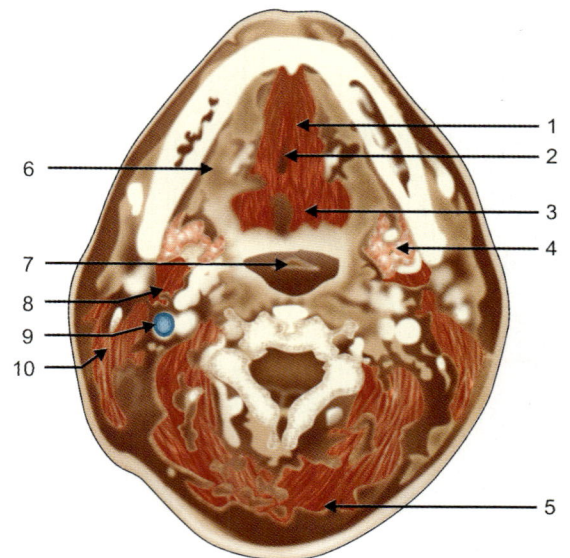

Figure 5.6

1. Genioglossus muscle	5. Trapezius muscle	9. IJV
2. Lingual septum	6. Mylohyoid	10. Sternocleidomastoid muscle
3. Hyoglossus muscle	7. Epiglottis	
4. Submandibular gland	8. Digastric muscle	

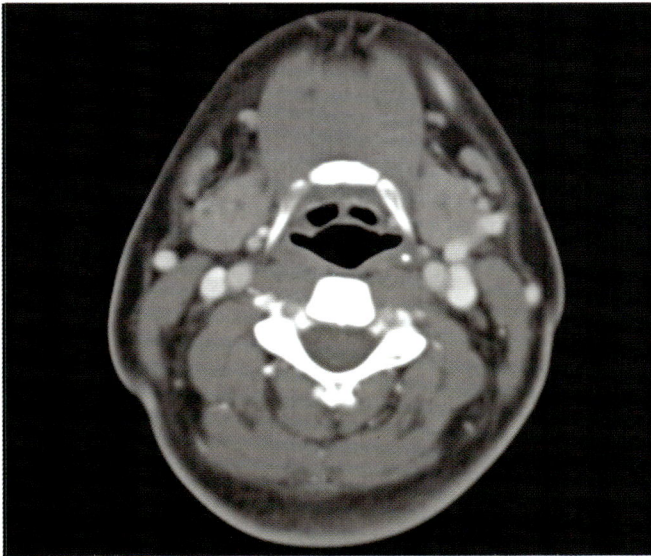

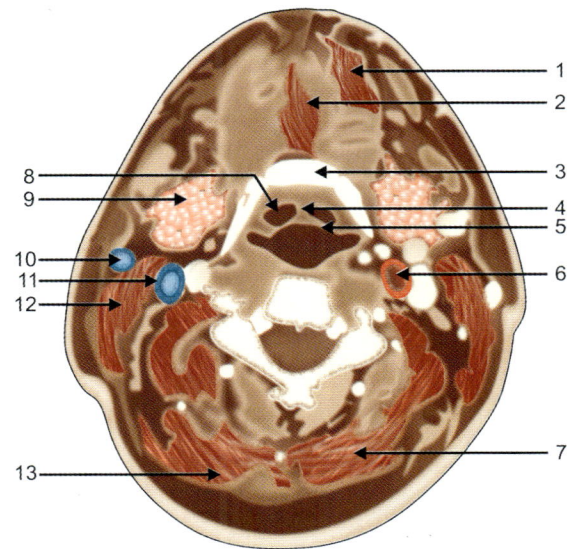

Figure 5.7

1. Digastric muscle	6. Carotid artery	11. Internal jugular vein
2. Mylohyoid muscle	7. Splenius muscle	12. Sternocleidomastoid muscle
3. Hyoid bone, body	8. Vallecula	13. Trapezius muscle
4. Median glosso-epiglottic fold	9. Submandibular gland	
5. Epiglottis	10. External jugular vein	

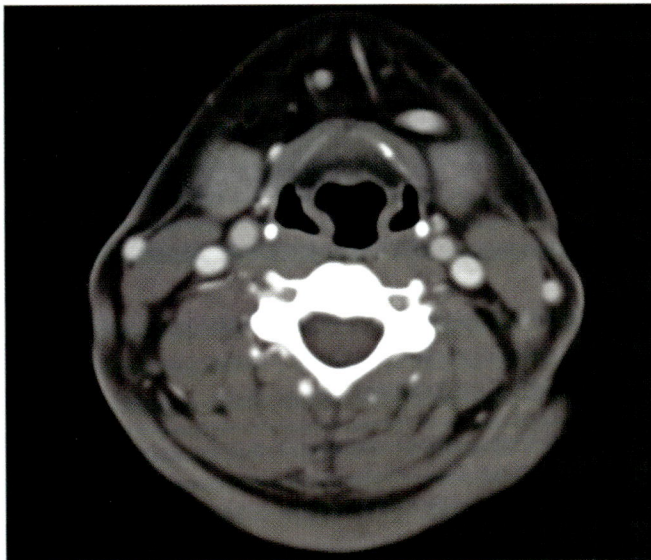

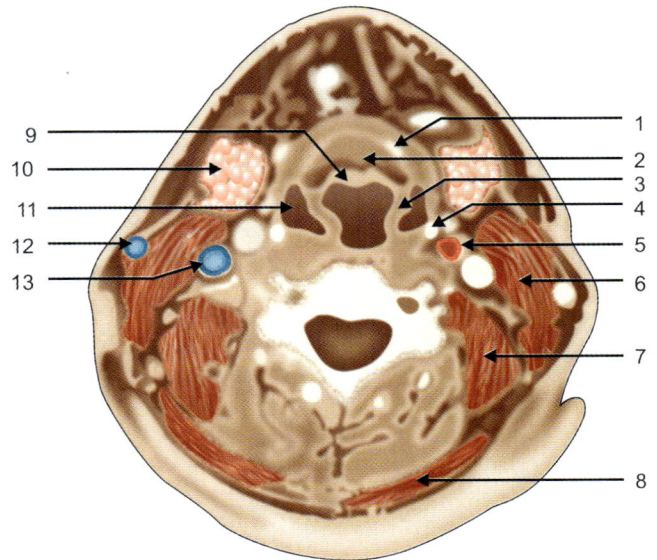

Figure 5.8

1. Thyroid cartilage	6. Sternocleidomastoid muscle	11. Pyriform sinus
2. Preepiglottic space	7. Levator scapulae	12. External jugular vein
3. Aryepiglottic fold	8. Trapezius	13. Internal jugular vein
4. Superior horn, thyroid cartilage	9. Epiglottis	
5. Common carotid artery	10. Submandibular gland	

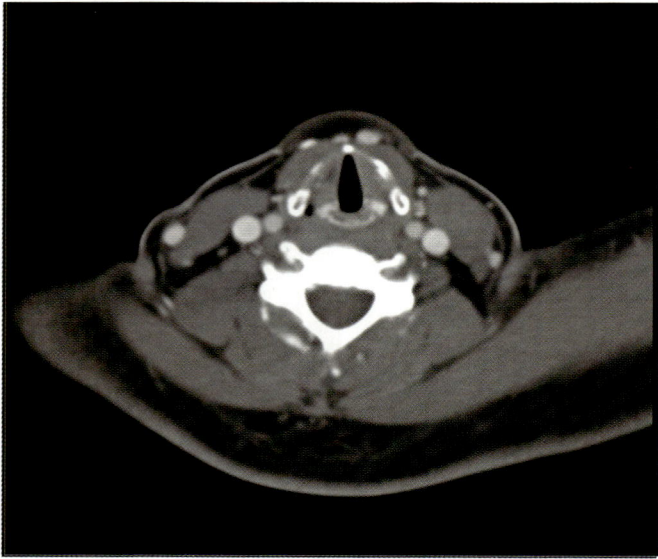

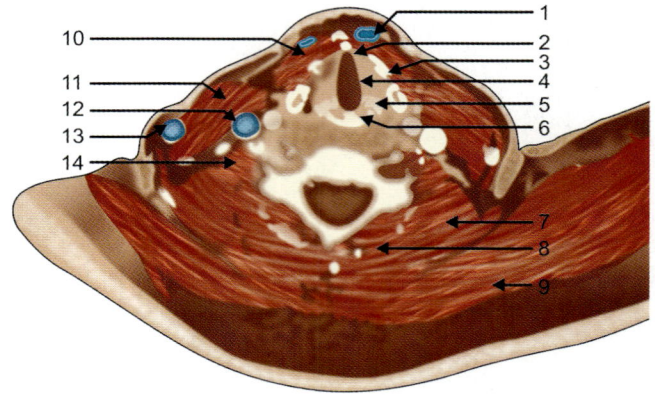

Figure 5.9

1. Anterior jugular vein	8. Paraspinal muscles
2. Anterior commissure	9. Trapezius muscle
3. Thyroid cartilage	10. Strap muscles
4. Vocal cord	11. Sternocleidomastoid muscle
5. Arytenoid cartilage	12. Internal jugular vein
6. Cricoid cartilage	13. External jugular vein
7. Levator scapulae	14. Middle scalene muscle

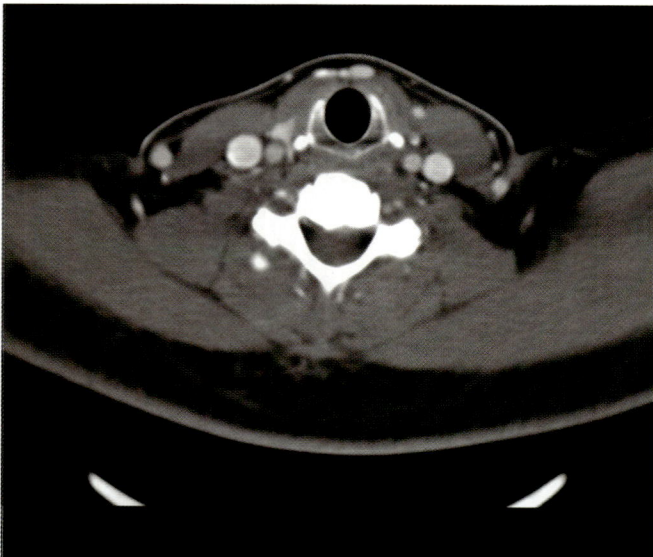

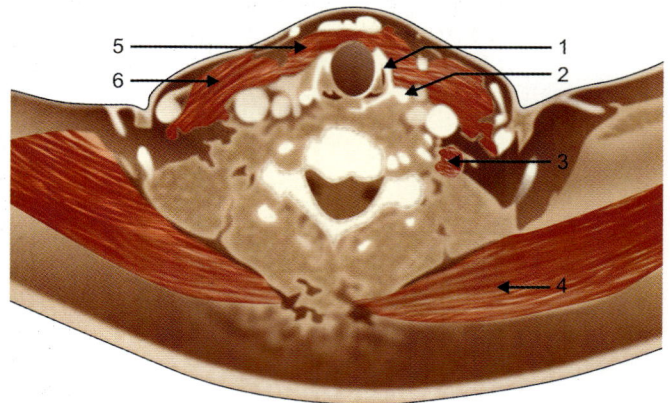

Figure 5.10

1. Cricoid cartilage	4. Trapezius muscle
2. Inferior horn of thyroid cartilage	5. Strap muscle
3. Middle scalene muscle	6. Sternocleidomastoid muscle

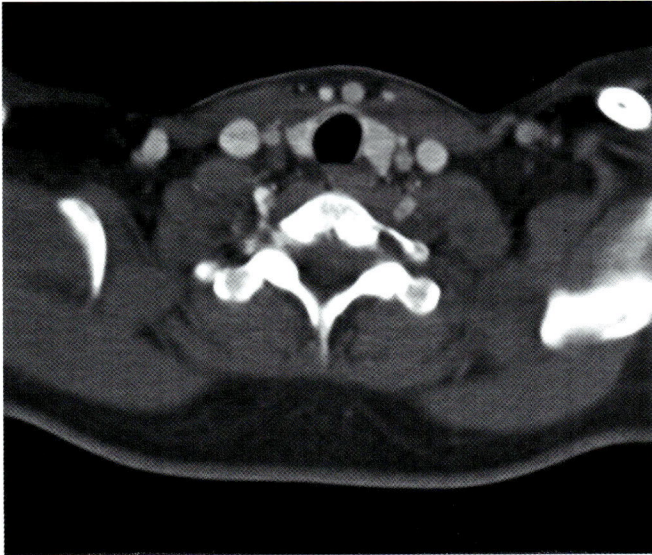

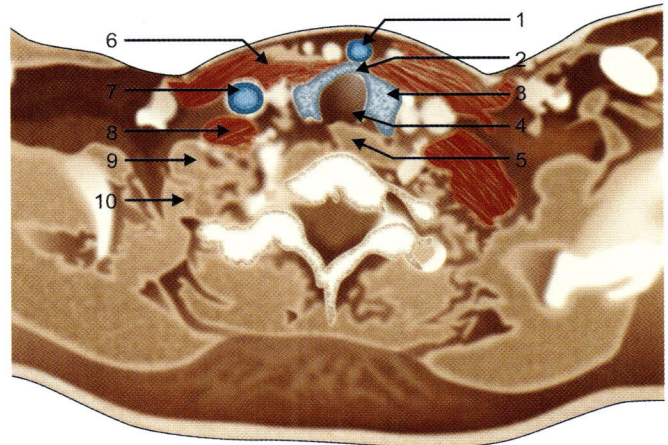

Figure 5.11

1. Anterior jugular vein	6. Sternocleidomastoid muscle
2. Thyroid isthmus	7. Internal jugular vein
3. Thyroid gland, left lobe	8. Scalene muscles, anterior
4. Trachea	9. Middle scalene muscle
5. Esophagus	10. Posterior scalene muscle

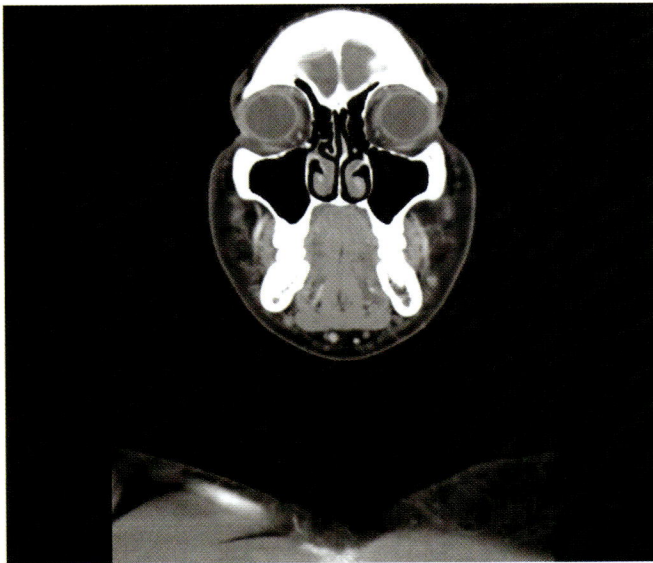

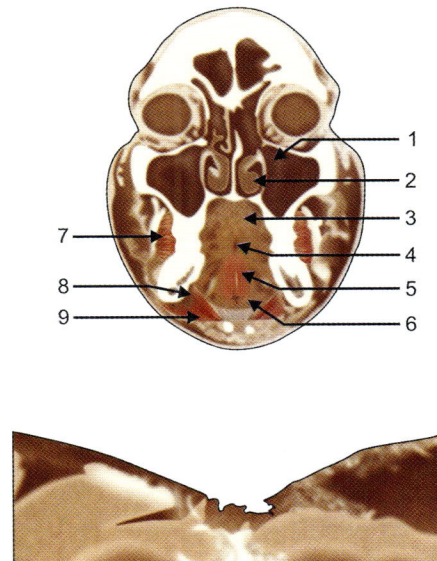

Figure 5.12

1. Maxillary antrum	6. Geniohyoid muscle
2. Inferior turbinate	7. Buccinator muscle
3. Tongue	8. Mylohyoid muscle
4. Lingual septum	9. Digastric muscle, anterior belly
5. Genioglossus muscle	

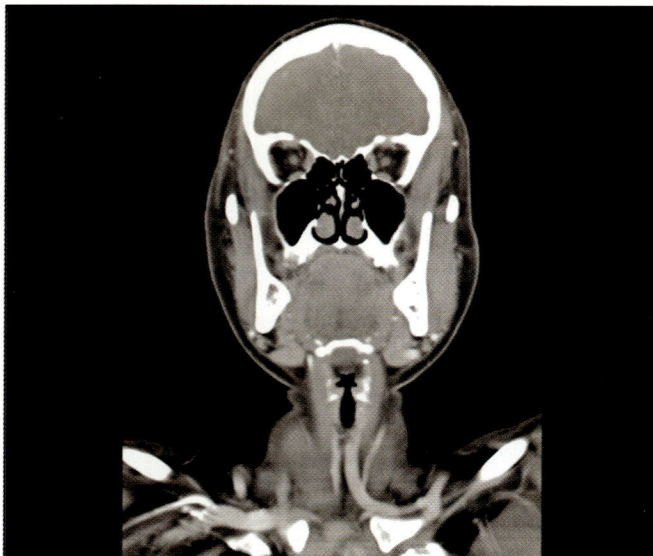

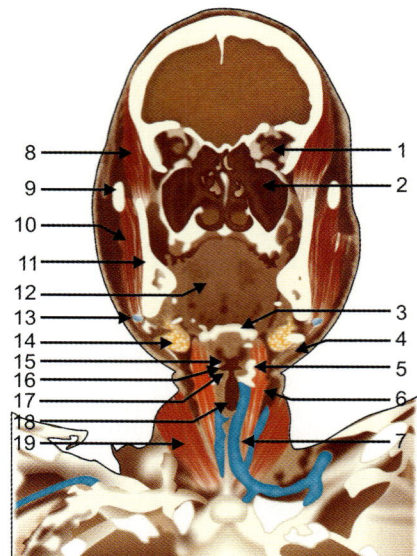

Figure 5.13

1. Optic nerve	6. Sternothyroid muscle	11. Mandible	16. Laryngeal ventricle
2. Maxillary antrum	7. Anterior jugular vein	12. Tongue	17. True vocal cord
3. Hyoid bone	8. Temporalis muscle	13. Facial vein	18. Trachea
4. Platysma	9. Zygomatic arch	14. Submandibular gland	19. Sternocleidomastoid muscle
5. Thyroid cartilage	10. Masseter muscle	15. False vocal cord	

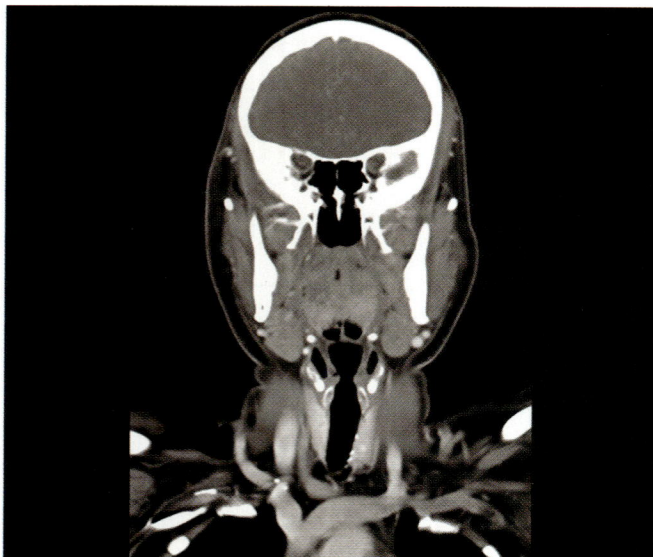

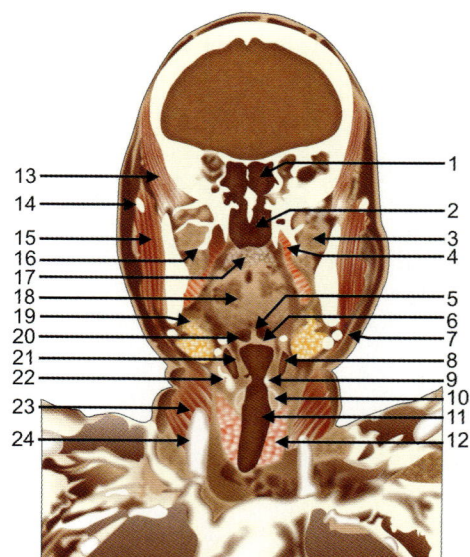

Figure 5.14

1. Ethmoid sinus	7. Platysma muscle	13. Temporalis muscle	19. Submandibular gland
2. Nasopharynx	8. Pyriform sinus	14. Zygomatic arch	20. Vallecula
3. Lateral pterygoid muscle	9. True vocal cord	15. Masseter muscle	21. Aryepiglottic fold
4. Medial pterygoid muscle	10. Cricoid cartilage	16. Lateral pterygoid plate	22. Thyroid cartilage
5. Median glossoepiglottic fold	11. Trachea	17. Soft palate	23. Sternocleidomastoid muscle
6. Epiglottis	12. Thyroid lobe	18. Tongue	24. Internal jugular vein

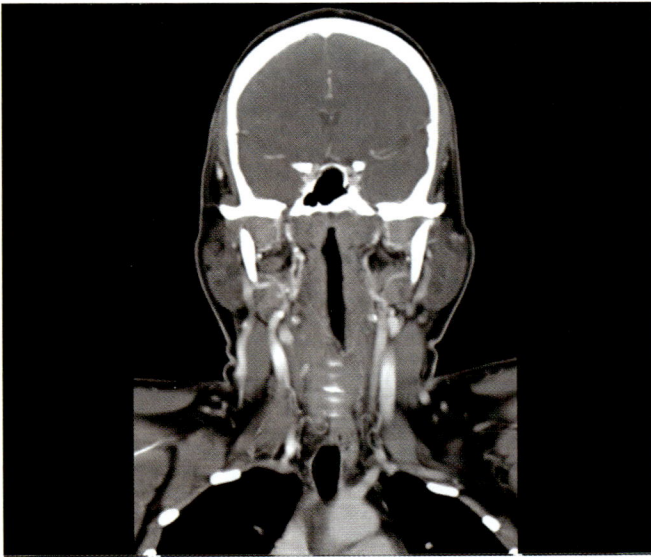

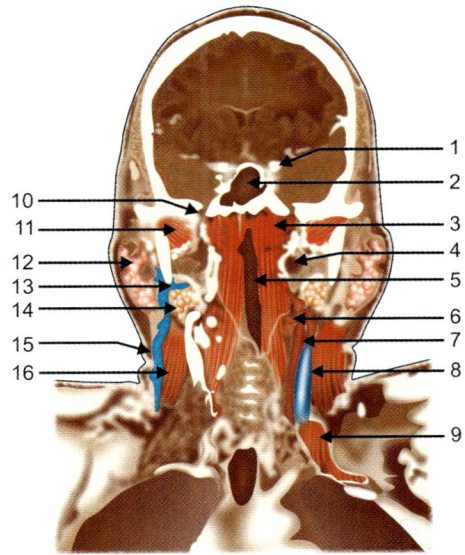

Figure 5.15

1. Anterior clinoid	5. Pharynx	9. Scalenus anterior muscle	13. Retromandibular vein
2. Sphenoid sinus	6. Hyoid bone, cornu	10. Foramen ovale	14. Submandibular gland
3. Longus capitis	7. Carotid artery	11. Lateral pterygoid muscle	15. External jugular vein
4. Parapharyngeal space	8. Internal jugular vein	12. Parotid gland	16. Sternocleidomastoid muscle

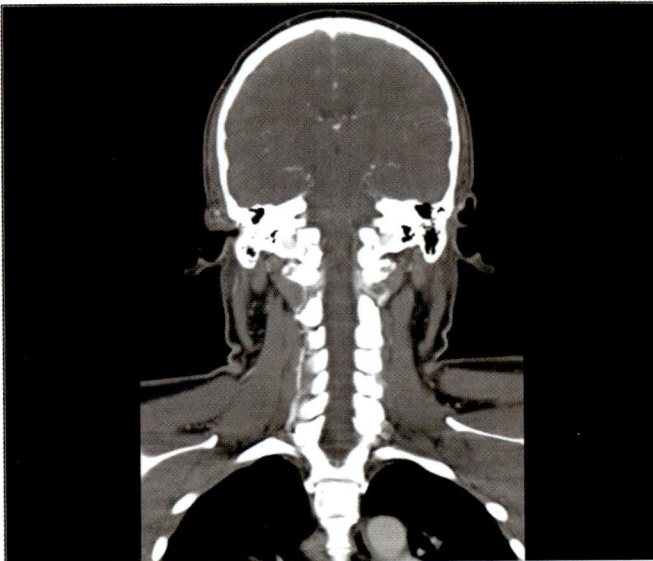

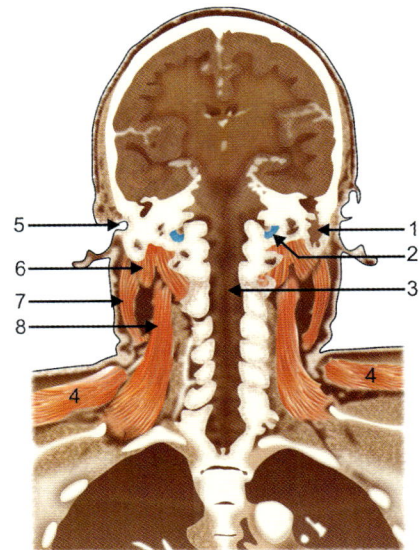

Figure 5.16

1. Mastoid sinus	5. External auditory canal
2. Internal Jugular vein	6. Digastric muscle
3. Spinal cord	7. Sternocleidomastoid muscle
4. Trapezius	8. Levator scapulae

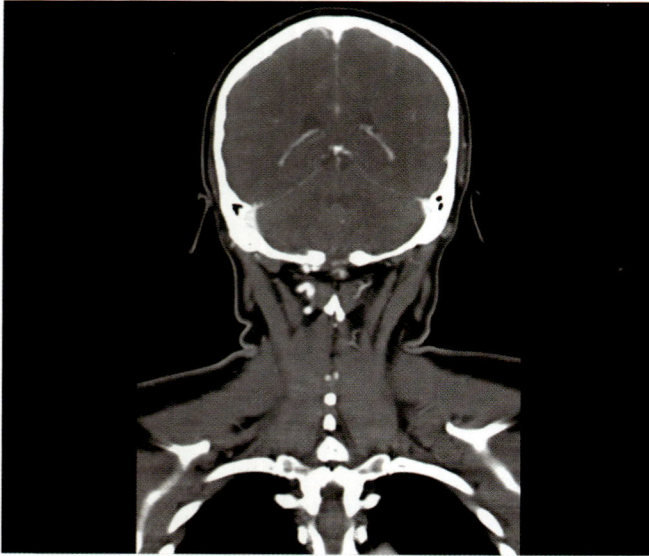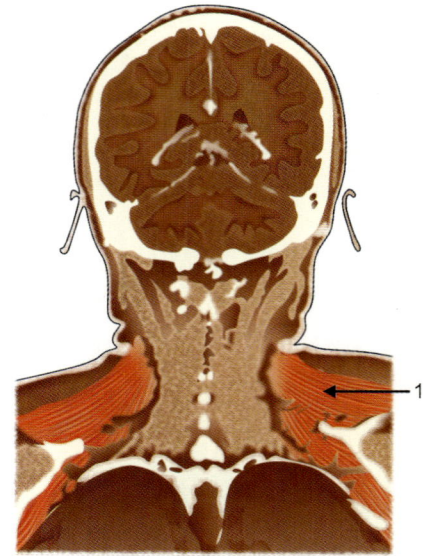

Figure 5.17

1. Trapezius

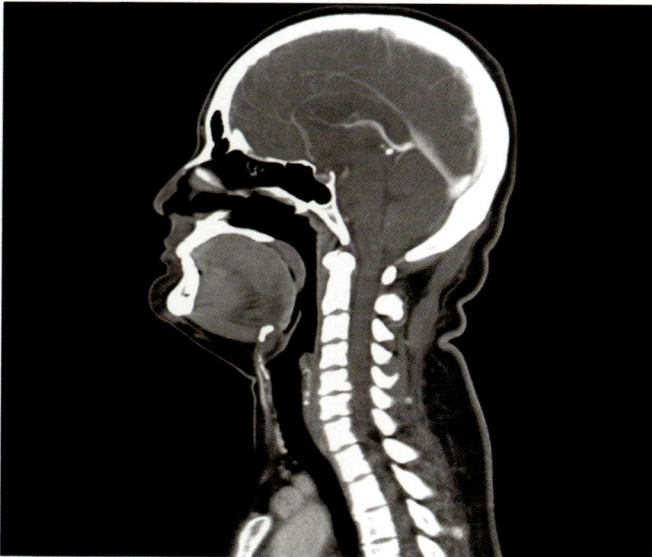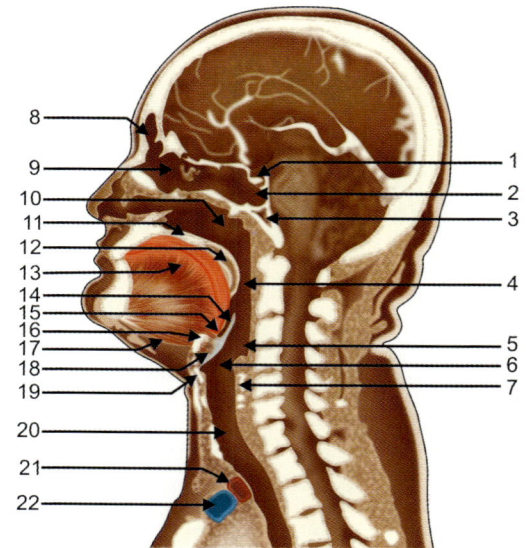

Figure 5.18

1. Pituitary gland	7. Cricoid cartilage	13. Tongue	19. Thyroid cartilage
2. Sphenoid sinus	8. Frontal sinus	14. Epiglottis	20. Trachea
3. Clivus	9. Ethmoid sinuses	15. Vallecula	21. Bracheocephalic artery
4. Oropharynx	10. Nasopharynx	16. Hyoid bone	22. Bracheocephalic vein
5. Hypopharynx	11. Hard palate	17. Mylohyoid muscle	
6. Larynx	12. Soft palate	18. Preepiglottic space	

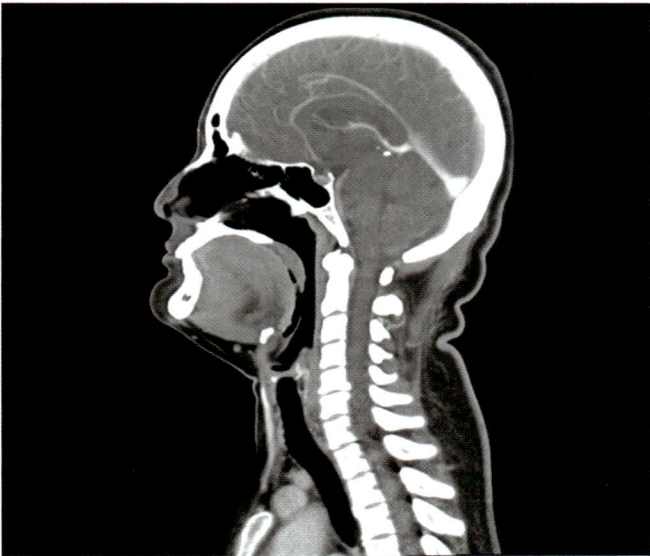

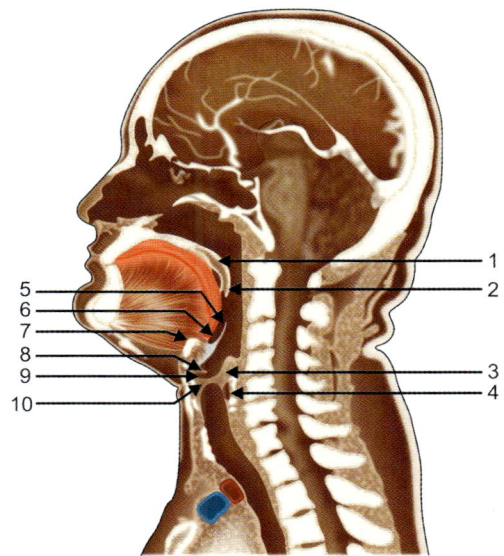

Figure 5.19

1. Soft palate	5. Epiglottis	9. Laryngeal ventricle
2. Uvula	6. Vallecula	10. True vocal cord
3. Arytenoid cartilage	7. Hyoid	
4. Cricoid cartilage	8. False vocal cord	

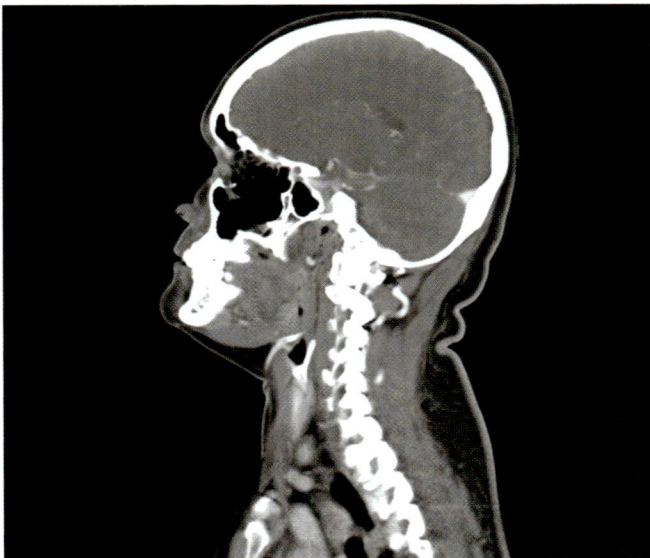

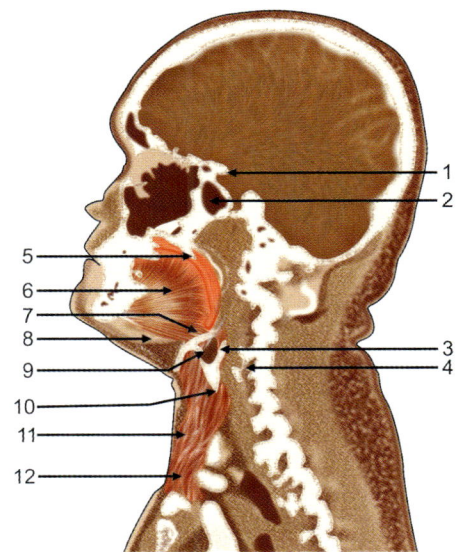

Figure 5.20

1. Anterior clinoid	4. Vertebral artery	7. Hyoid bone	10. Thyroid cartilage
2. Sphenoid sinus	5. Hard palate	8. Mylohyoid muscle	11. Strap muscles
3. Superior horn, thyroid cartilage	6. Tongue	9. Pyriform sinus	12. Sternocleidomastoid muscle

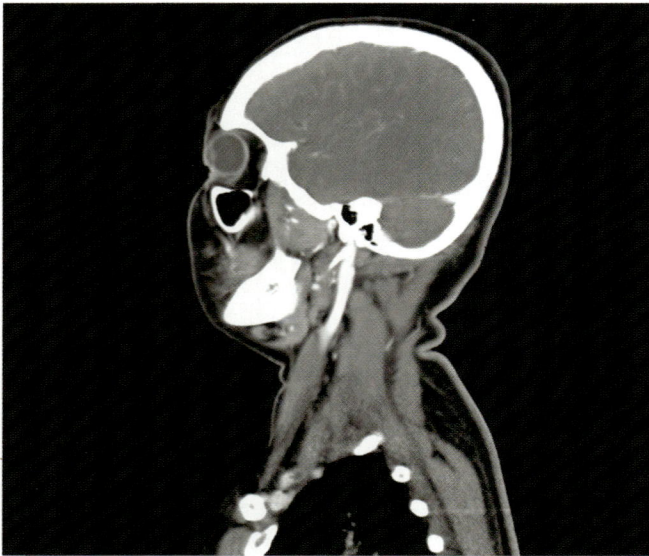

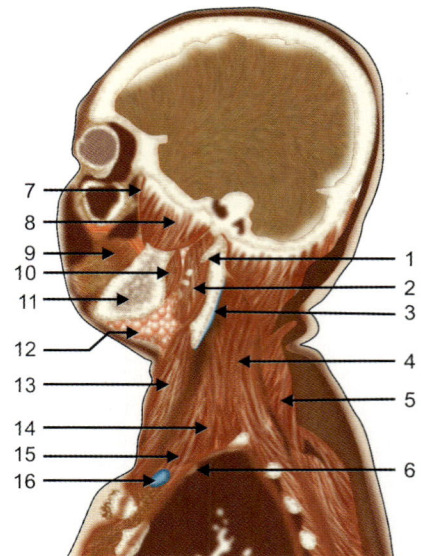

Figure 5.21

1. Styloid process	9. Buccinator muscle
2. Digastric muscle	10. Medial pterygoid muscle
3. Internal jugular vein	11. Mandible
4. Levator scapulae	12. Submandibular gland
5. Trapezius muscle	13. Sternocleidomastoid muscle
6. Subclavian artery	14. Scalenus medius muscle
7. Temporalis muscle	15. Scalenus anterior muscle
8. Lateral pterygoid muscle	16. Subclavian vein

Section 2

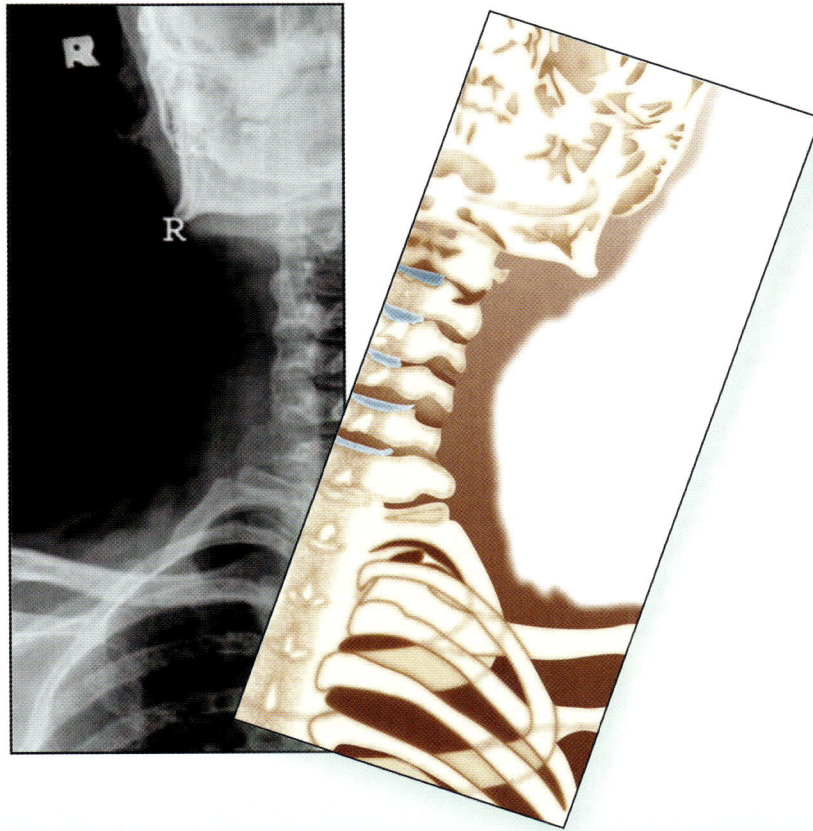

Spine

- Spine

CHAPTER 6

Spine

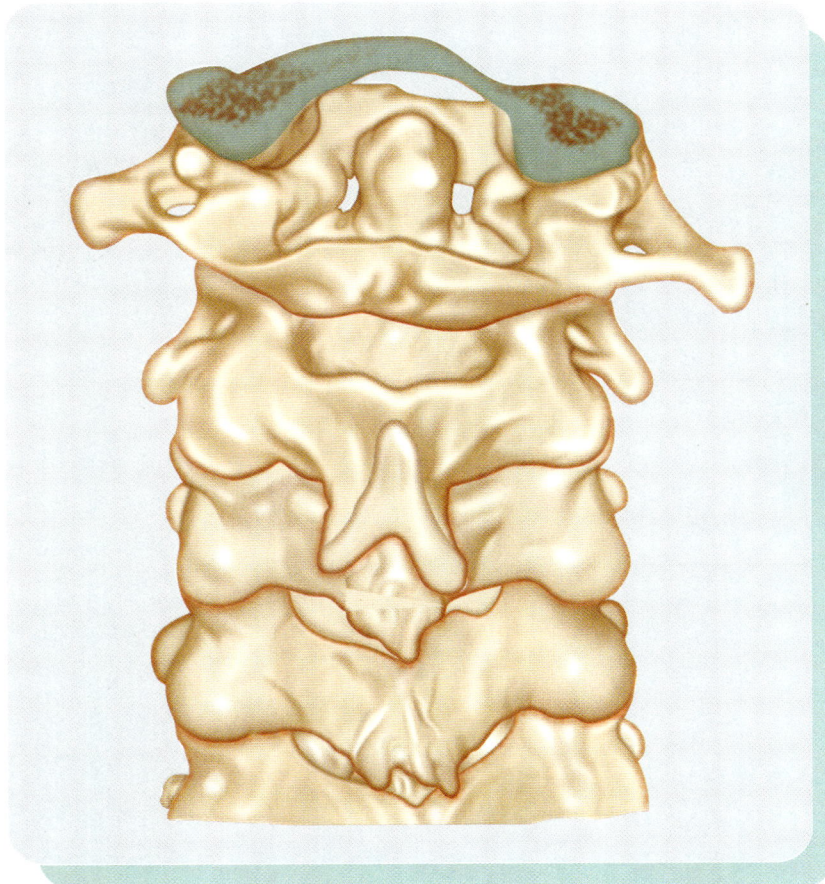

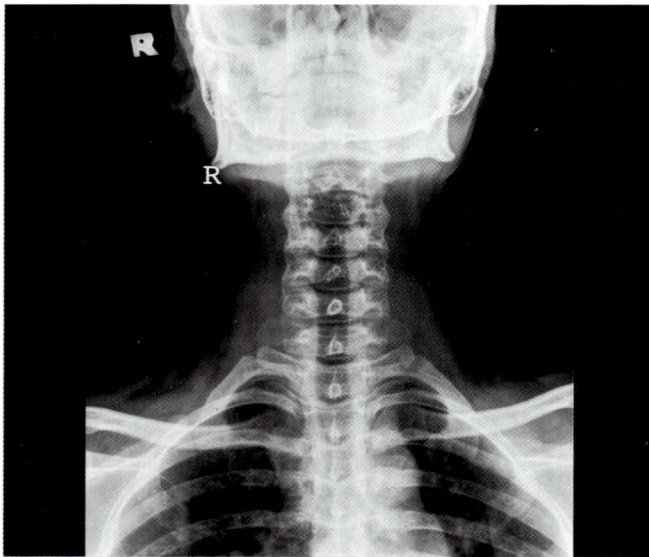

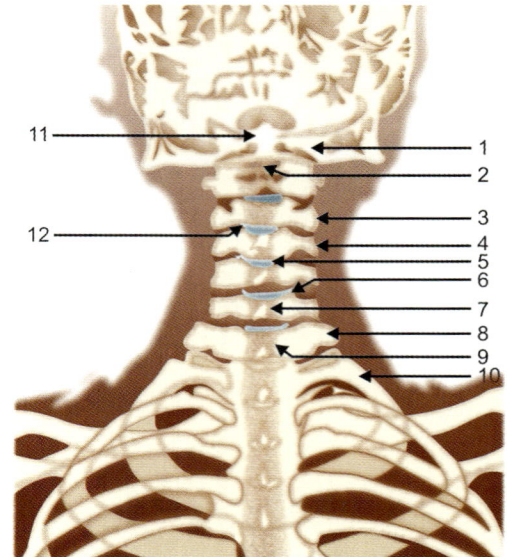

Figure 6.1

1. Lateral mass of atlas	4. Transverse process	7. Spinous process	10. First rib
2. C2 body	5. Disk space	8. C7 transverse process	11. Dens
3. Facet joint	6. Uncinate process	9. Trachea	12. Uncovertebral joint

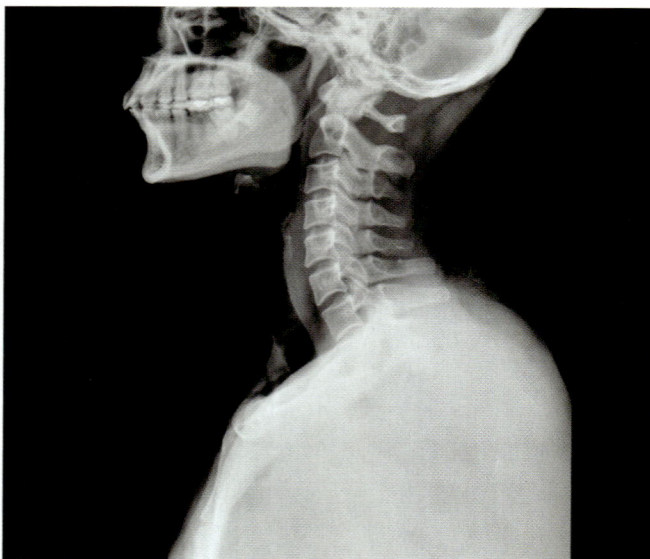

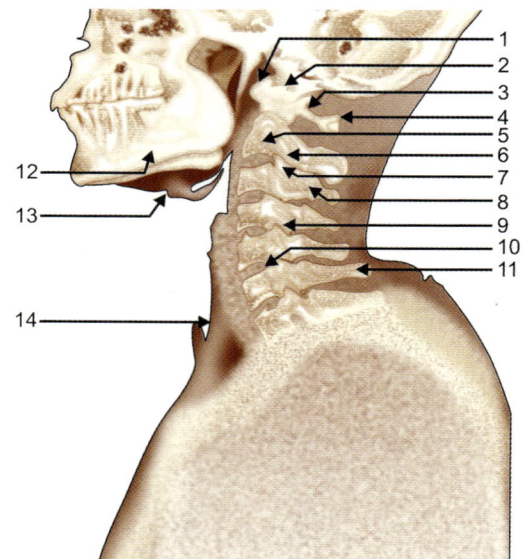

Figure 6.2

1. Anterior tubercle of atlas	5. C2 vertebra	9. Facet joint	13. Hyoid
2. Dens	6. Inferior facet	10. Disk space	14. Trachea
3. Posterior arch of atlas	7. Superior facet	11. Spinous process	
4. Posterior tubercle of atlas	8. Spinolaminar line	12. Mandible	

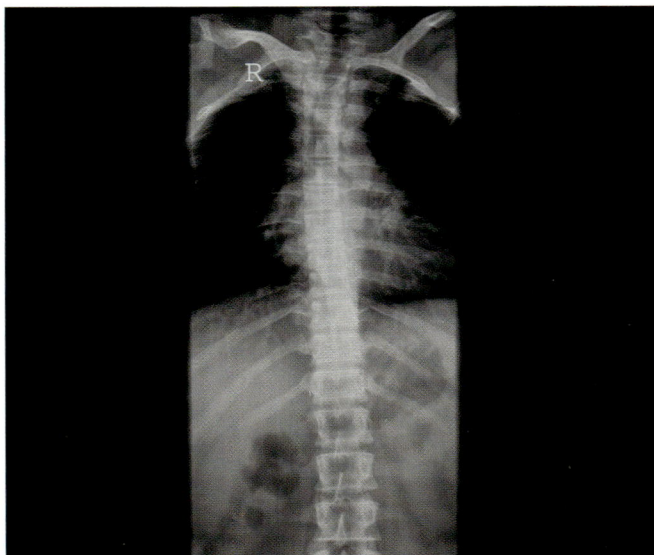

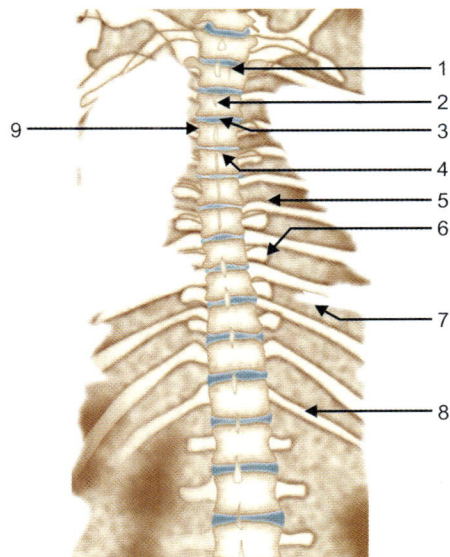

Figure 6.3

1. Trachea	6. Transverse process
2. Spinous process	7. Left diaphragm
3. Disk space	8. 12th rib
4. Carina	9. Pedicle
5. Aortic shadow	

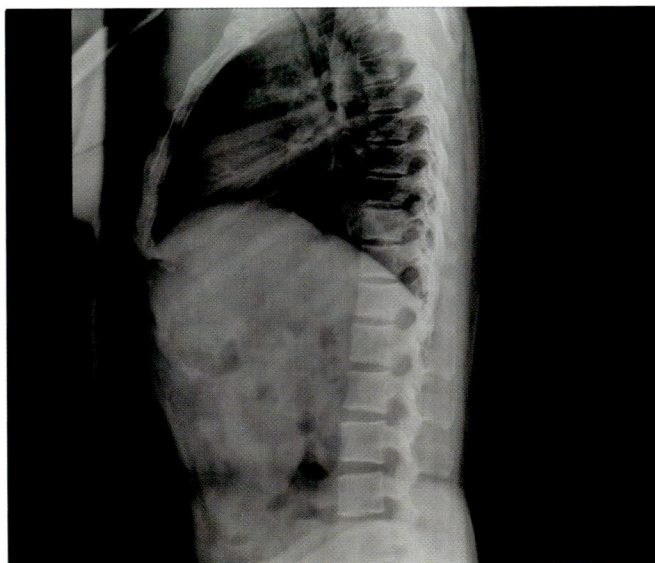

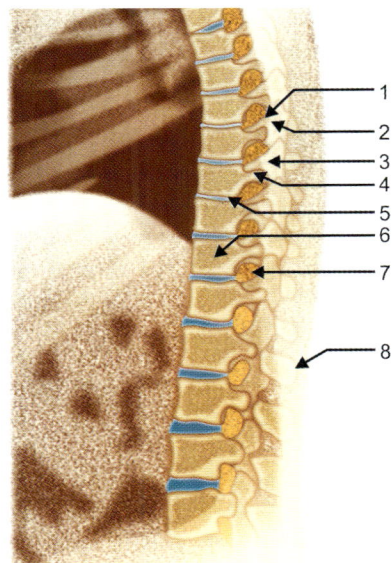

Figure 6.4

1. Superior facet	5. Disk space
2. Inferior facet	6. Vertebral body
3. Facet joint	7. Intervertebral foramen
4. Pedicle	8. Spinous process

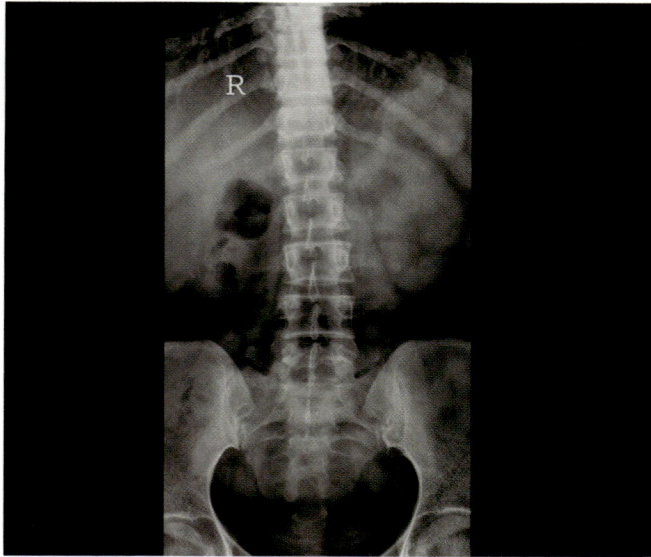

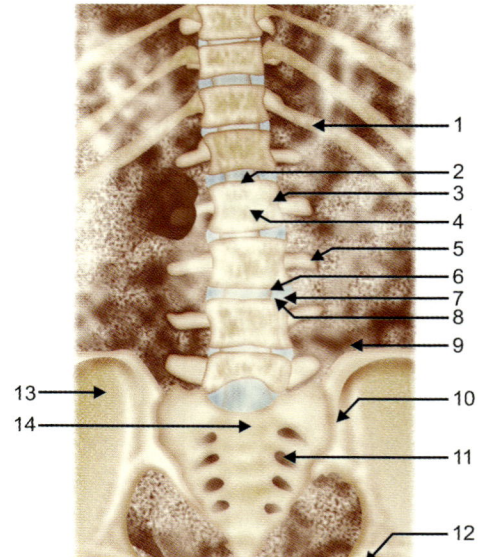

Figure 6.5

1. Twelfth rib	5. Transverse process	9. Psoas	13. Ileum
2. Spinous process L1	6. Inferior facet	10. SI joint	14. Sacrum
3. Pedicle	7. Superior facet	11. Sacral foramen	
4. Lamina L2	8. Facet joint	12. Hip joint	

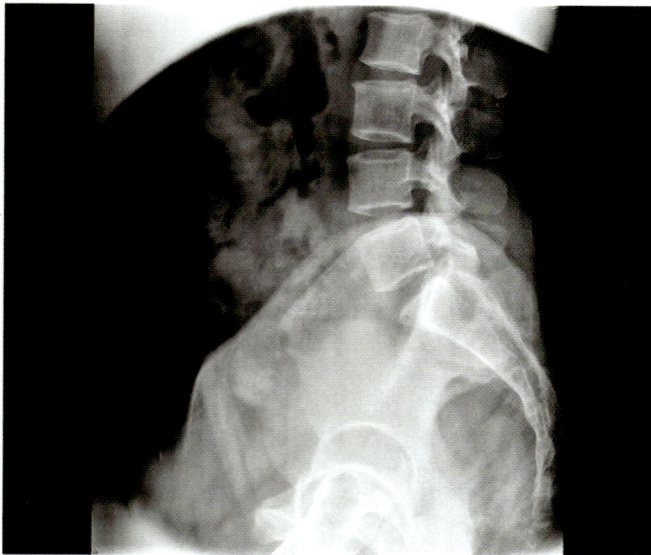

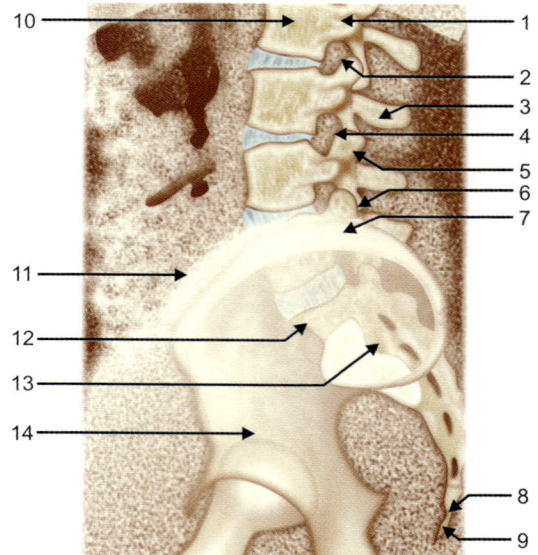

Figure 6.6

1. Pedicle	5. Inferior facet L3	9. Coccyx	13. S2
2. Intervertebral foramen	6. Facet joint	10. L2 body	14. Hip joint
3. Spinous process	7. Pars interarticularis	11. Iliac crest	
4. Superior facet L4	8. Sacrococcygeal joint	12. Sacral promontory	

CERVICAL SPINE CT

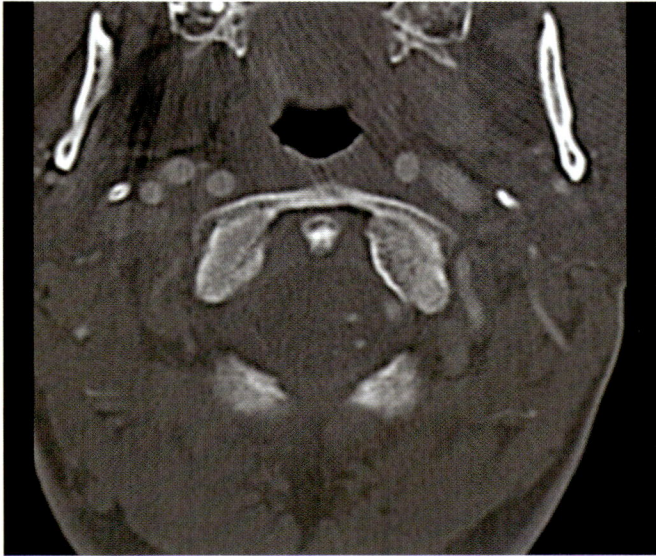

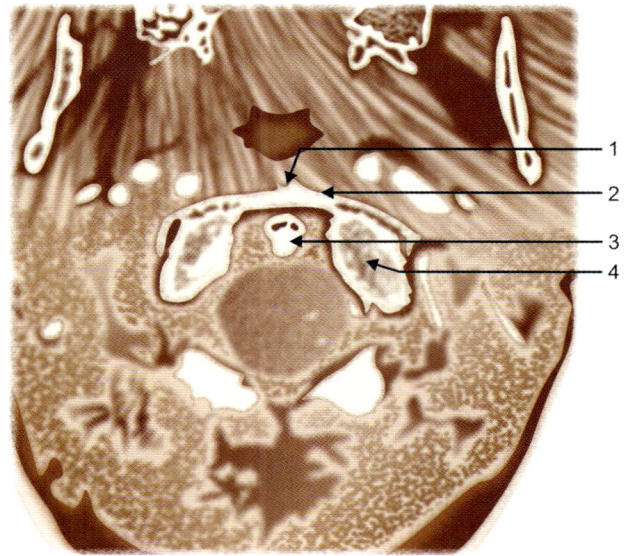

Figure 6.7

1. Anterior tubercle of atlas	3. Dens
2. Anterior arch of atlas	4. Occipital condyle

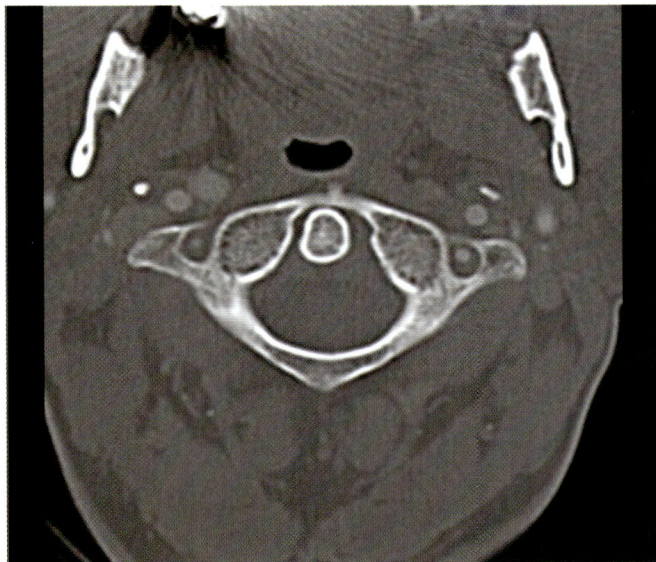

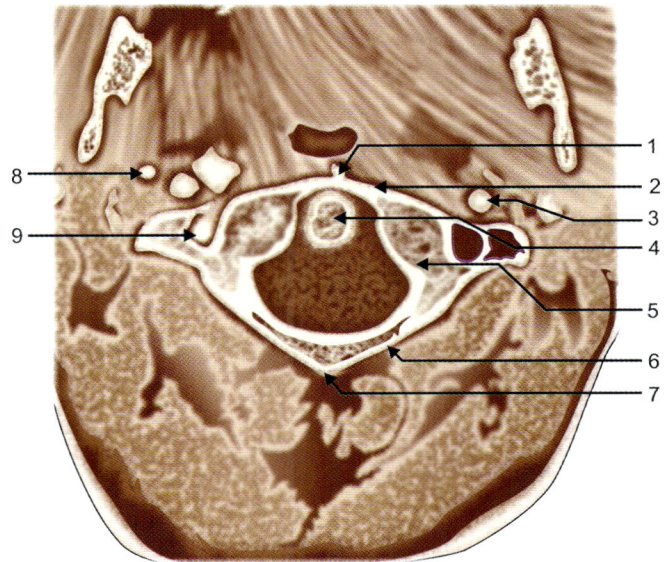

Figure 6.8

1. Anterior tubercle C1	6. Posterior arch of atlas
2. Anterior arch of atlas	7. Posterior tubercle
3. ICA	8. Styloid process
4. Dens	9. Vertebral artery
5. Lateral mass C1	

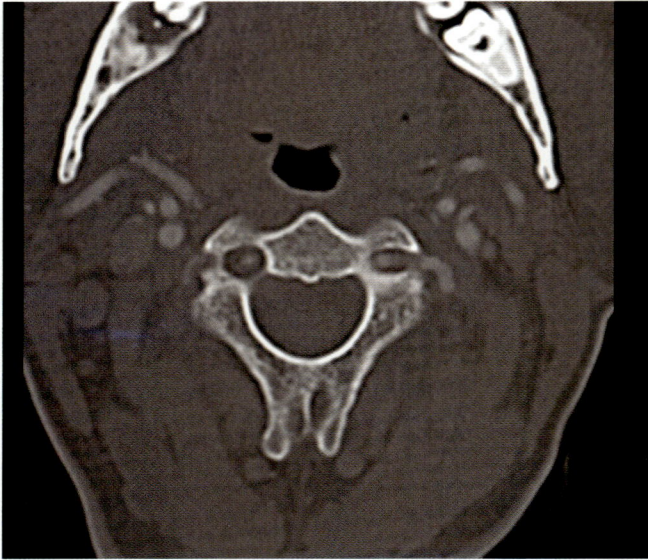

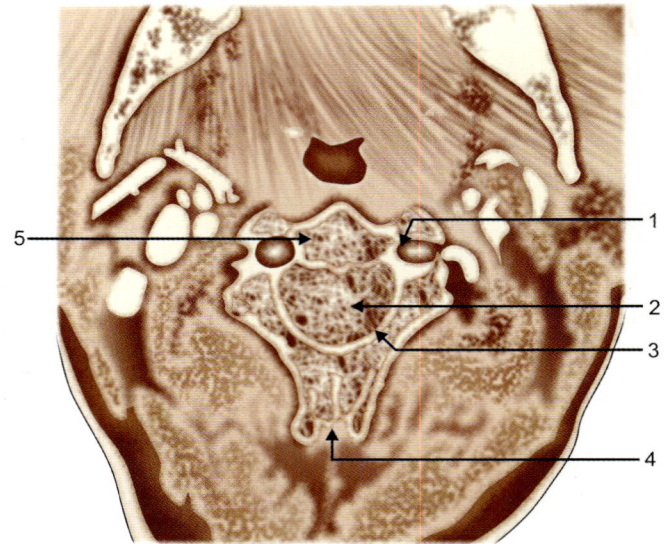

Figure 6.9

1. Vertebral artery in transverse foramen
2. Spinal canal
3. Lamina
4. Spinous process
5. C2 body

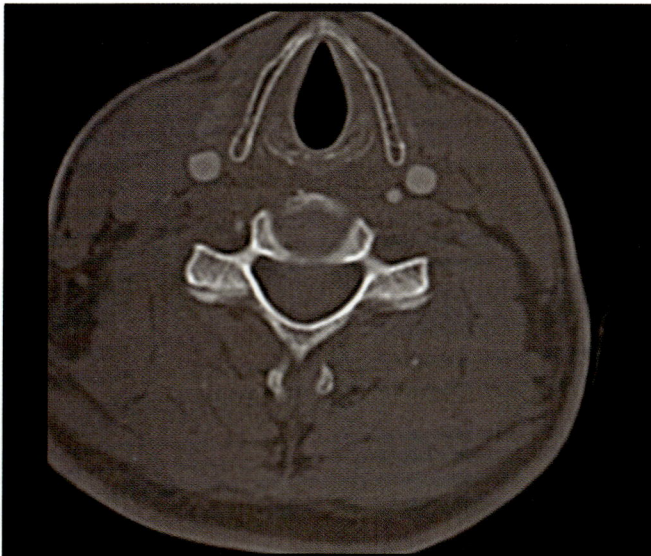

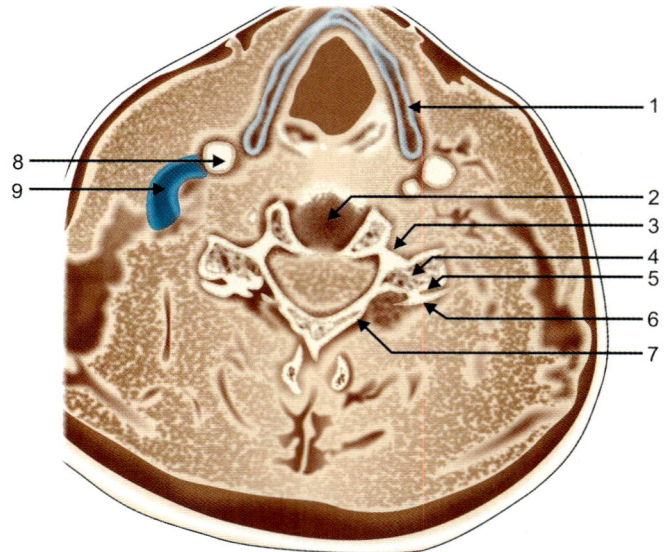

Figure 6.10

1. Thyroid cartilage
2. Intervertebral disk
3. Pedicle
4. Superior facet
5. Facet joint
6. Inferior facet
7. Lamina
8. Common carotid artery
9. Internal jugular vein

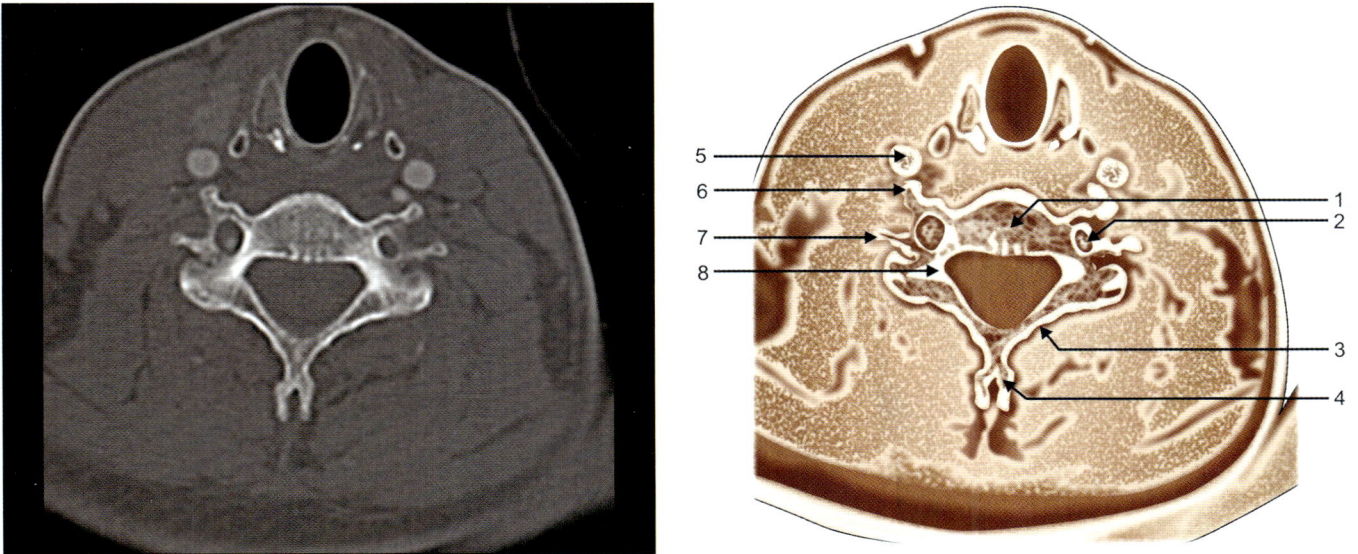

Figure 6.11

1. Vertebral body	5. CCA
2. Foramen transversarium	6. Anterior tubercle of transverse process
3. Lamina	7. Posterior tubercle of transverse process
4. Spinous process	8. Pedicle

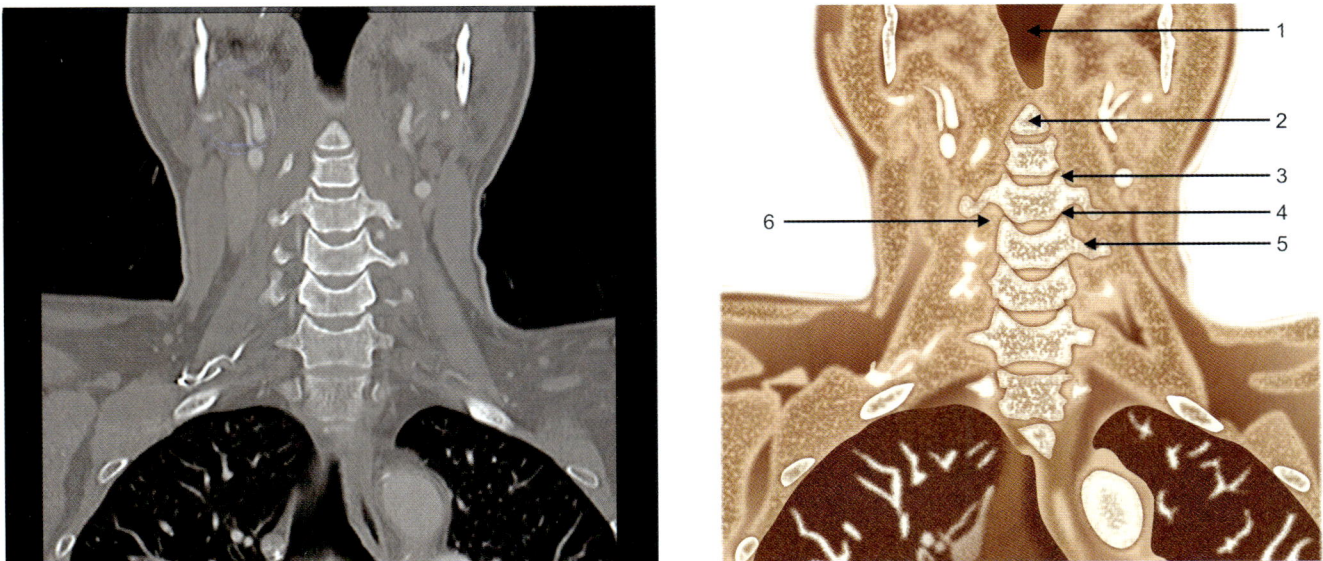

Figure 6.12

1. Pharynx	4. Uncovertebral joint
2. C2 body	5. Transverse process
3. Uncinate process	6. Vertebral artery

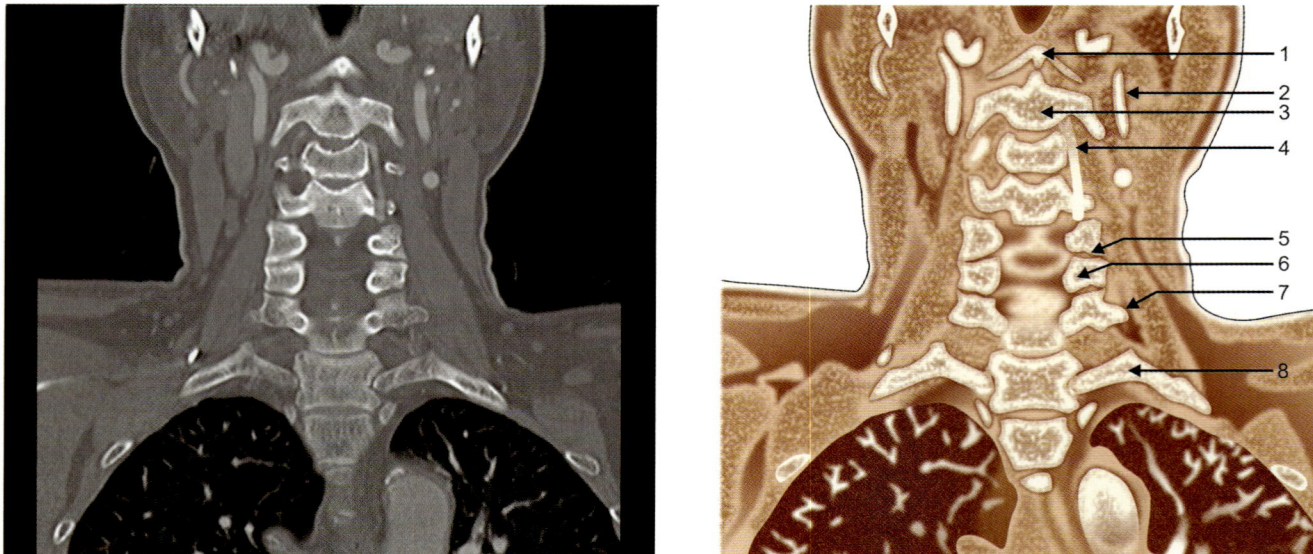

Figure 6.13

1. Anterior tubercle of atlas
2. ICA
3. C2
4. Vertebral artery
5. Facet joint
6. Pedicle
7. Transverse process C7
8. First rib

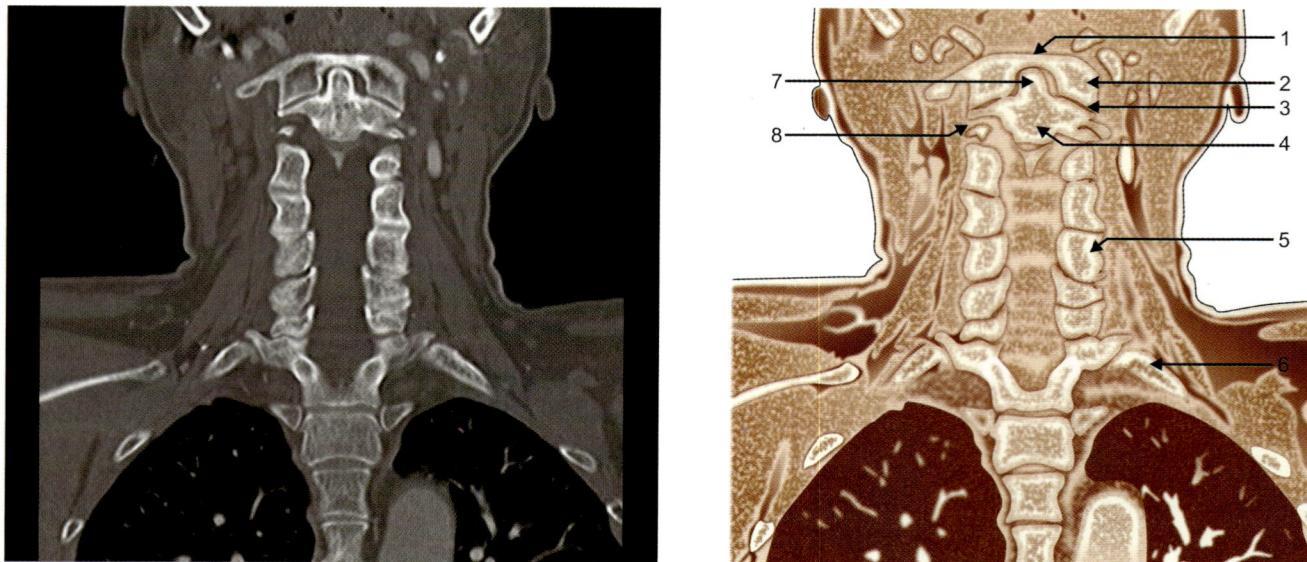

Figure 6.14

1. Anterior arch of atlas
2. Lateral mass of atlas
3. Atlantoaxial joint
4. C2
5. Articular pillar
6. First rib
7. Dens
8. Vertebral artery

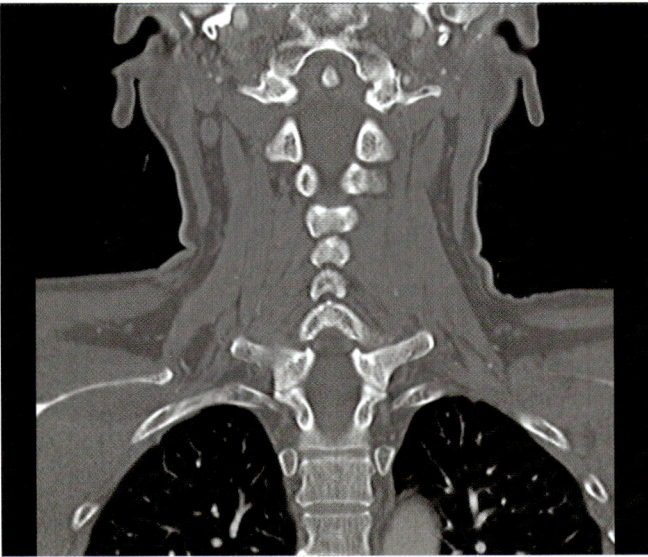

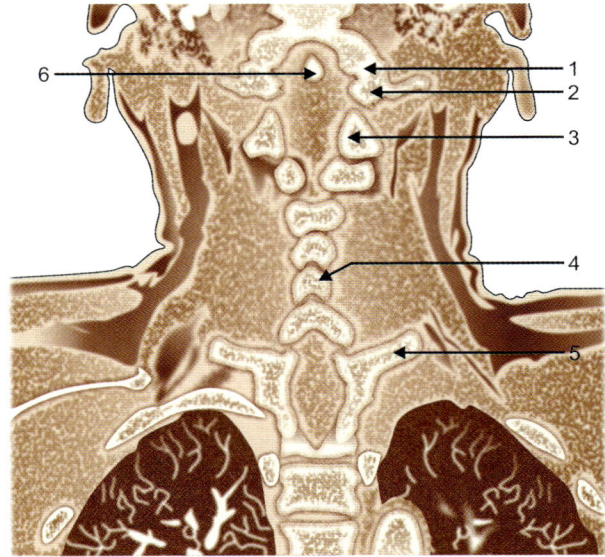

Figure 6.15

1. Atlantoaxial joint	4. Spinous process
2. C2	5. T1 transverse process
3. C3 lamina	6. Dens

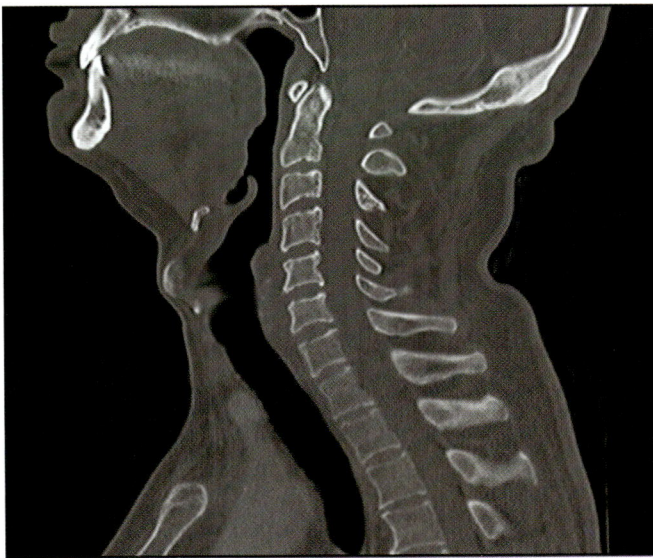

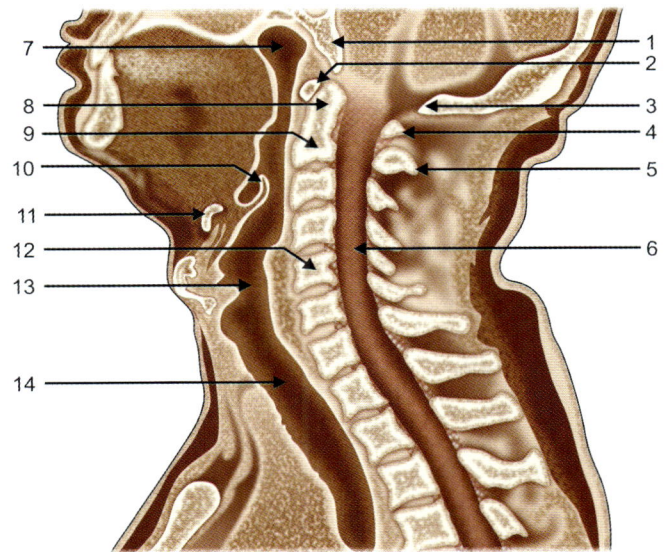

Figure 6.16

1. Clivus	8. Dens
2. Anterior tubercle of atlas	9. C2 body
3. Posterior margin of foramen magnum	10. Epiglottis
4. Posterior tubercle of atlas	11. Hyoid
5. C2 spinous process	12. C5 vertebra
6. Spinal canal	13. Glottis
7. Nasopharynx	14. Trachea

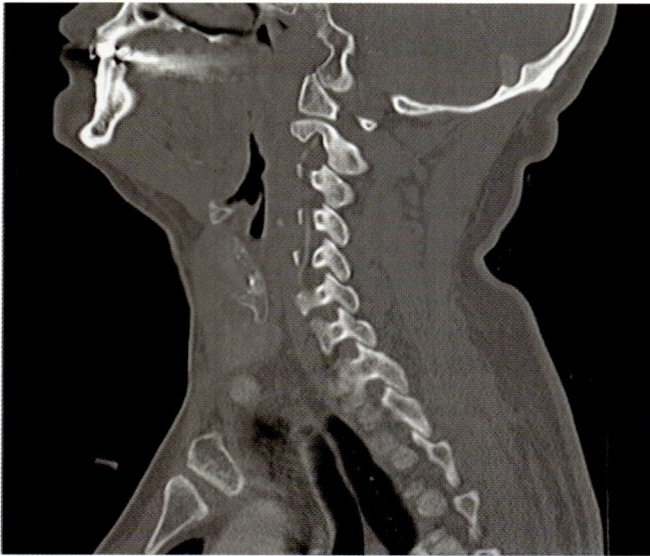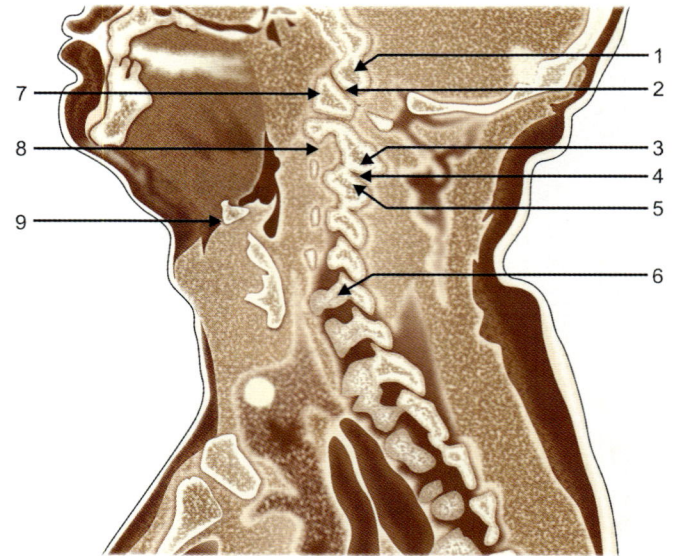

Figure 6.17

1. Occipital condyle	6. Pedicle
2. Atlanto-occipital joint	7. Lateral mass of atlas
3. Inferior facet	8. Vertebral artery in transverse foramen
4. Facet joint	9. Hyoid
5. Superior facet	

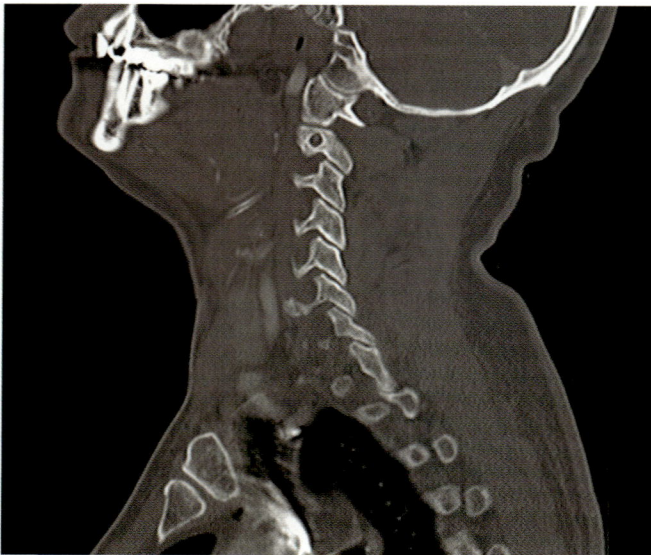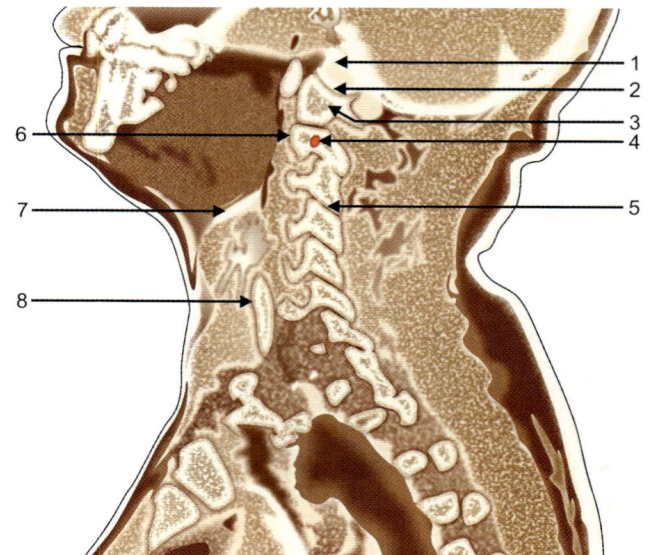

Figure 6.18

1. Occipital condyle	5. Facet joint
2. Atlanto-occipital joint	6. C2 vertebra
3. Lateral mass of atlas	7. Hyoid
4. Vertebral artery in transverse foramen	8. Common carotid artery

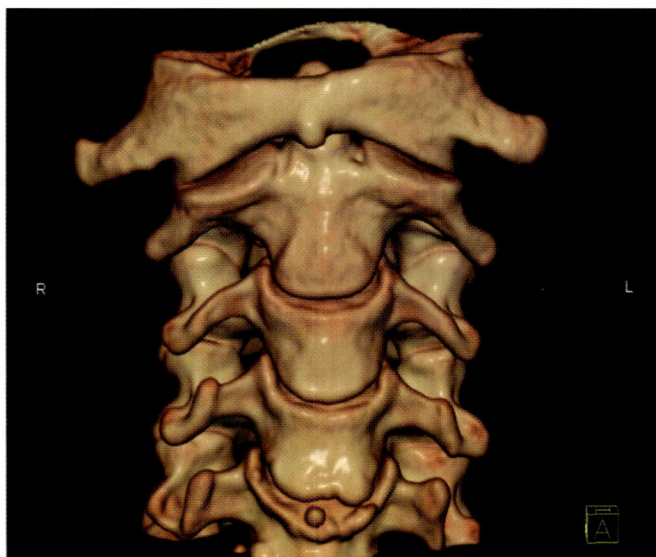

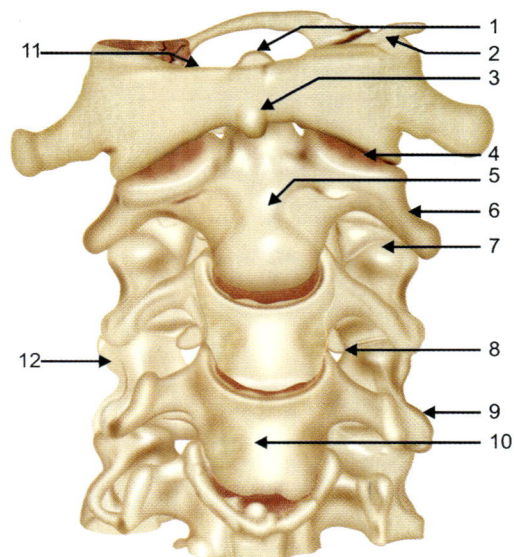

Figure 6.19

Anterior view
1. Dens
2. Atlanto-occipital joint
3. Anterior tubercle of atlas
4. Atlanto-axial joint
5. C2 body
6. Transverse process
7. Facet joint
8. Intervertebral foramen
9. Transverse process C4
10. C4 body
11. Anterior arch of atlas
12. Articular pillar

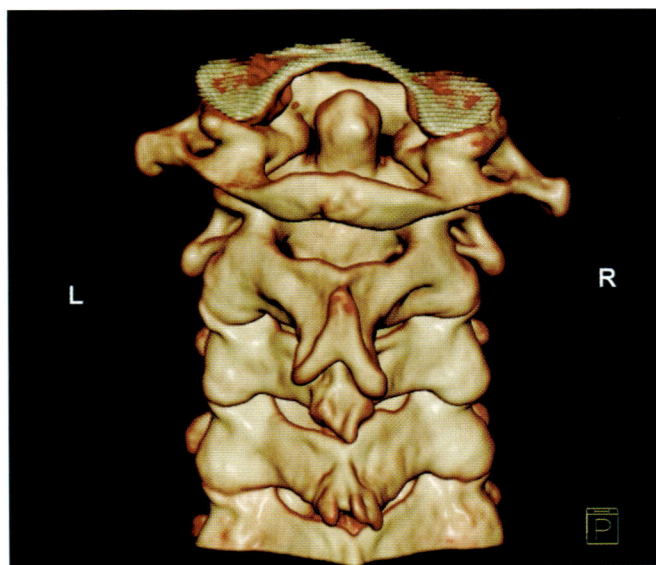

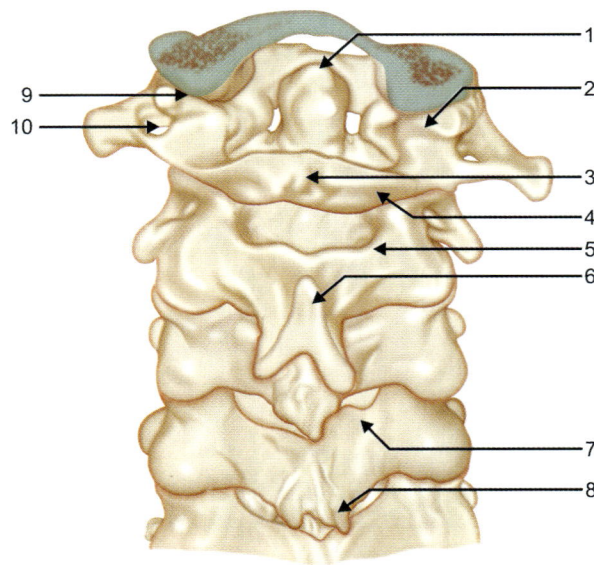

Figure 6.20

Posterior view
1. Dens
2. Lateral mass of atlas
3. Posterior tubercle of atlas
4. Posterior arch of atlas
5. C2 lamina
6. C2 spinous process
7. C4 lamina
8. C4 spinous process
9. Atlanto-occipital joint
10. Transverse foramen

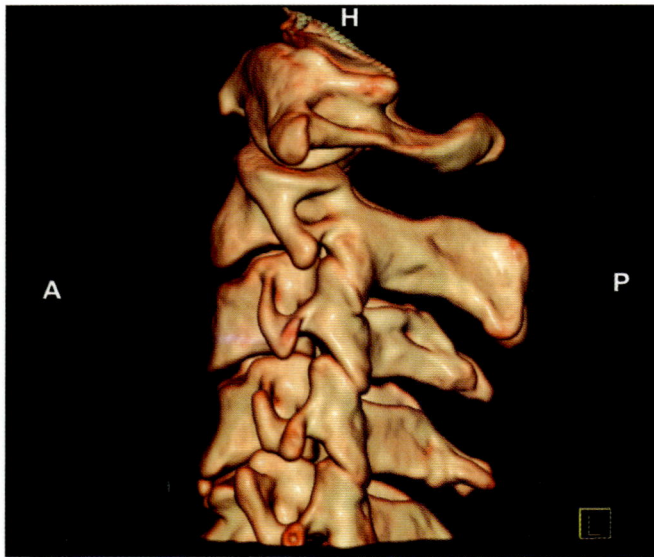

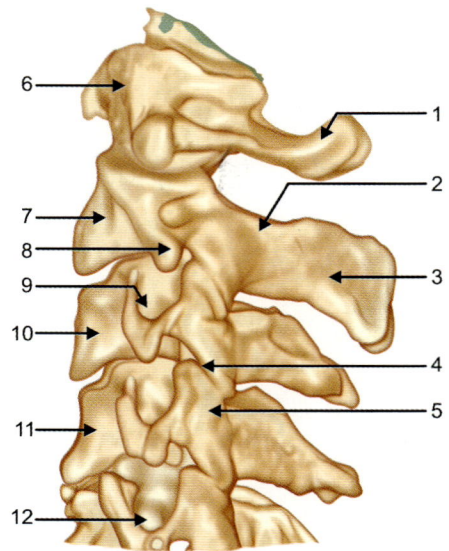

Figure 6.21

Lateral view	5. Articular pillar	10. C3 vertebra
1. Posterior arch of atlas	6. C1 vertebra	11. C4 vertebra
2. Lamina	7. C2 vertebra	12. Transverse foramen of C5
3. Spinous process C2	8. Transverse process of C2	
4. Facet joint	9. Foramen transversarium	

CERVICAL SPINE MR

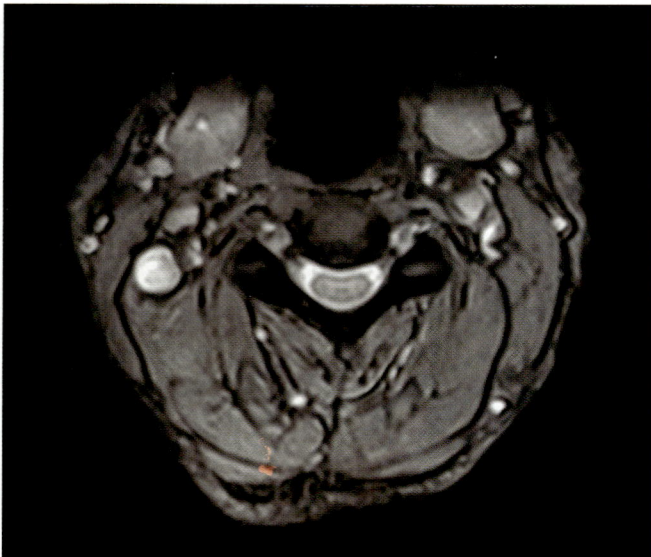

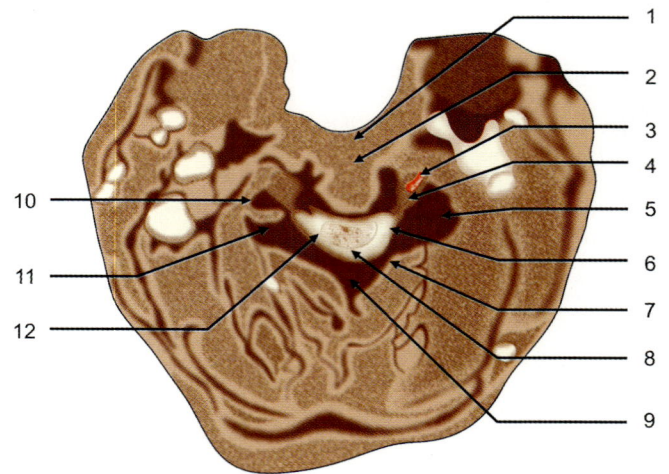

Figure 6.22

1. Anterior longitudinal ligament	7. Lamina
2. Intervertebral disk	8. Spinal cord
3. Vertebral artery	9. Spinolaminar junction
4. Dorsal root ganglion	10. Superior facet
5. Facet joint	11. Inferior facet
6. Posterior root	12. CSF

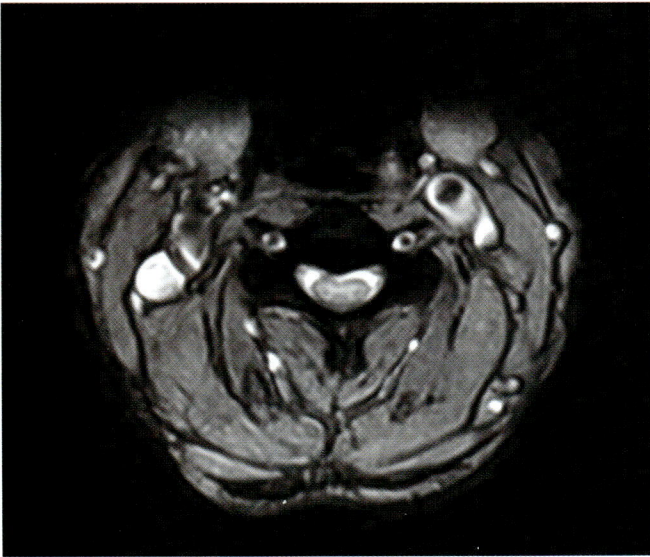
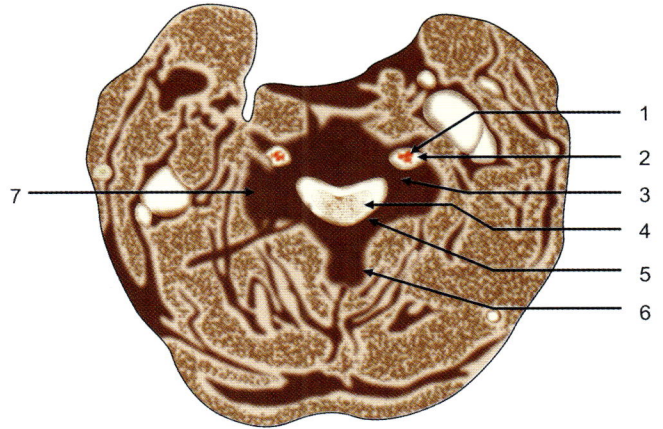

Figure 6.23

1. Vertebral artery	5. Ligamentum flavum
2. Transverse foramen	6. Spinous process
3. Pedicle	7. Articular pillar
4. Spinal cord	

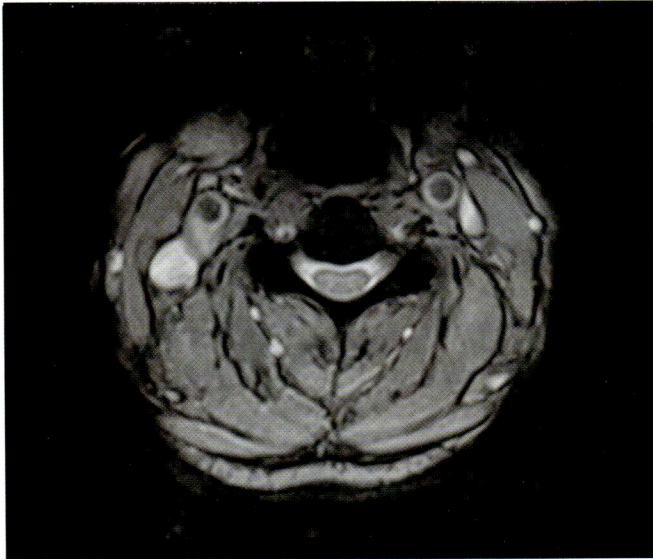
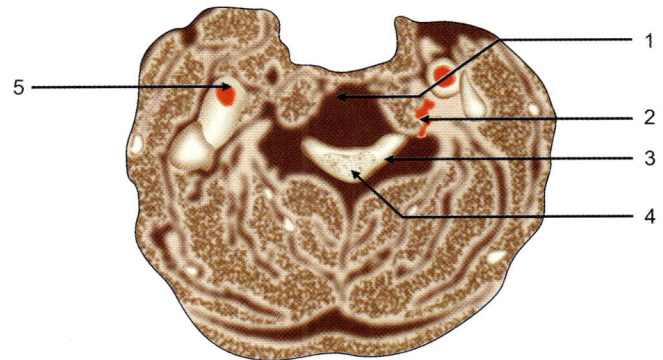

Figure 6.24

1. Cervical vertebral body
2. Vertebral artery
3. Posterior root
4. Spinal gray matter
5. Carotid artery

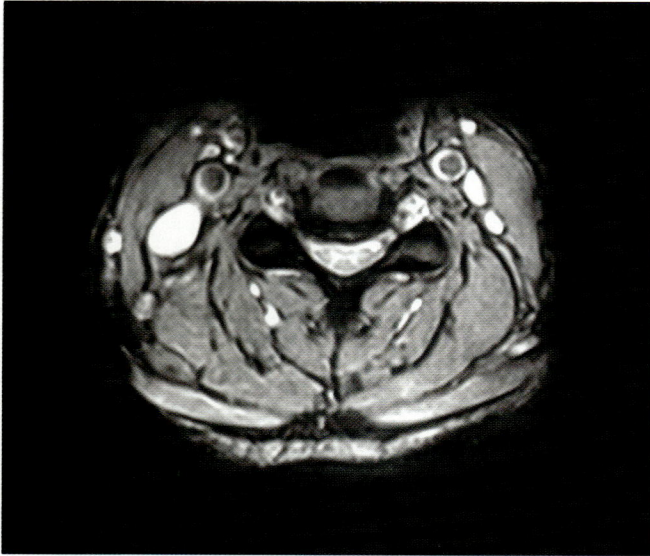
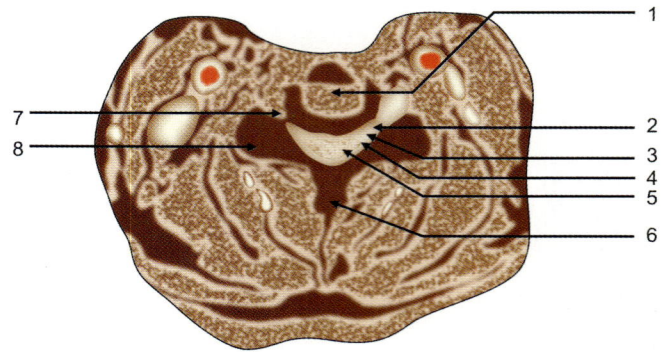

Figure 6.25

1. Intervertebral disk	5. H shaped spinal gray matter
2. Uncinate process	6. Spinous process
3. Dorsal root ganglion	7. Intervertebral foramen
4. Posterior root	8. Facet joint

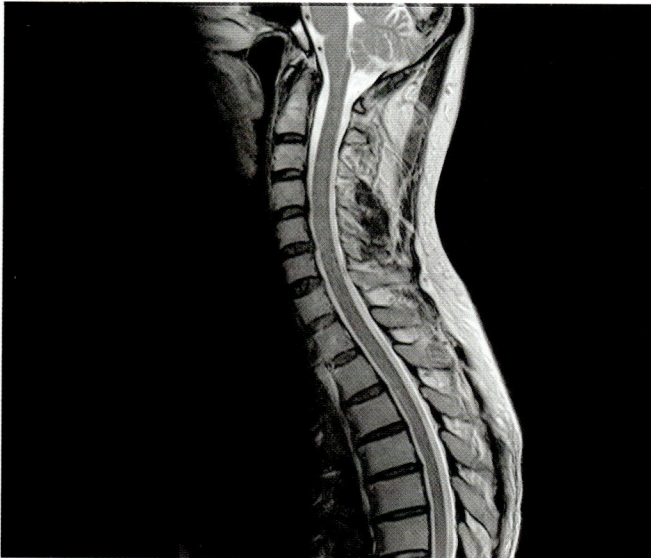
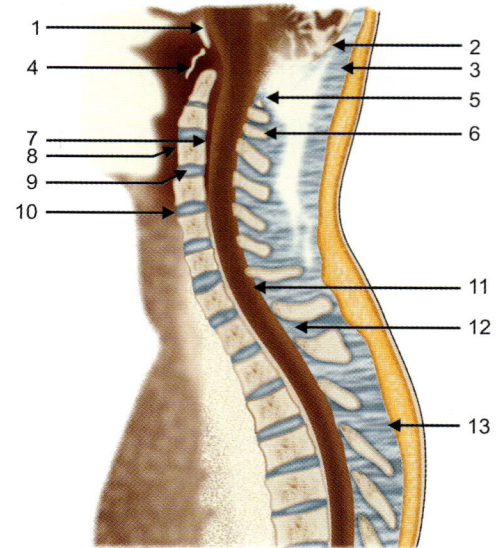

Figure 6.26

1. Clivus	6. Spinous process of C2	9. Nucleus pulposis
2. Occipital bone	7. Posterior longitudinal ligament	10. Annulus fibrosis
3. Ligamentum nuchae	8. Anterior longitudinal ligament	11. Spinal cord
4. Ant tubercle of atlas dens		12. Ligamentum flavum
5. Posterior tubercle of C1		13. Supraspinatous ligament

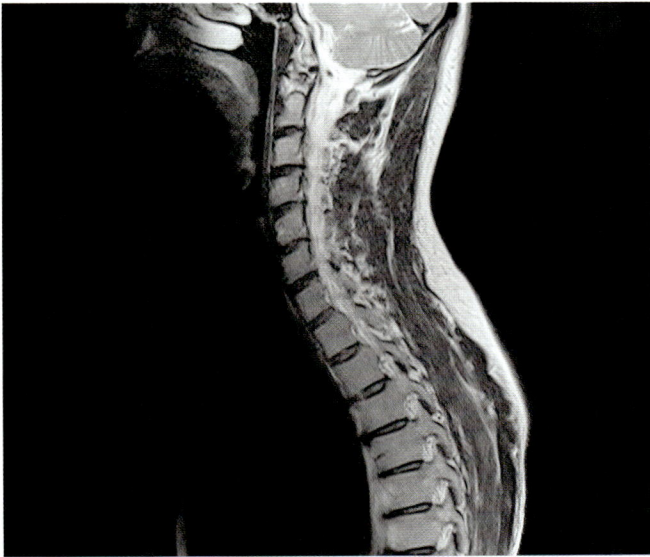

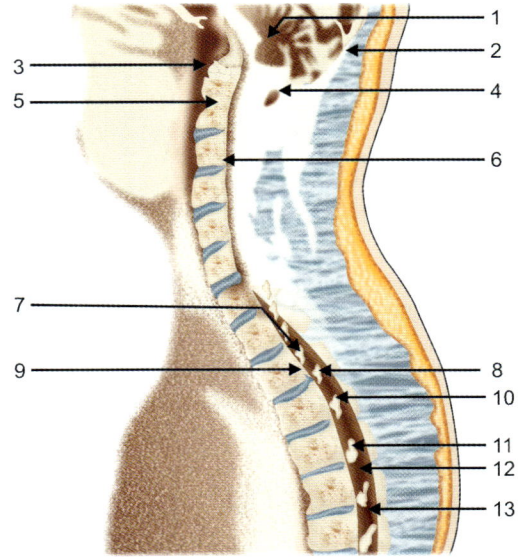

Figure 6.27

1. Cerebellum	8. Ligamentum flavum
2. Occipital bone	9. Ventral nerve root
3. Anterior arch of C1	10. Intervertebral foramen
4. Posterior arch of C1	11. Nerve root
5. Dens	12. Pedicle
6. Intervertebral disk	13. Facet joint
7. Dorsal nerve root	

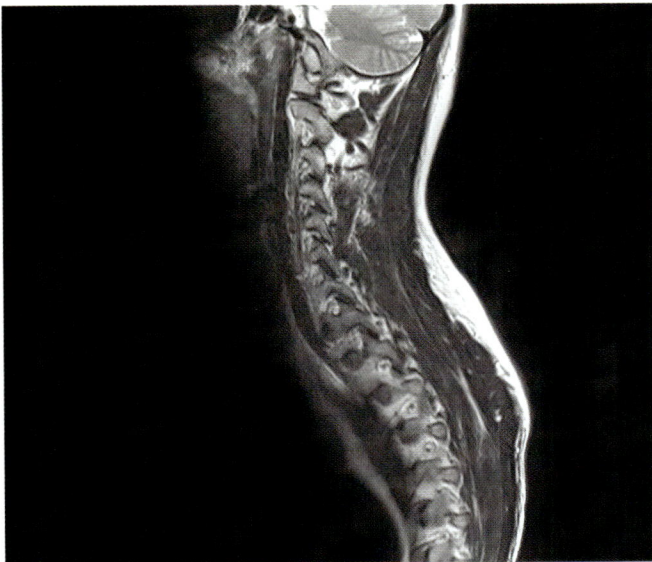

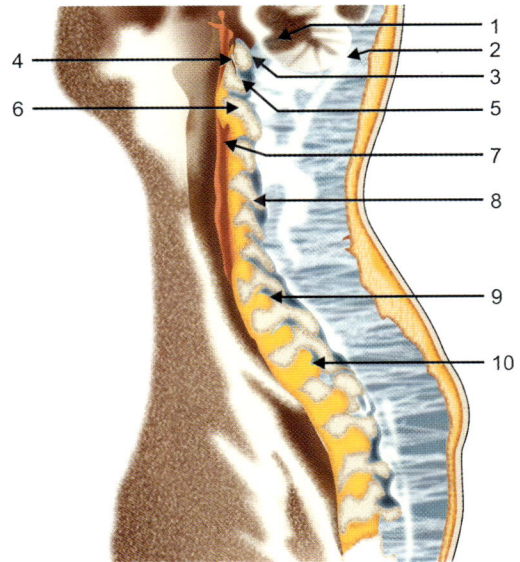

Figure 6.28

1. Cerebellum	6. C2 vertebra
2. Occipital bone	7. Vertebral artery
3. Occipital condyle	8. Facet joint
4. Atlanto-occipital joint	9. Intervertebral foramen
5. Lateral mass of atlas	10. Dorsal root ganglion

LUMBAR SPINE CT

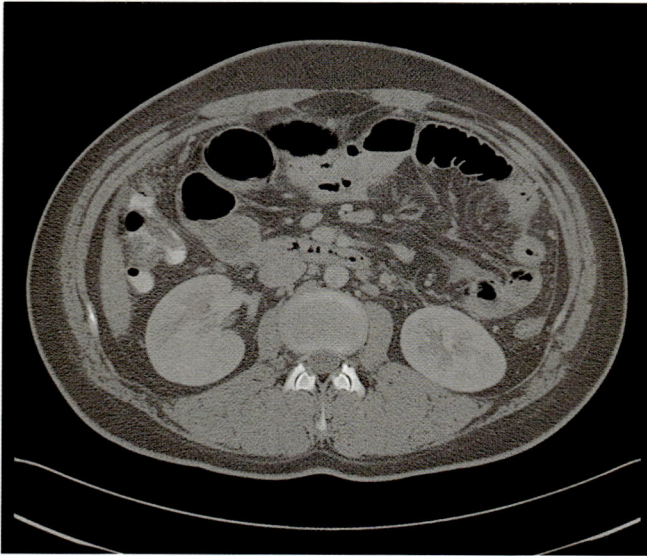

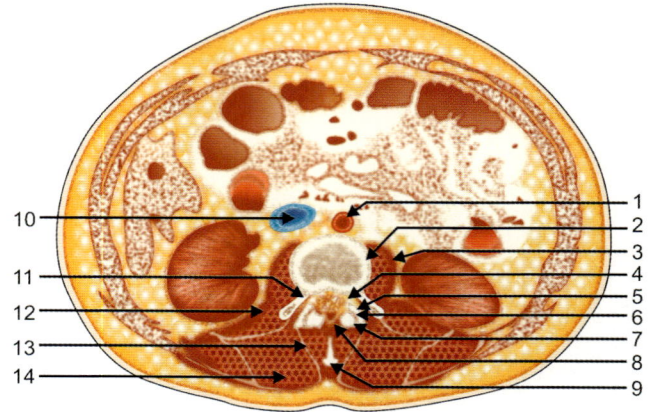

Figure 6.29

1. Aorta	6. Facet joint	11. Intervertebral foramen
2. Intervertebral disk	7. Inferior facet	12. Quadratus lumborum
3. Psoas muscle	8. Ligamentum flavum	13. Multifidus
4. Thecal sac	9. Spinous process	14. Erector spinae
5. Superior facet	10. IVC	

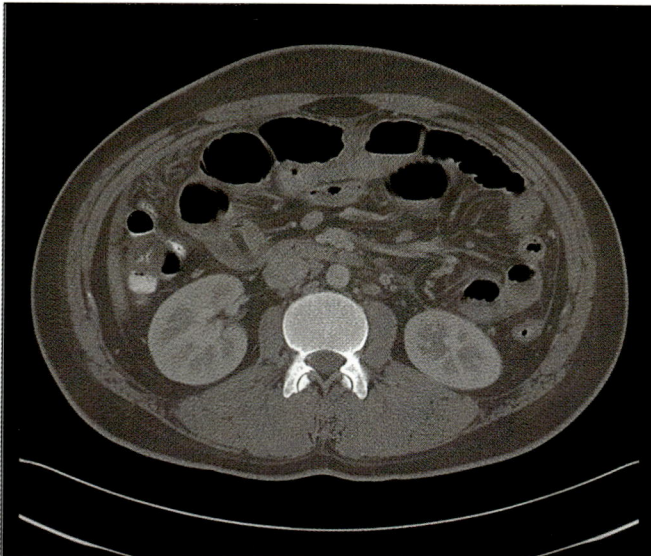

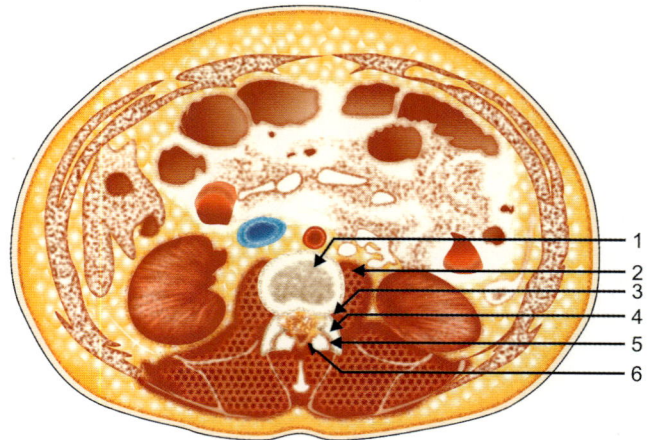

Figure 6.30

1. Vertebral body
2. Psoas muscle
3. Pedicle
4. Superior facet
5. Facet joint
6. Ligamentum flavum

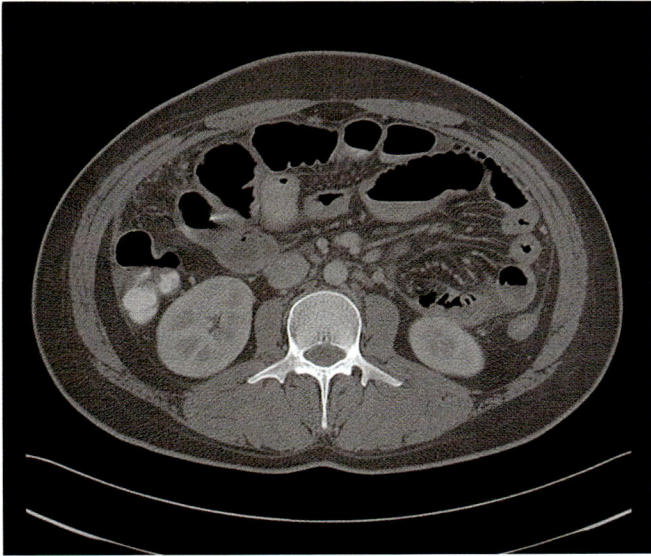

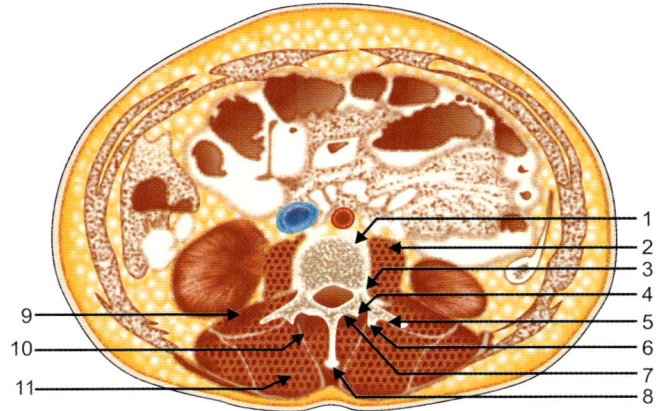

Figure 6.31

1. Vertebral body	6. Mammillary process
2. Psoas muscle	7. Lamina
3. Pedicle	8. Spinous process
4. Accessory tubercle	9. Quadratus lumborum
5. Transverse process	10. Multifidus muscle
	11. Erector spinae

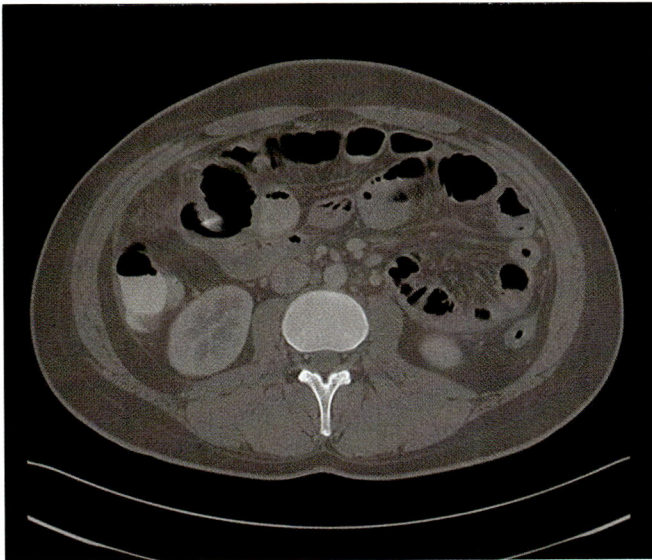

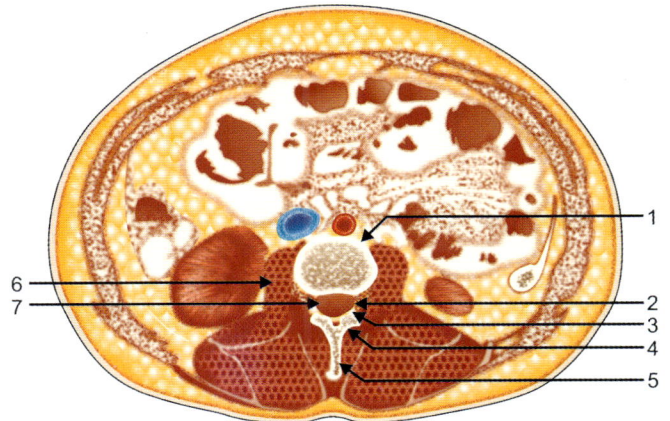

Figure 6.32

1. Vertebral body
2. Intervertebral foramen
3. Ligamentum flavum
4. Lamina
5. Spinous process
6. Psoas muscle
7. Thecal sac

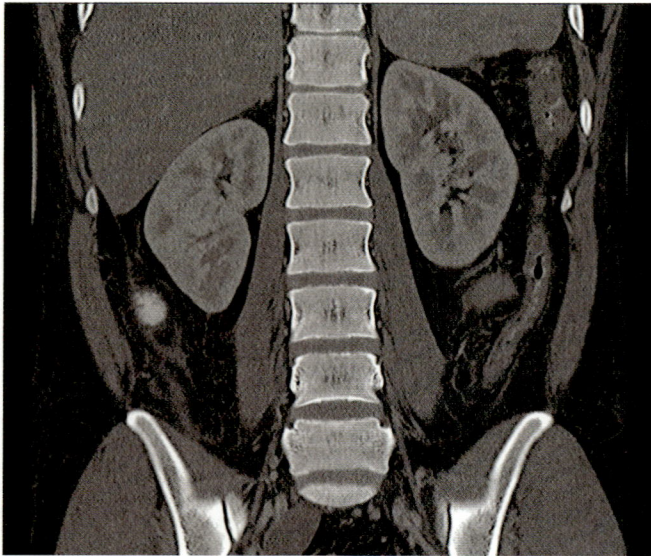

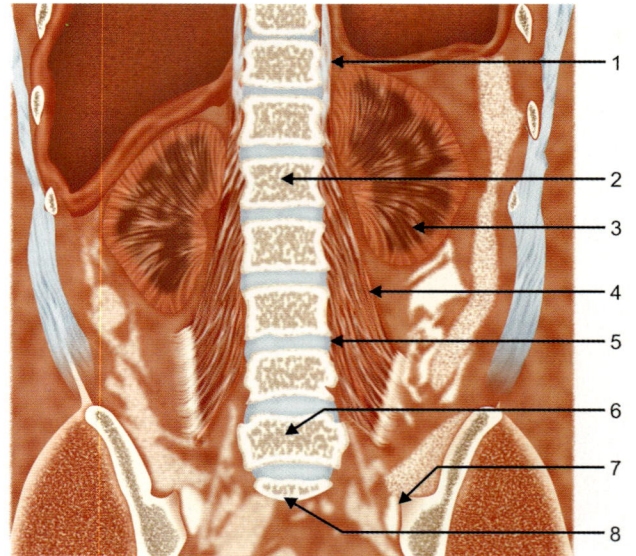

Figure 6.33

1. Crus of diaphragm	5. Intervertebral disk
2. L1	6. L5 body
3. Left Kidney	7. Sacroiliac joint
4. Psoas muscle	8. Sacral promontory

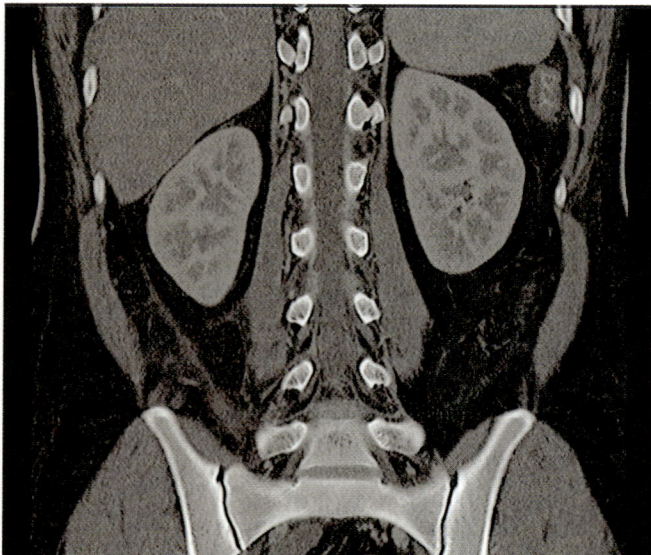

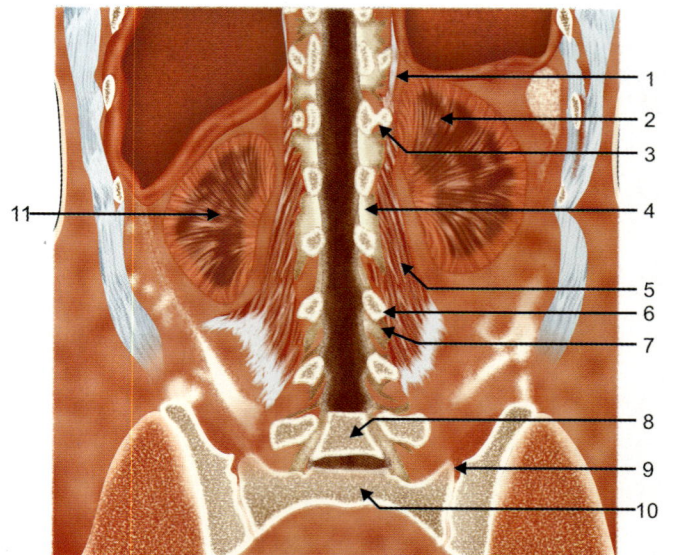

Figure 6.34

1. Left crus of diaphragm	7. Nerve root
2. Left kidney	8. L5
3. Costovertebral joint	9. Sarcoiliac joint
4. Intervertebral foramen	10. Sacrum
5. Psoas muscle	11. Right kidney
6. Pedicle	

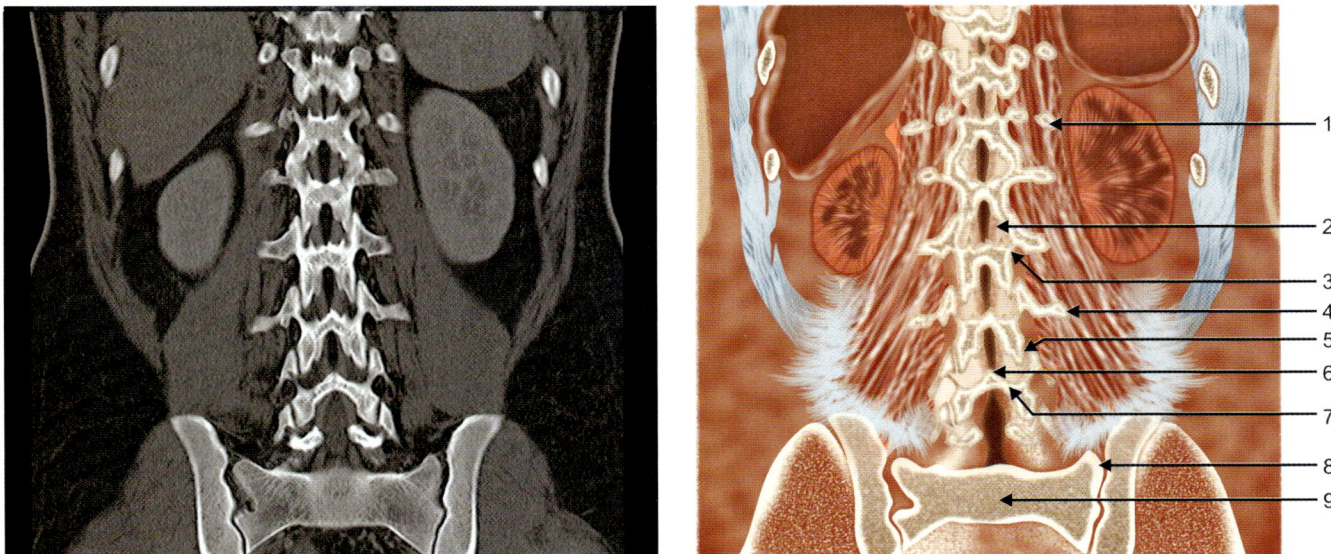

Figure 6.35

1. Twelfth rib	6. Spinolaminar junction
2. Ligamentum flavum	7. Lamina
3. Pars interarticularis	8. Sacroiliac joint
4. Transverse process	9. Sacrum
5. Facet joint	

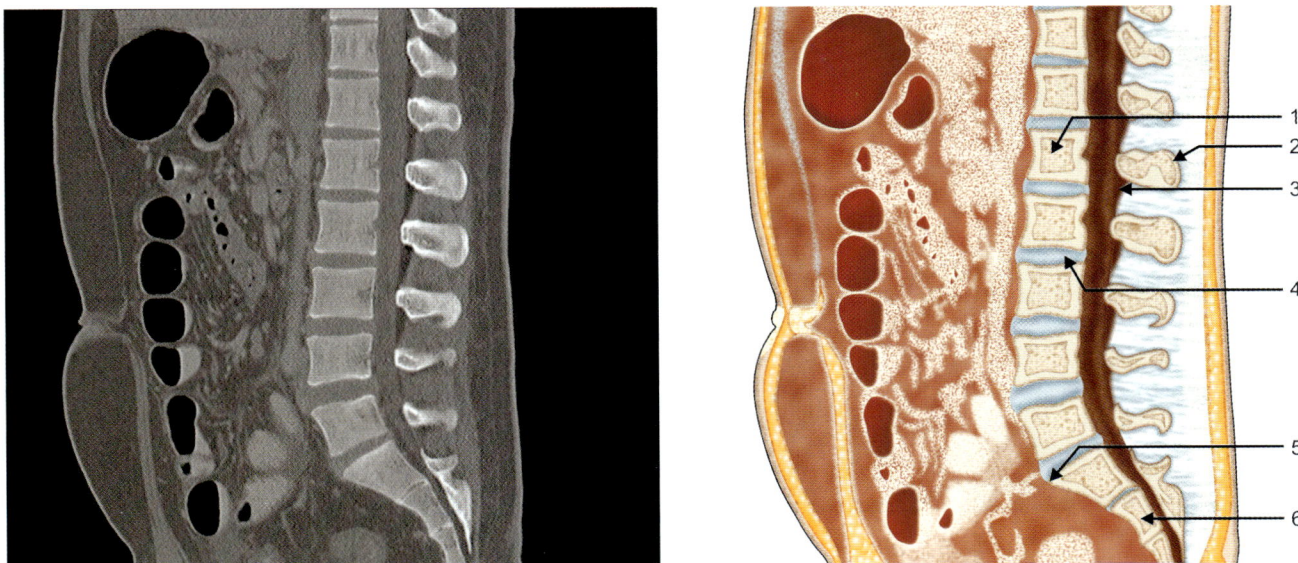

Figure 6.36

1. L1	4. Intervertebral disk
2. Spinous process	5. Sacral promontory
3. Thecal sac	6. S2

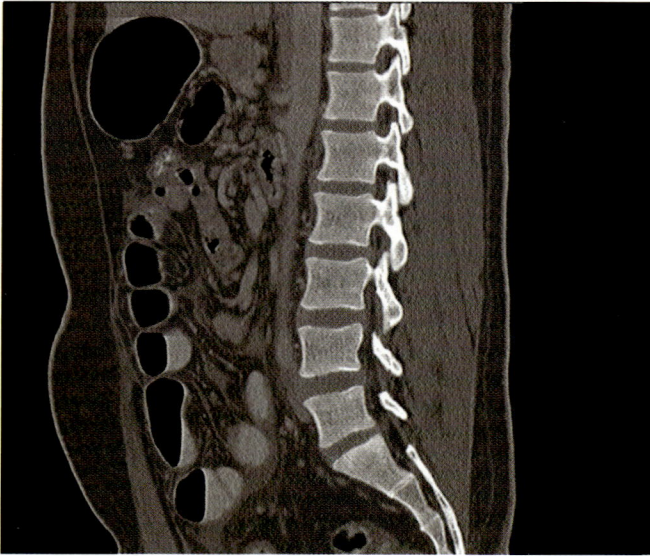

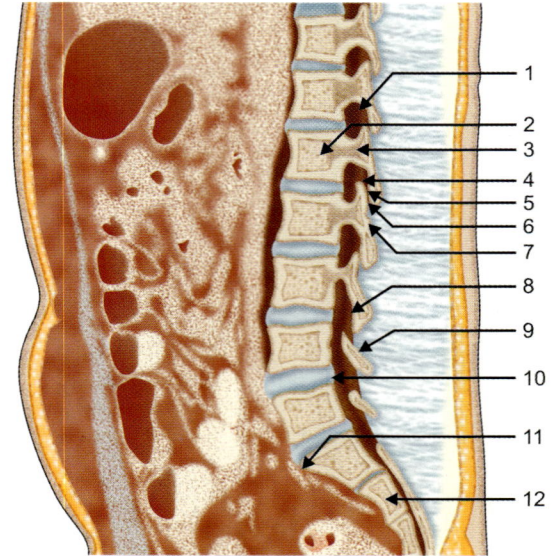

Figure 6.37

1. Intervertebral foramen	7. Pars interarticularis
2. L1 body	8. Ligamentum flavum
3. Pedicle	9. Lamina
4. Superior facet	10. Intervertebral disk
5. Facet joint	11. Sacral promontory
6. Inferior facet	12. S2

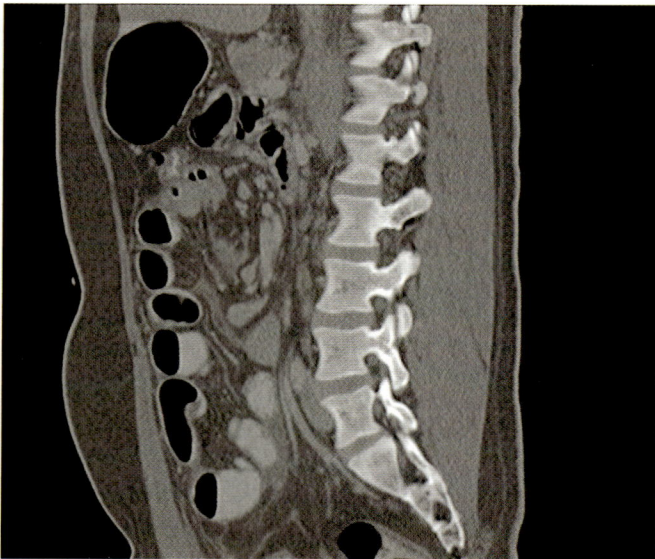

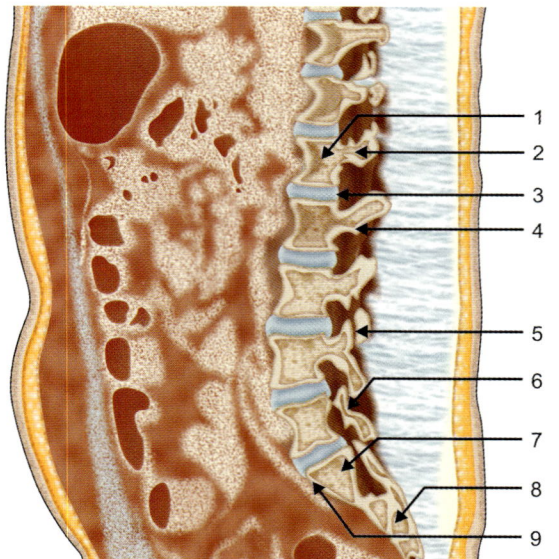

Figure 6.38

1. L1	6. Pars interarticularis
2. Pedicle	7. S1
3. Intervertebral disk	8. Sacral foramen
4. Accessory tubercle	9. Sacral promontory
5. Facet joint	

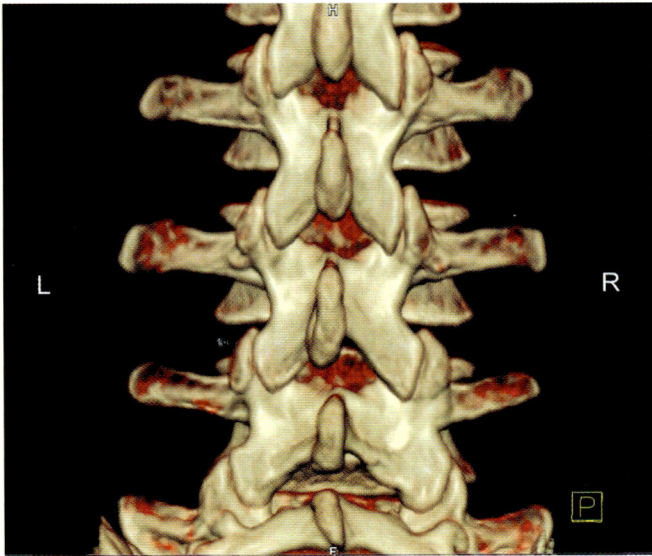

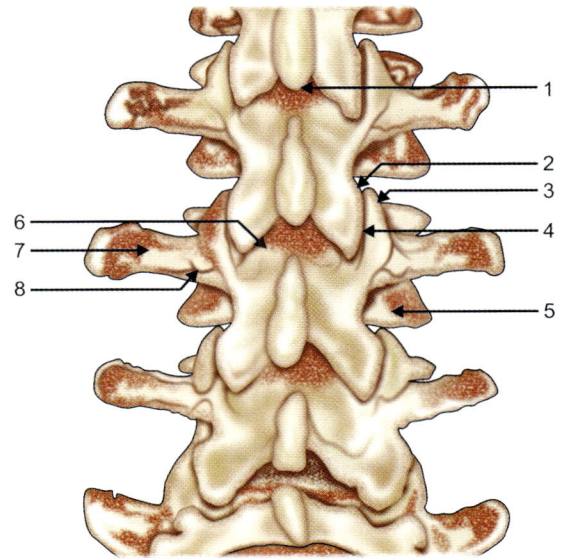

Figure 6.39

Posterior view	5. Inferior margin of vertebra
1. Spinous process	6. Lamina
2. Inferior facet	7. Transverse process
3. Superior facet	8. Accessory tubercle
4. Facet joint	

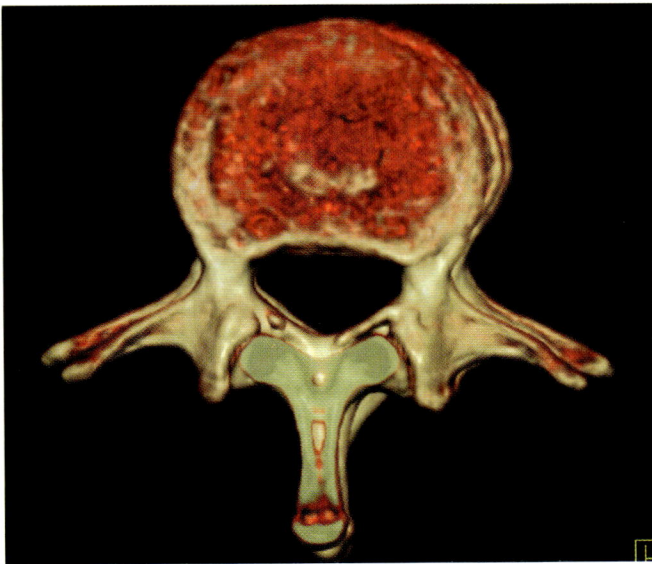

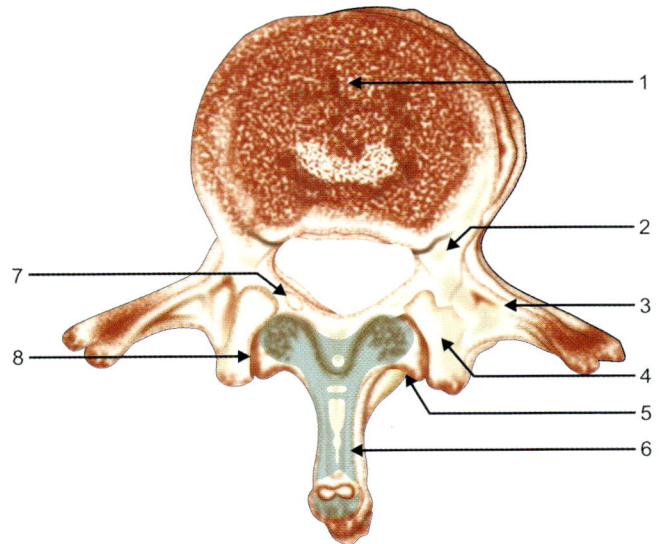

Figure 6.40

Superior view	5. Inferior facet
1. Vertebral body	6. Spinous process
2. Pedicle	7. Lamina
3. Transverse process	8. Facet joint
4. Superior facet	

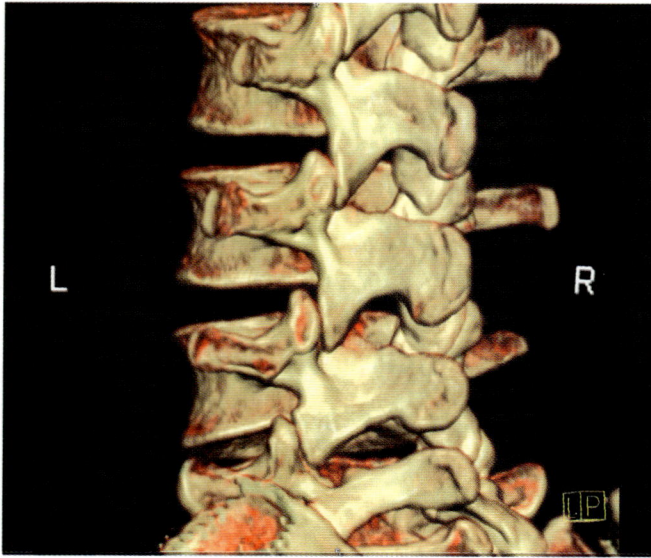

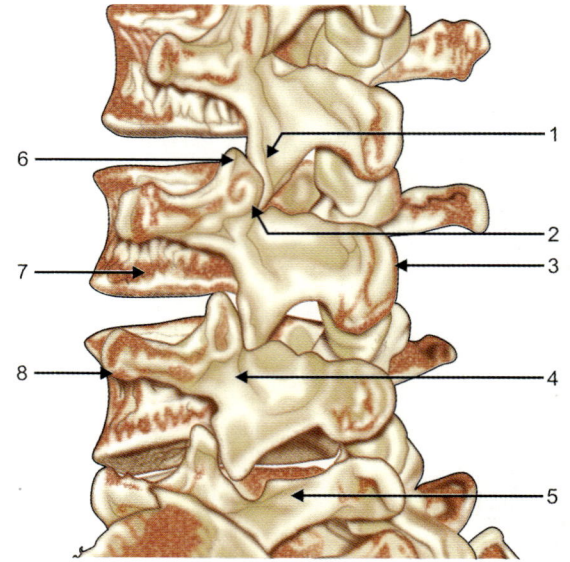

Figure 6.41

Lateral view	
1. Inferior facet	5. Lamina
2. Facet joint	6. Superior facet
3. Spinous process	7. Vertebral body
4. Pars interarticularis	8. Transverse process

LUMBAR SPINE MR

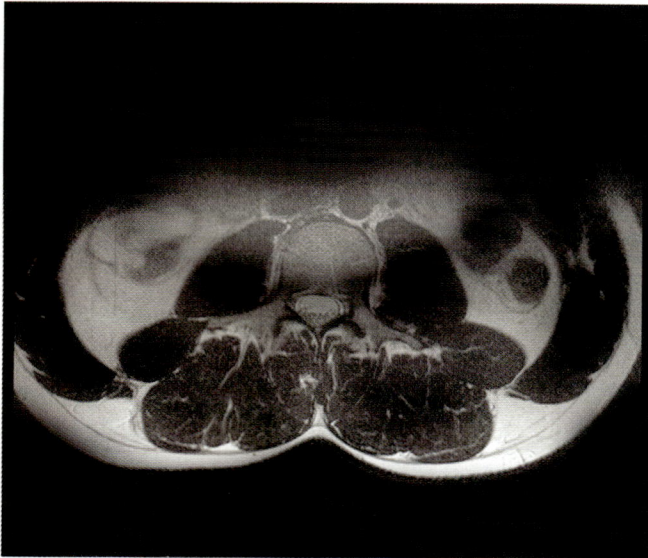

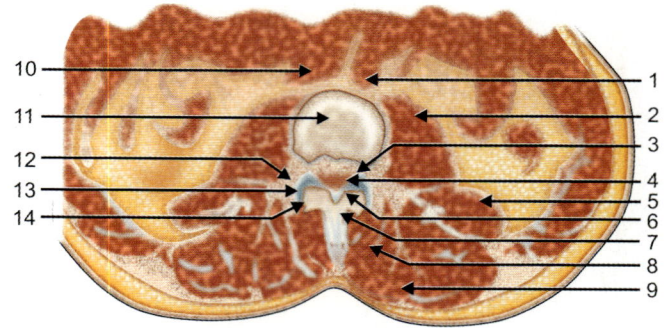

Figure 6.42

1. Aorta	8. Multifidus muscle
2. Psoas muscle	9. Erector spinae
3. Dura	10. IVC
4. Nerve roots	11. Vertebral body
5. Quadratus lumborum	12. Superior facet
6. Ligamentum flavum	13. Facet joint
7. Interspinous ligament	14. Inferior facet

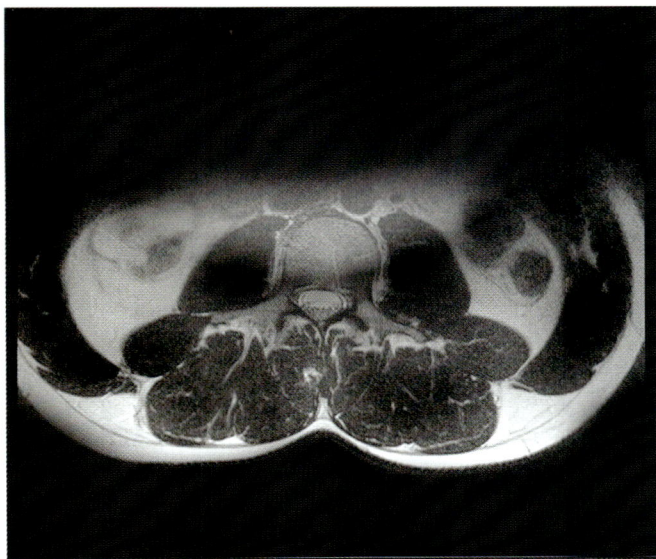

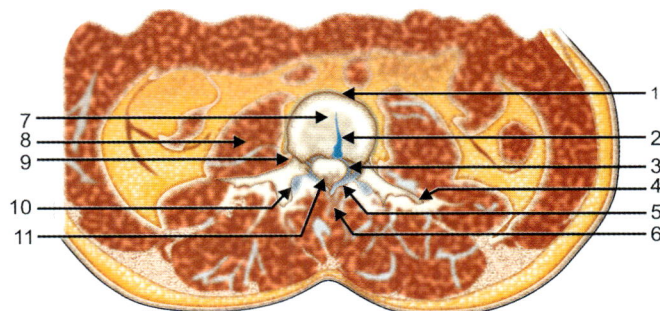

Figure 6.43

1. Anterior longitudinal ligament	5. Ligamentum flavum	9. Pedicle
2. Basivertebral vein	6. Interspinous ligament	10. Facet joint
3. Dural sac	7. Vertebral body	11. Nerve roots
4. Transverse process	8. Psoas	

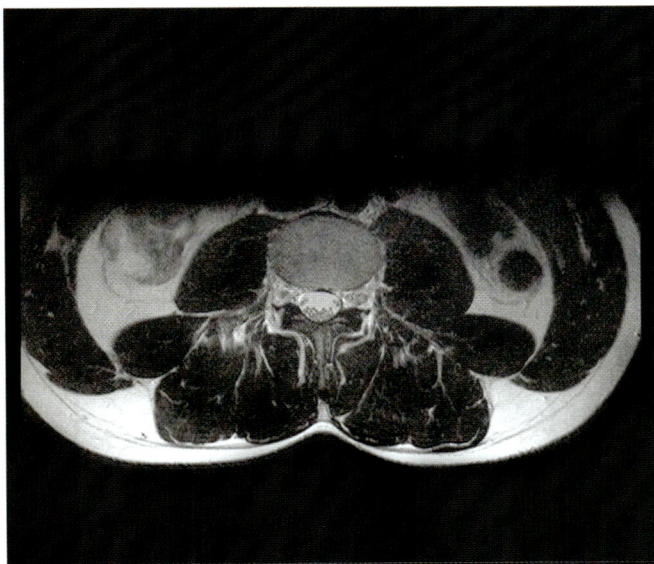

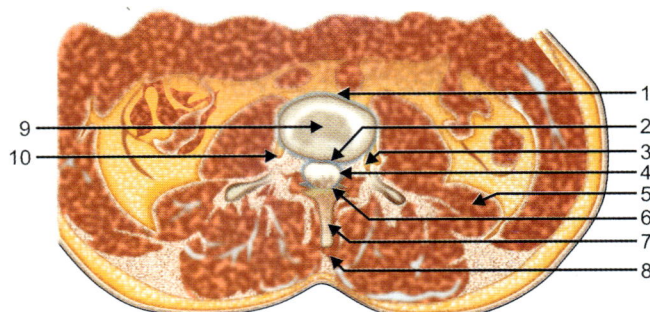

Figure 6.44

1. Anterior longitudinal ligament	4. Dura	7. Spinous process
2. Posterior longitudinal ligament	5. Quadratus lumborum	8. Supraspinatous ligament
3. Dorsal root ganglion	6. Lamina	9. Vertebral body
		10. Intervertebral foramen

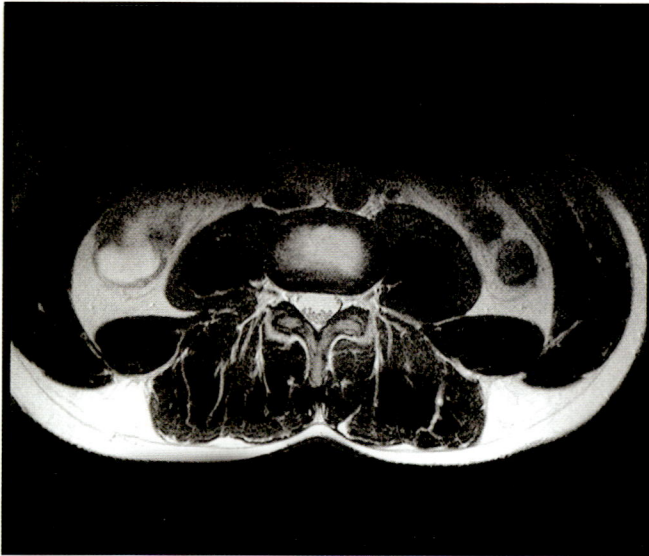

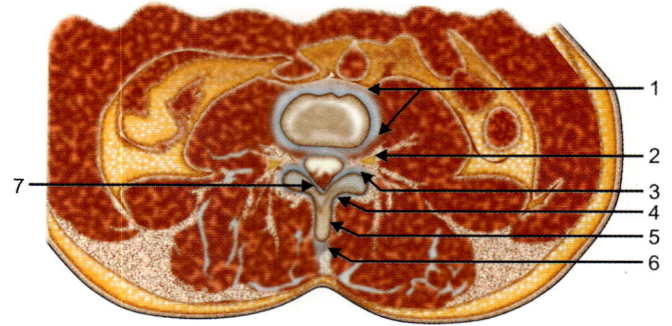

Figure 6.45

1. Intervertebral disk	5. Spinous process
2. Nerve roots	6. Supraspinatous ligament
3. Facet joint	7. Ligamentum flavum
4. Lamina	

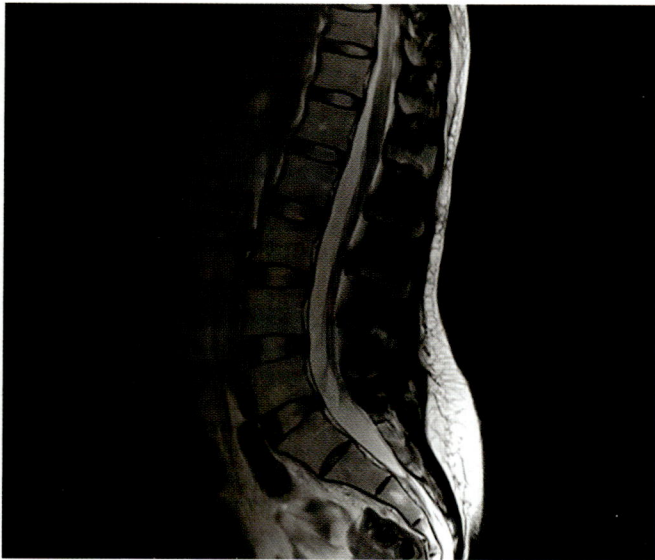

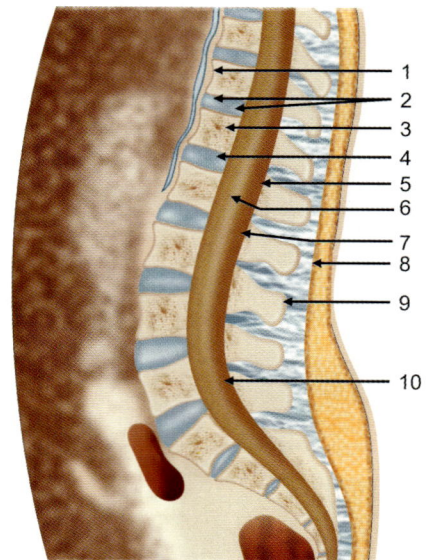

Figure 6.46

1. Anterior longitudinal ligament	6. Conus medullaris
2. Annular fibrosis	7. Cauda equina
3. Vertebral body	8. Supraspinatous ligament
4. Nucleus pulposis	9. Spinous process
5. Dura	10. Nerve roots

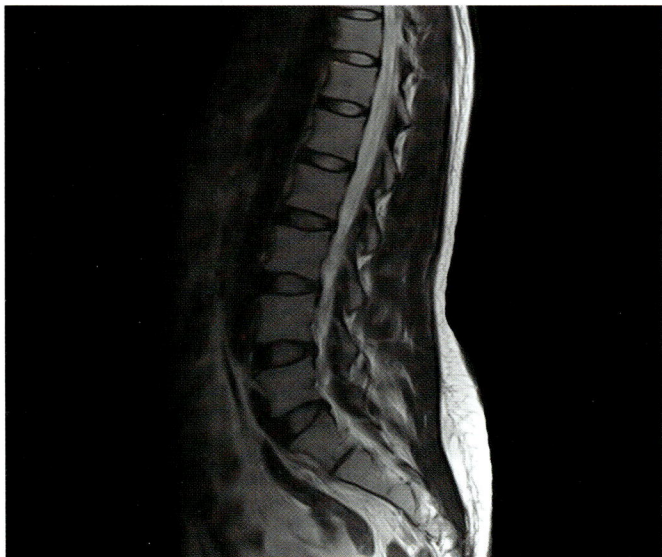

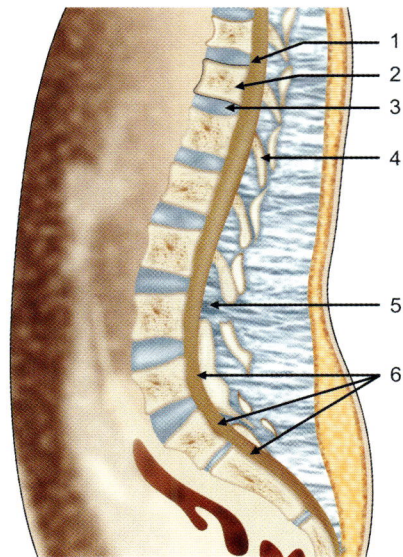

Figure 6.47

1. Annulus fibrosus	4. Lamina
2. Vertebral body	5. Ligamentum flavum
3. Nucleus pulposus	6. Nerve roots

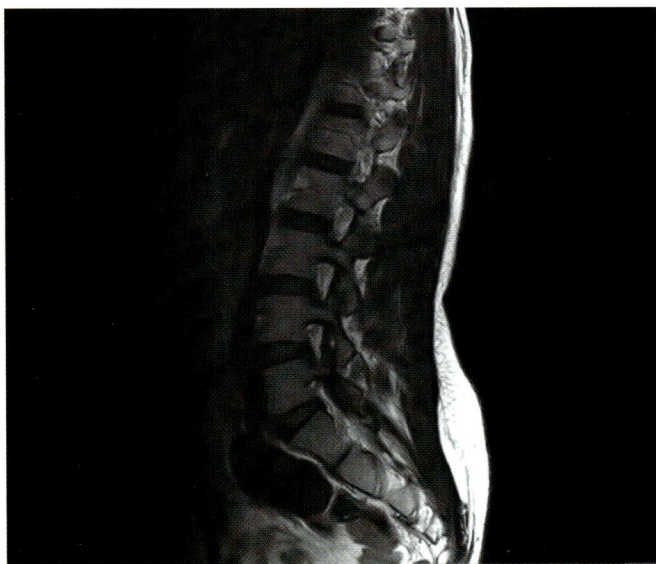

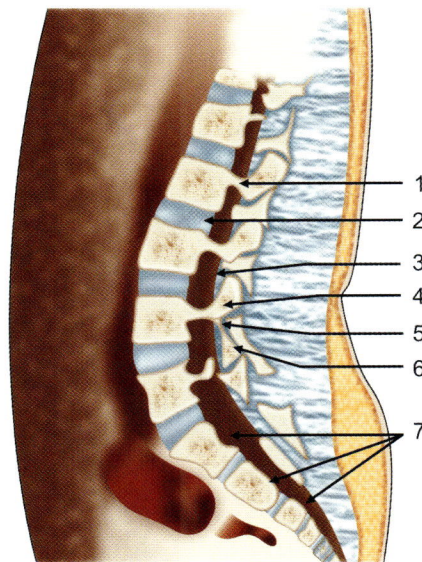

Figure 6.48

1. Pedicle	5. Pars interarticularis
2. Intervertebral disk	6. Inferior facet
3. Intervertebral foramen	7. Nerve roots
4. Superior facet	

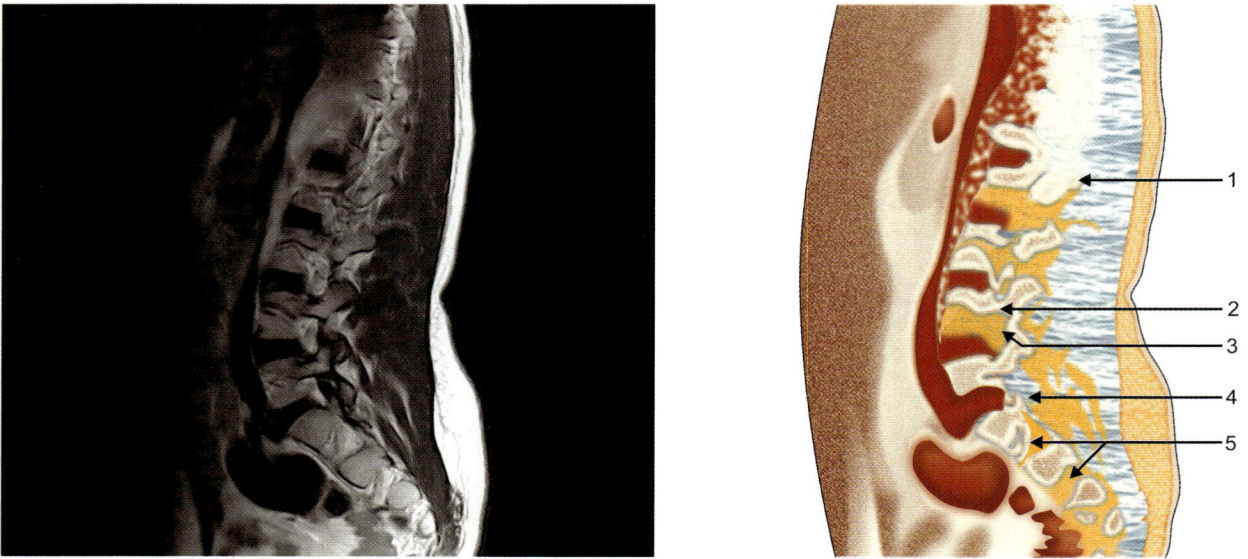

Figure 6.49

1. Transverse process
2. Pedicle
3. Intervertebral foramen
4. Facet joint
5. Sacral nerve roots

Section 3

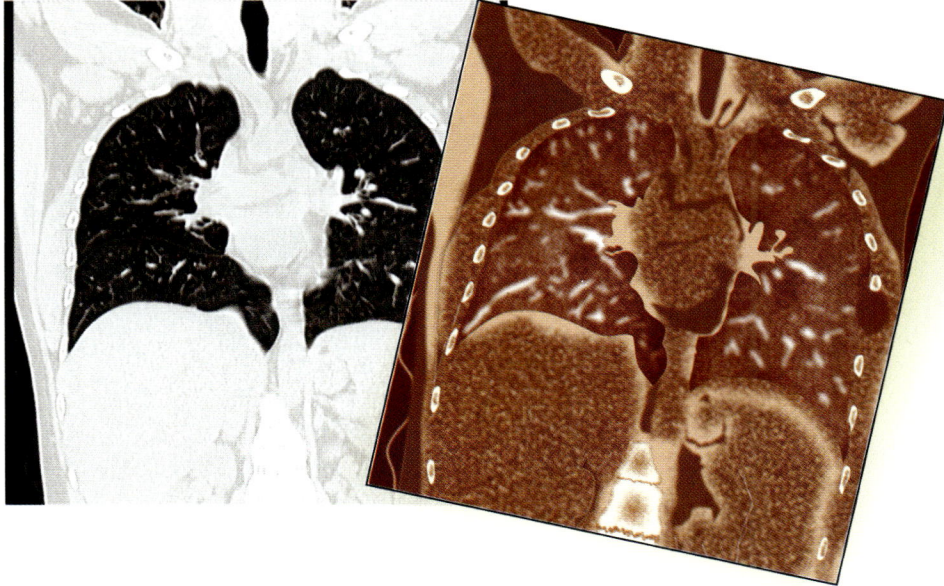

Trunk

- **Chest**
- **Abdomen**
- **Pelvis**

CHAPTER 7

Chest

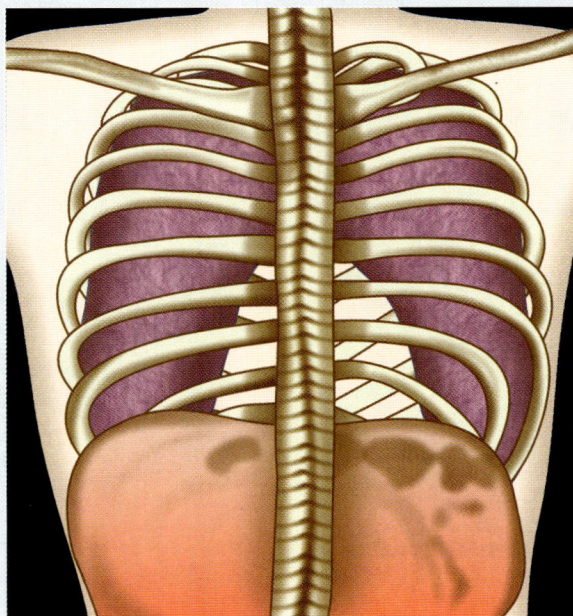

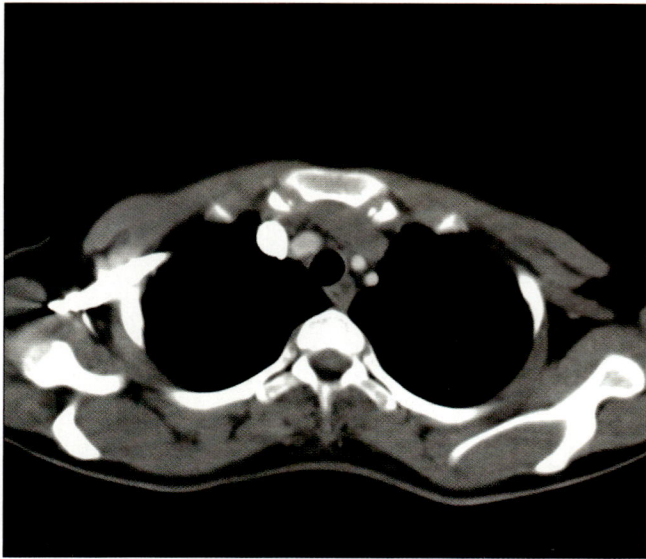

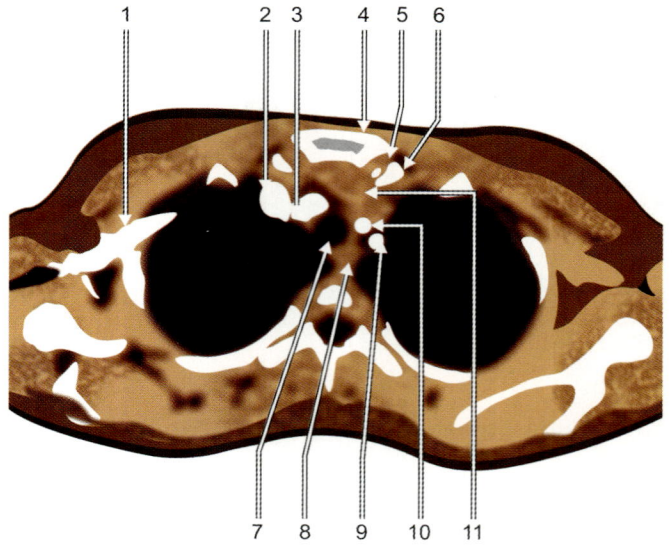

Figure 7.1

1. Right subclavian vein	5. Sternoclavicular joint	9. Left subclavian artery
2. Right brachiocephalic vein	6. Clavicle	10. Left carotid artery
3. Right brachiocephalic artery	7. Trachea	11. Left brachiocephalic vein
4. Sternum	8. Esophagus	

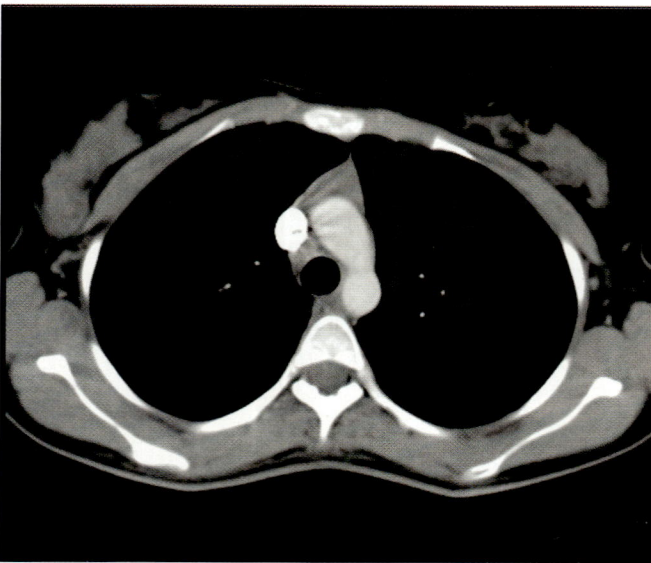

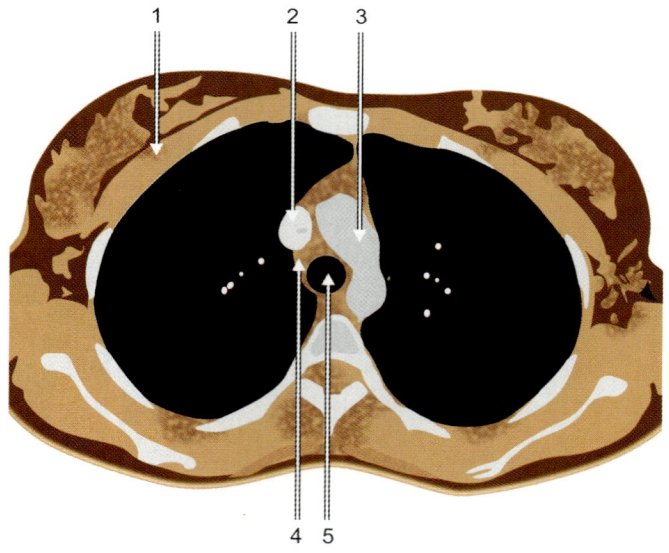

Figure 7.2

1. Pectoral muscles	4. Azygos vein
2. SVC	5. Trachea
3. Arch of aorta	

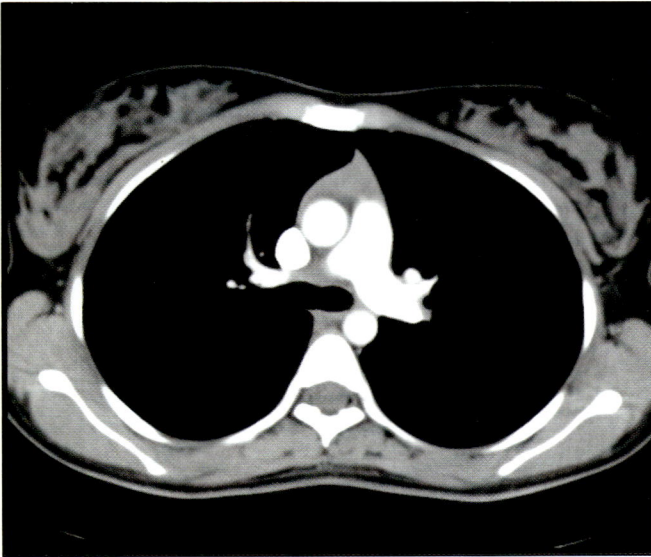

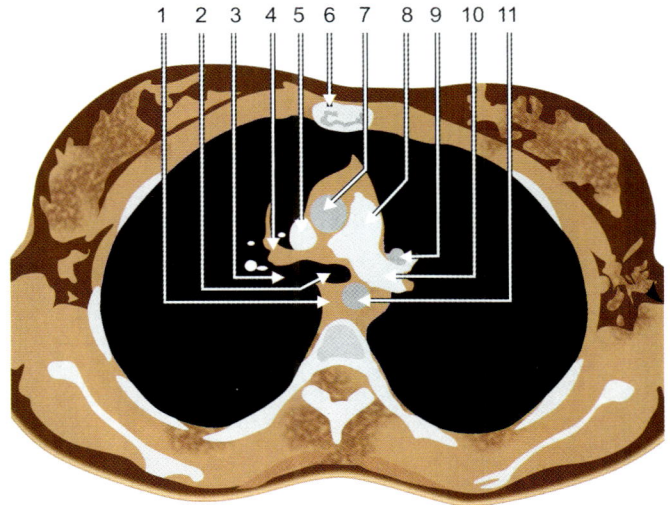

Figure 7.3

1. Esophagus
2. Left main bronchus
3. Right main bronchus
4. Right superior pulmonary artery
5. SVC
6. Sternum
7. Ascending aorta
8. Main pulmonary artery
9. Left superior pulmonary vein
10. Left pulmonary artery
11. Descending aorta

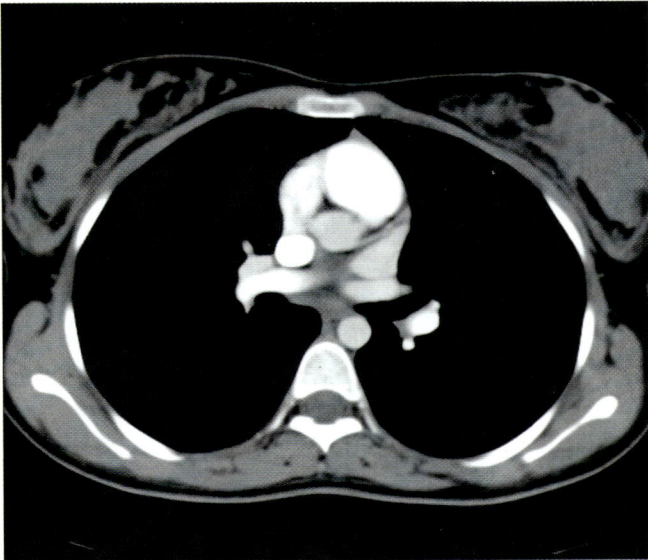

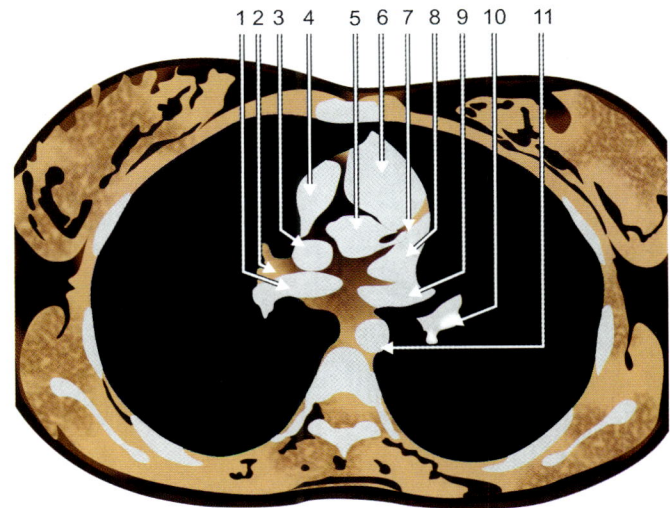

Figure 7.4

1. Right pulmonary artery
2. Rt Superior pulmonary vein
3. SVC
4. Right atrial appendage
5. Aortic root
6. Right ventricular outflow tract
7. Left coronary artery
8. Left atrial appendage
9. Left superior pulmonary vein
10. Left inferior pulmonary artery
11. Descending aorta

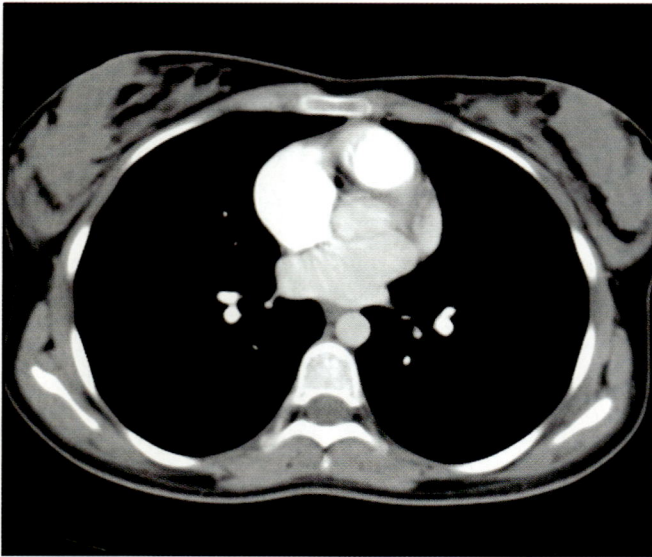

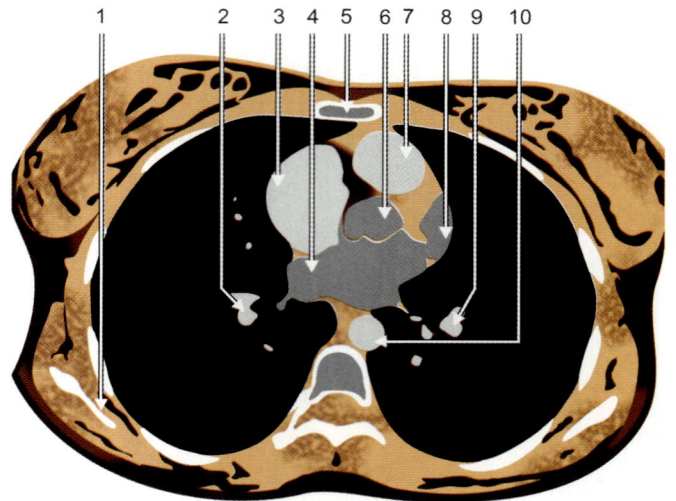

Figure 7.5

1. Scapula	6. Aortic root
2. Right inferior pulmonary artery	7. Infundibulum of right ventricle
3. Right atrium	8. Left atrial appendage
4. Left atrium	9. Left inferior pulmonary artery
5. Sternum	10. Descending aorta

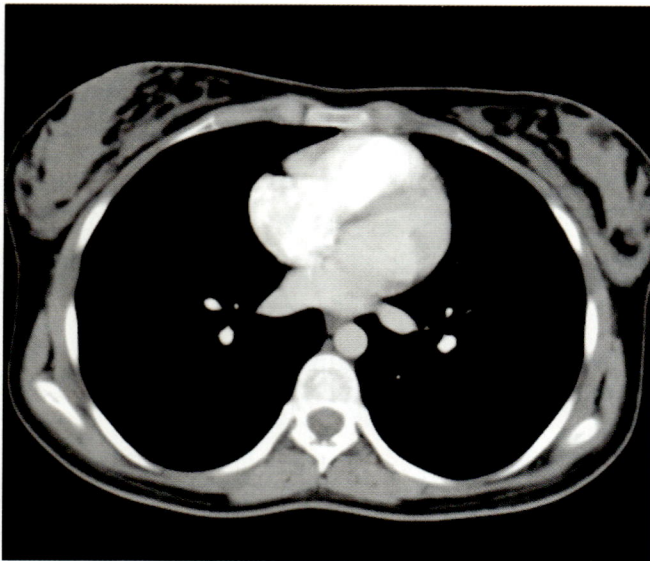

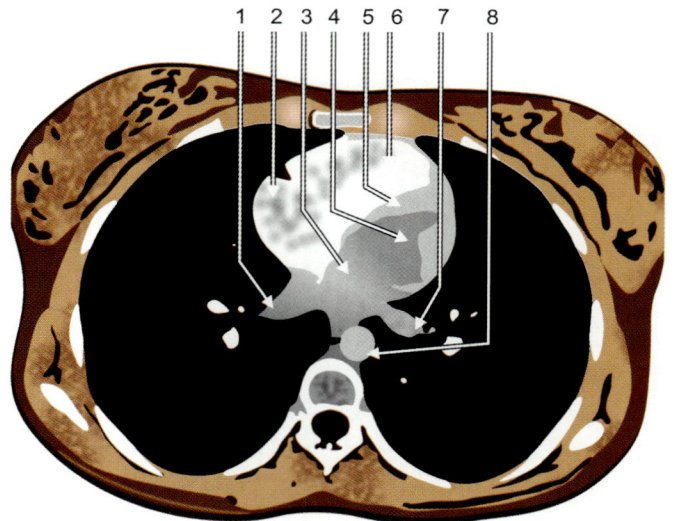

Figure 7.6

1. RT inferior pulmonary vein	5. Interventricular septum
2. Right atrium	6. Right ventricle
3. Left atrium	7. Left inferior pulmonary vein
4. Left ventricle	8. Descending aorta

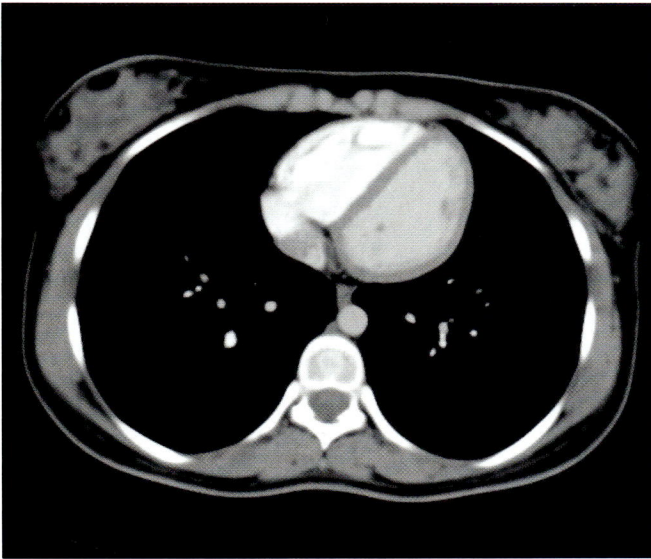

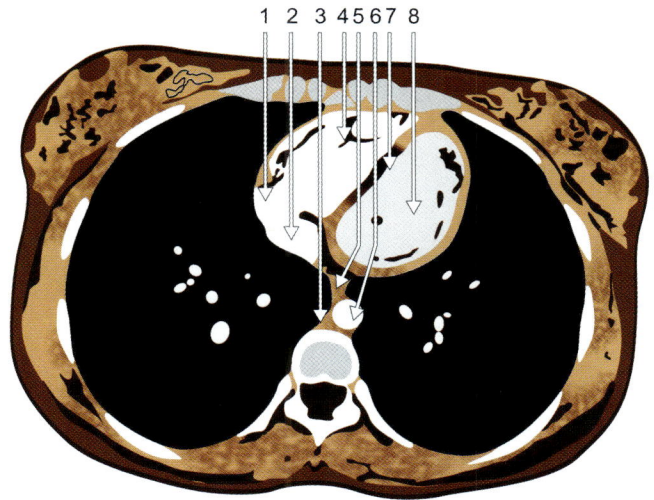

Figure 7.7

1. Right atrium	5. Esophagus
2. IVC opening into RA	6. Descending aorta
3. Azygos vein	7. Interventricular septum
4. Right ventricle	8. Left ventricle

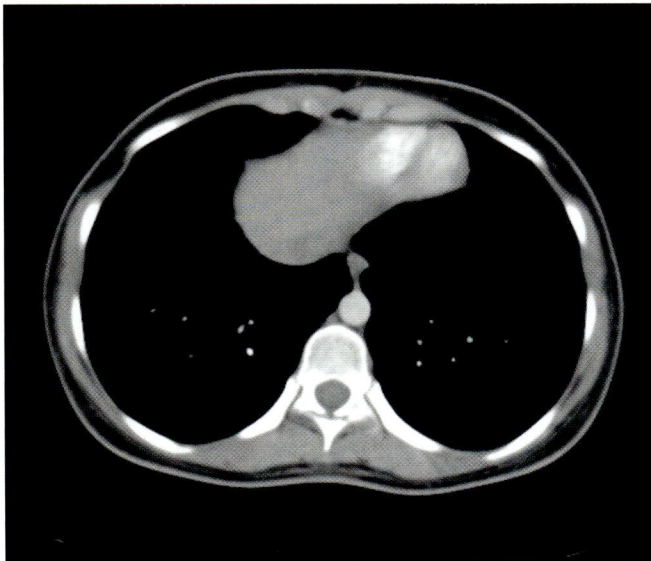

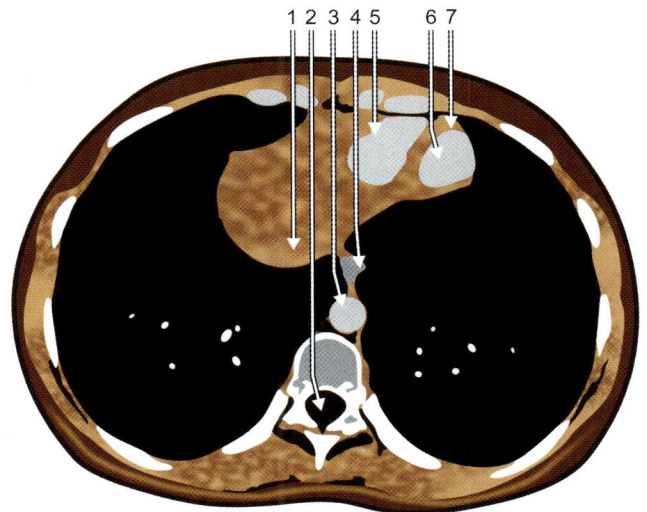

Figure 7.8

1. IVC	5. Right ventricle
2. Spinal cord	6. Left ventricle
3. Aorta	7. Cardiac apex
4. Esophagus	

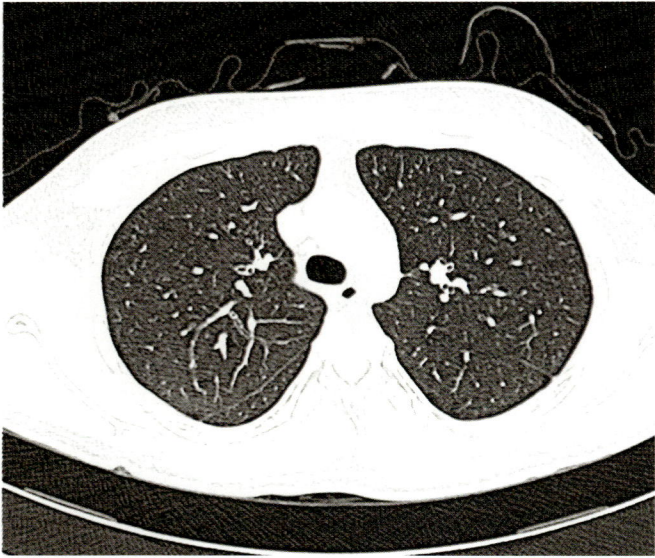 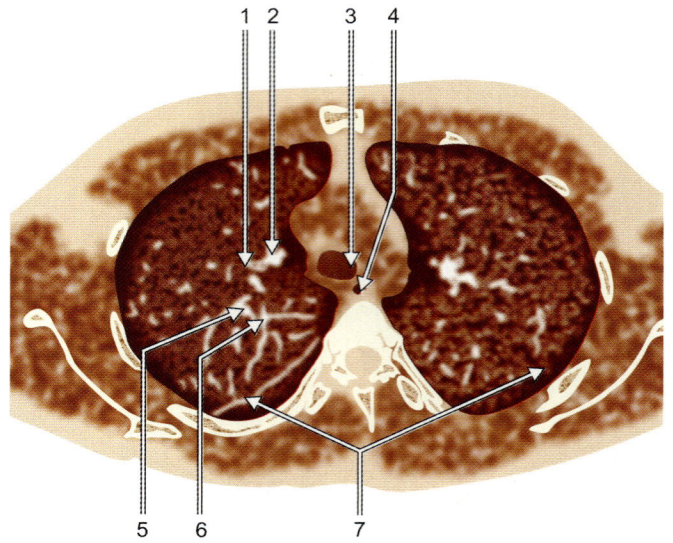

Figure 7.9

1. Bronchus
2. Apical segment vessels
3. Trachea
4. Esophagus
5. Bronchovascular structures
6. Posterior segment
7. Major fissure

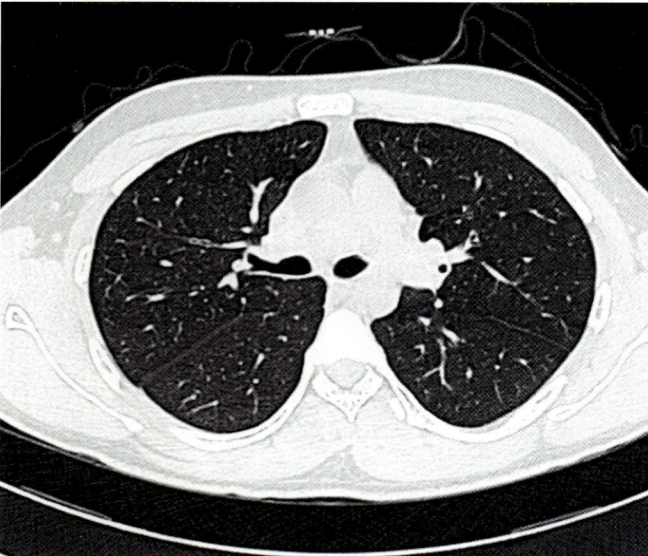 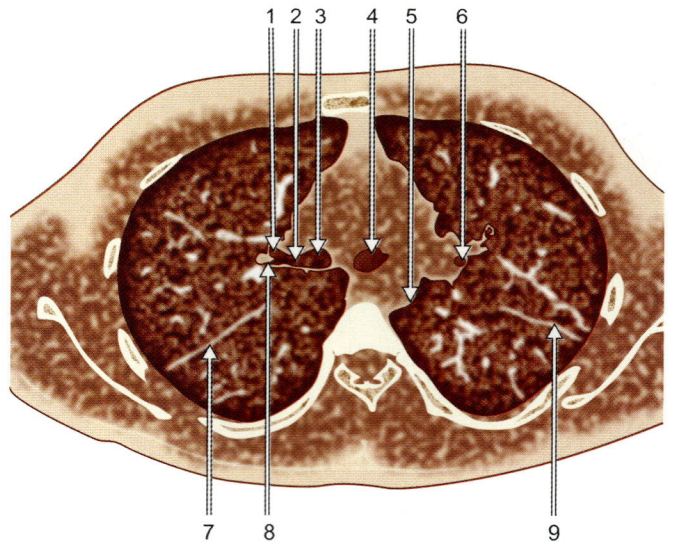

Figure 7.10

1. Anterior segment
2. Right upper lobe bronchus
3. Right mainstem bronchus
4. Left mainstem bronchus
5. Descending aorta
6. Apicoposterior bronchus
7. Major fissure
8. Posterior segment bronchus
9. Major fissure

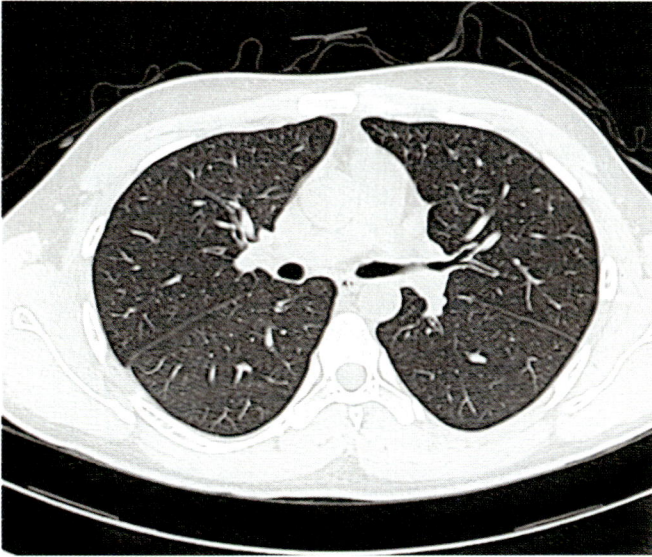

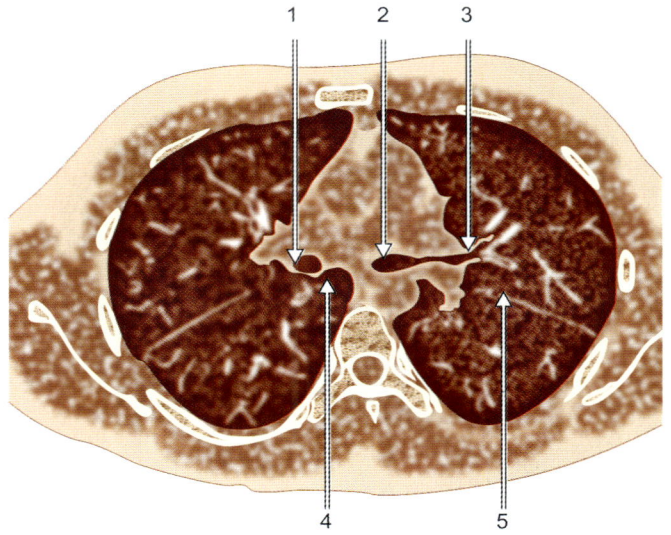

Figure 7.11

1. Bronchus intermedius
2. Left mainstem bronchus
3. Anterior segment bronchus
4. Azygoesophageal recess
5. Major fissure

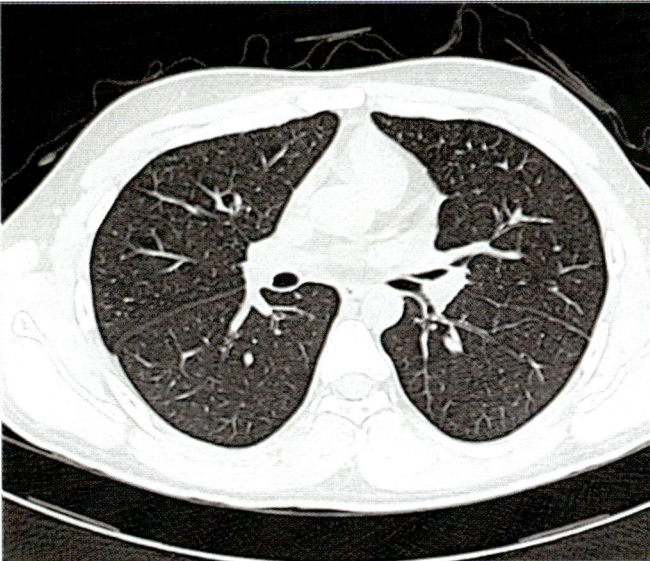

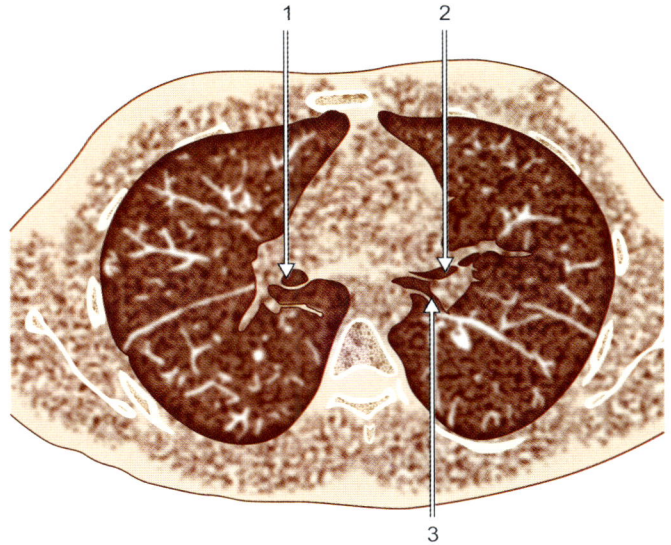

Figure 7.12

1. Bronchus intermedius
2. Lingular lobe bronchus
3. Superior basal segment bronchus

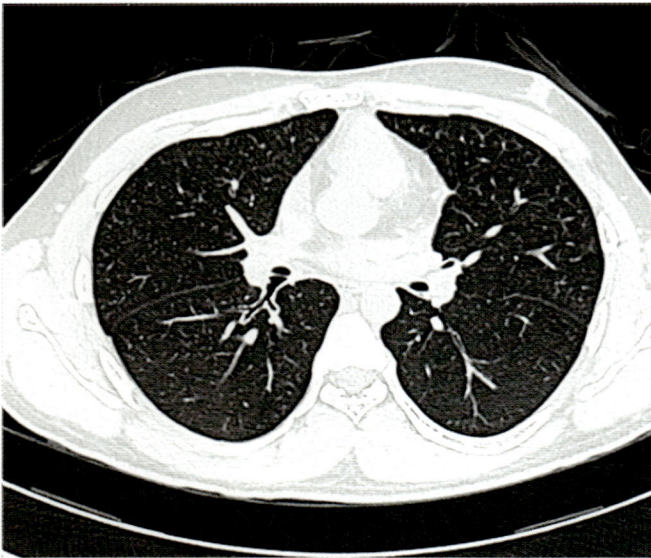

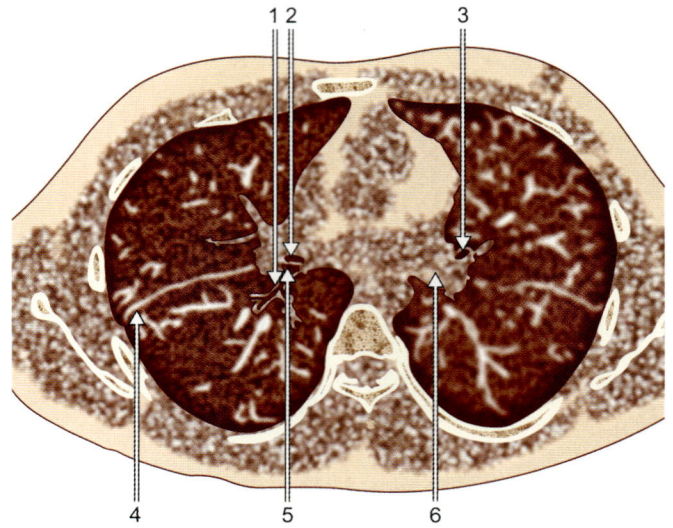

Figure 7.13

1. Superior basal segment bronchus
2. Middle lobe bronchus
3. Lingular lobe bronchus
4. Major fissure
5. Lower lobe bronchus
6. Lower lobe bronchus

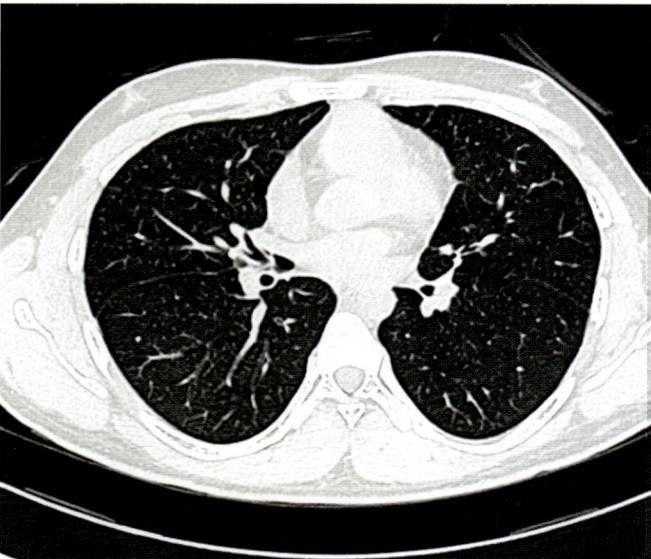

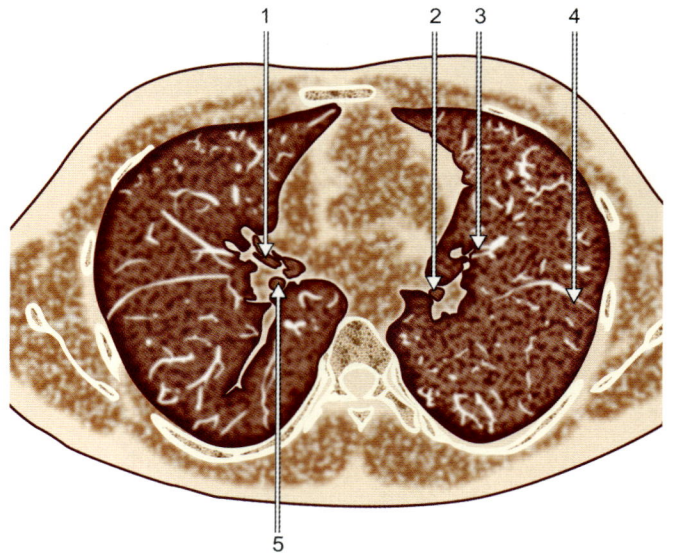

Figure 7.14

1. Middle lobe bronchus
2. Left lower lobe bronchus
3. Lingular lobe bronchus
4. Major fissure
5. Lower lobe bronchus

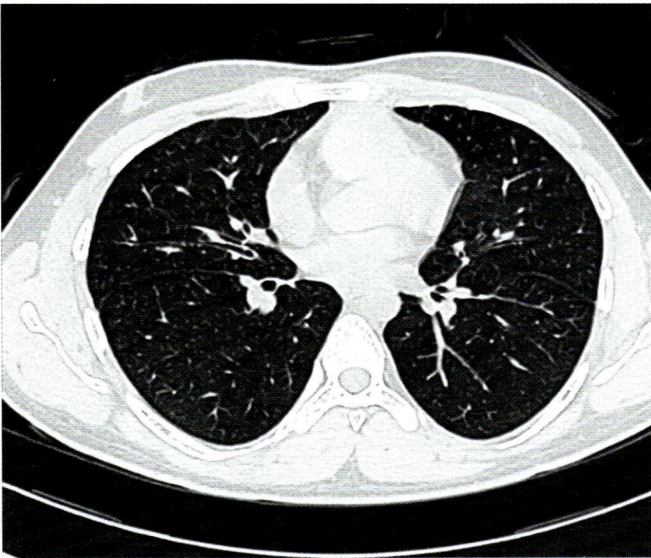

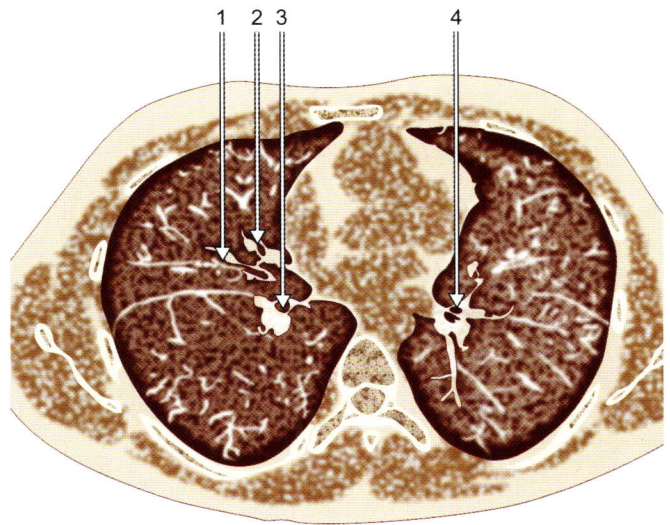

Figure 7.15

1. Bronchus of lateral segment of right middle lobe
2. Bronchus of medial segment of RML
3. Lower lobe bronchus
4. Left lower lobe bronchi

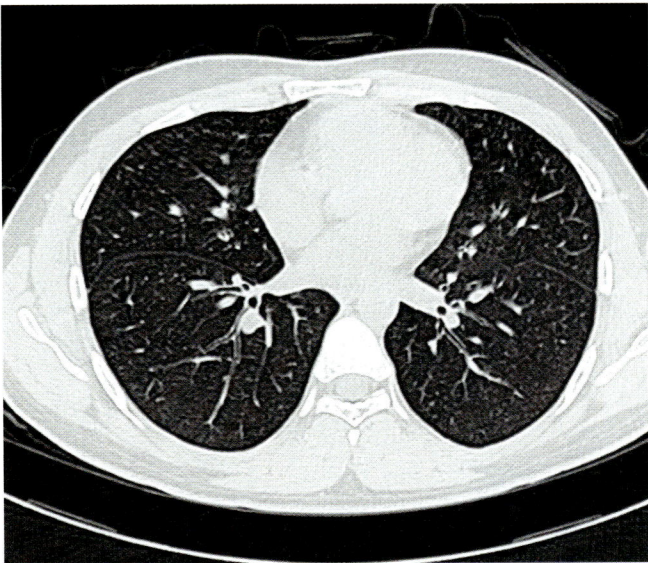

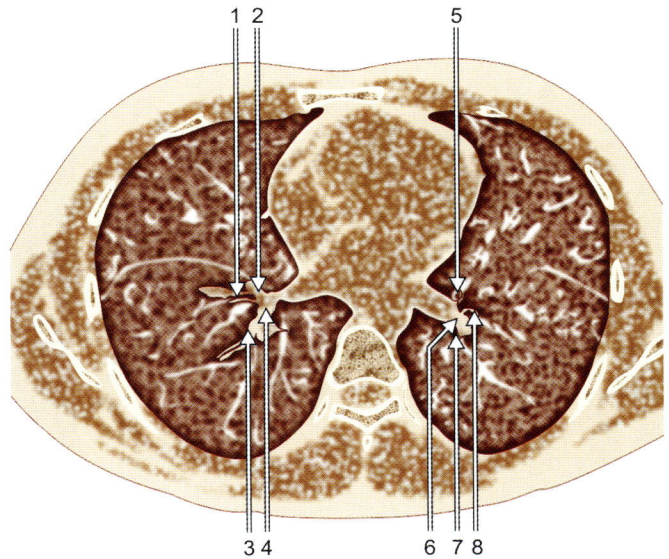

Figure 7.16

Segmental bronchi	Lower lobe Segmental bronchi
1. Anterior basal	5. Medial basal
2. Medial basal	6. Lateral basal
3. Lateral basal	7. Posterior basal
4. Posterior basal	8. Anterior basal

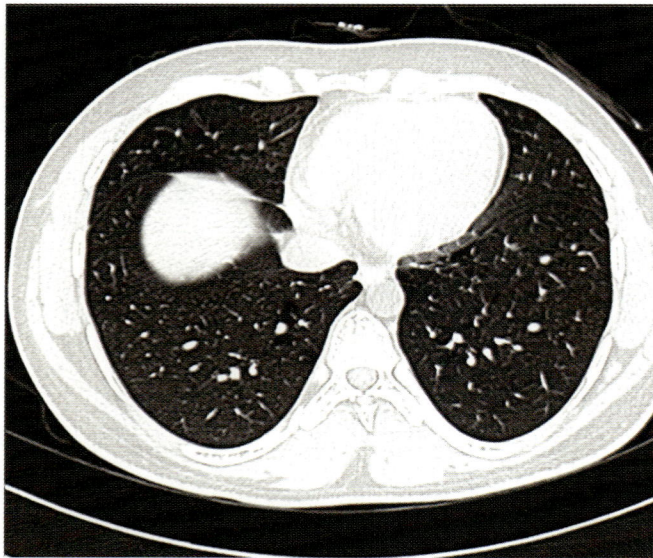

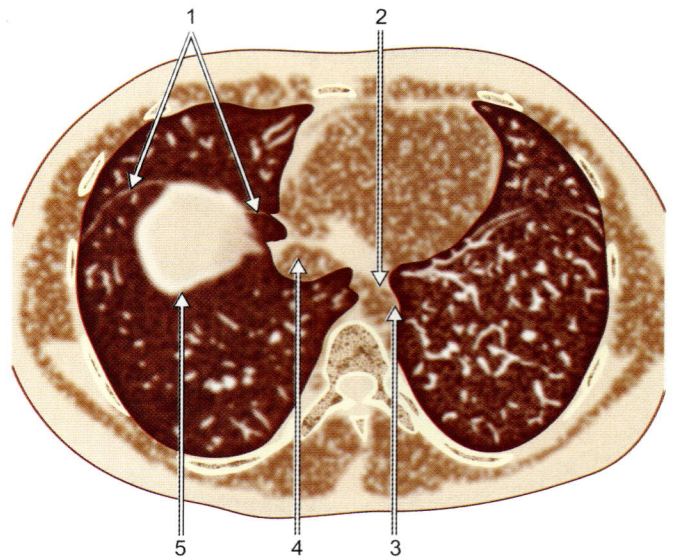

Figure 7.17

1. Major fissure
2. Esophagus
3. Descending aorta
4. IVC
5. Liver

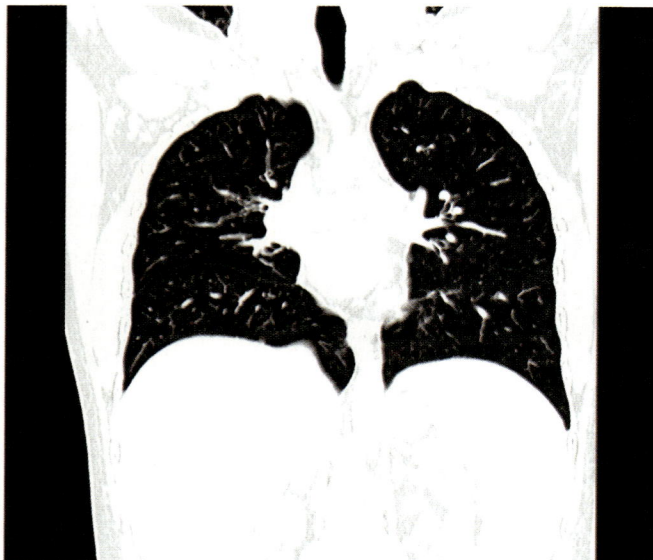

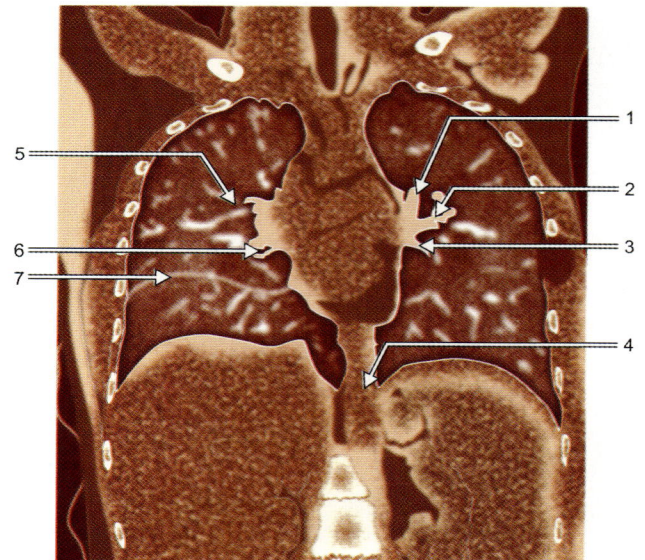

Figure 7.18

1. Left superior pulmonary vein
2. Anterior segment bronchus
3. Lingular lobe bronchi
4. Descending aorta
5. Anterior segment bronchi
6. Middle lobe bronchus
7. Major fissure

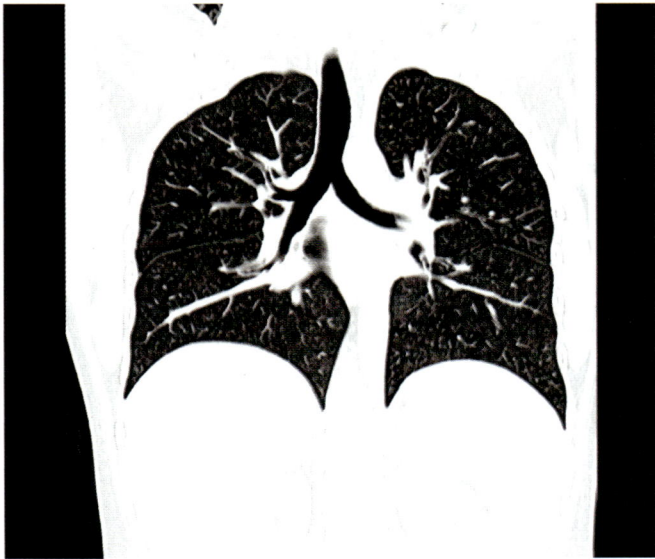
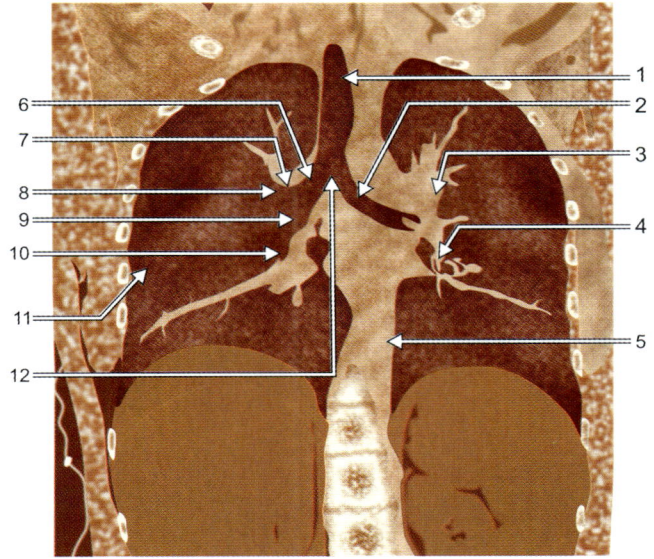

Figure 7.19

1. Trachea	5. Descending aorta	9. Posterior segment bronchi
2. Left mainstem bronchus	6. Right mainstem bronchus	10. Bronchus intermedius
3. Apicoposterior segment bronchus	7. Right upper lobe bronchus	11. Major fissure
4. Lower lobe bronchi	8. Apical segment bronchus	12. Carina

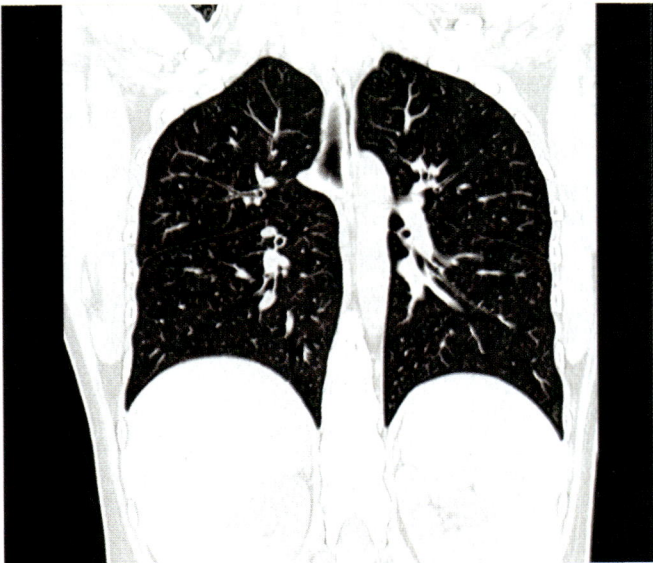
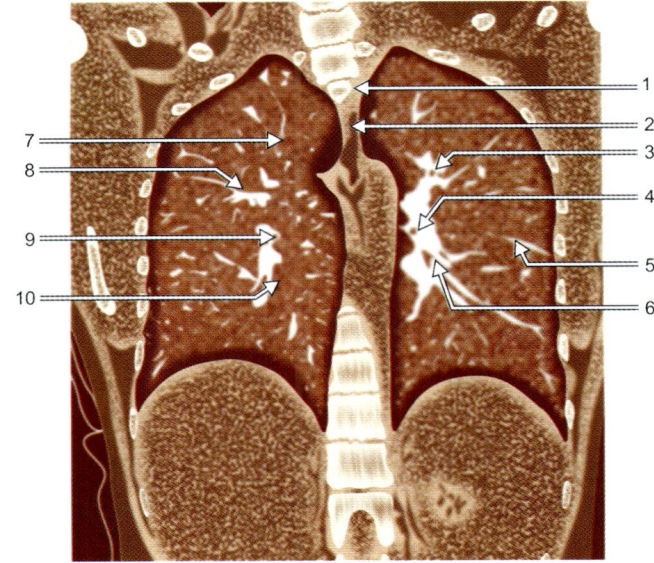

Figure 7.20

1. Air in the esophagus	4. Superior basal segment bronchus	8. Posterior segment bronchus
2. Trachea	5. Major fissure	9. Superior basal segment bronchus
3. Apicoposterior segment bronchus	6. Lower lobe segment bronchus	10. Lower lobe segment bronchus
	7. Apical segment bronchus	

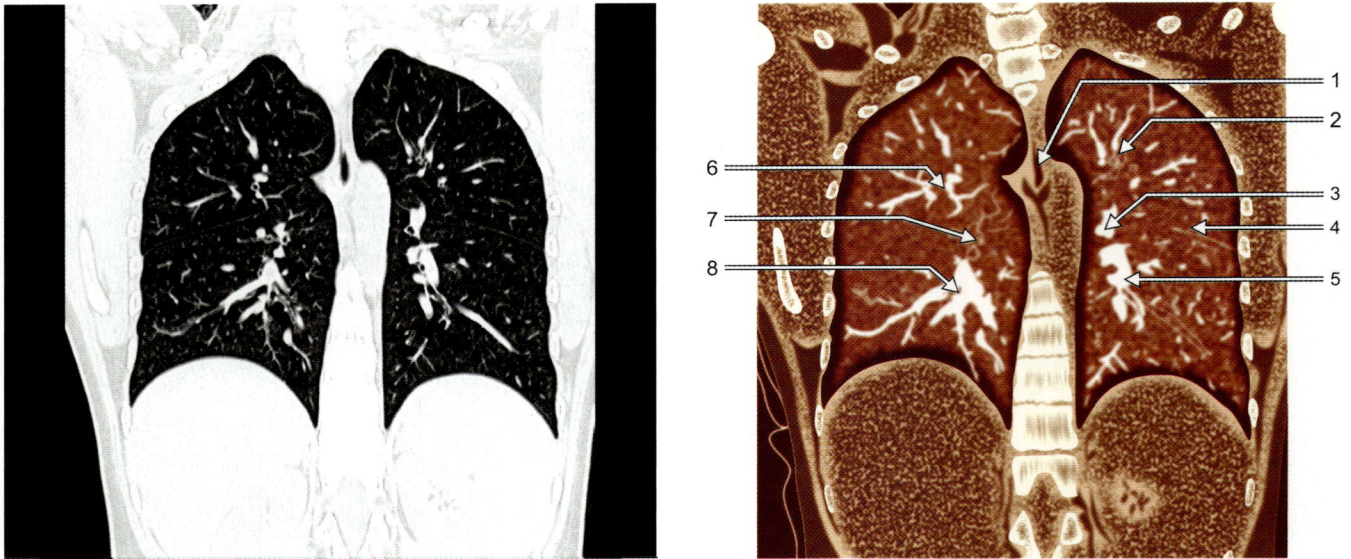

Figure 7.21

1. Air in the esophagus	5. Lower lobe segment bronchus
2. Apicoposterior segment bronchus	6. Posterior segment bronchus
3. Superior basal segment bronchus	7. Superior basal segment bronchus
4. Major fissure	8. Lower lobe segment bronchus

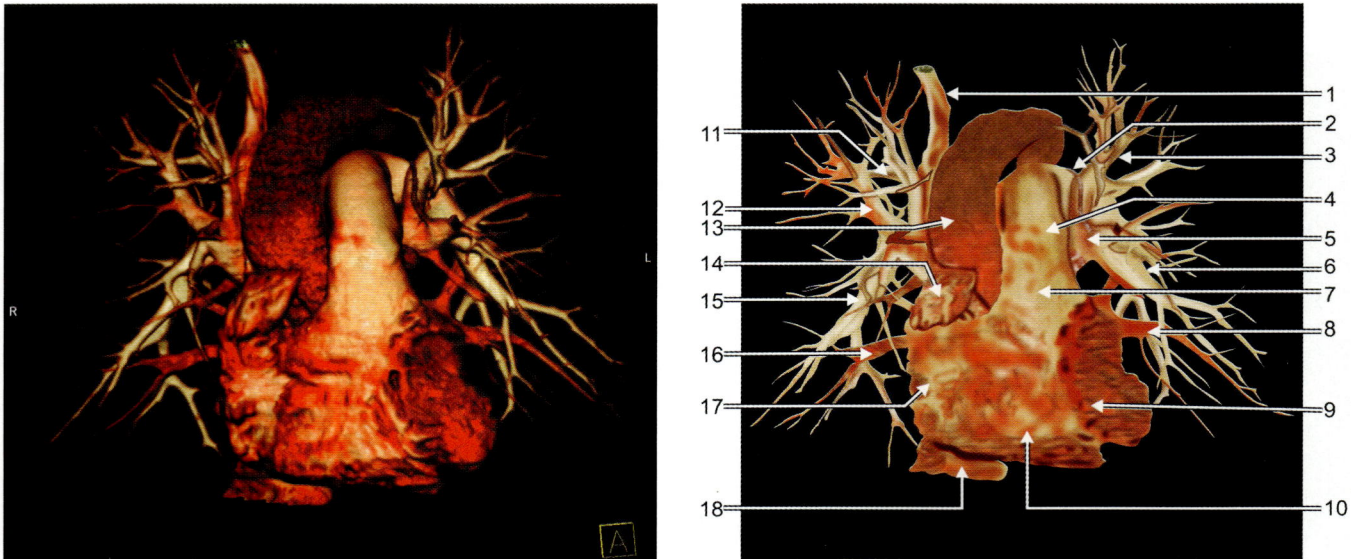

Figure 7.22

1. SVC	7. Infundibulum	13. Aorta
2. Left pulmonary artery	8. Inf. pulmonary vein	14. RAA
3. Sup. pulmonary artery	9. Left ventricle	15. Inf. pulmonary artery
4. Main pulmonary artery	10. Right ventricle	16. Inf. pulmonary vein
5. Sup. pulmonary vein	11. Sup. pulmonary artery	17. Right atrium
6. Inf. pulmonary artery	12. Sup. pulmonary vein	18. IVC

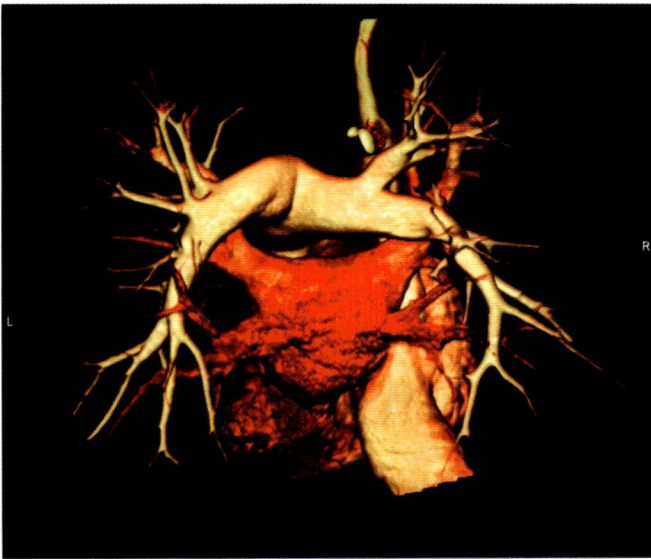

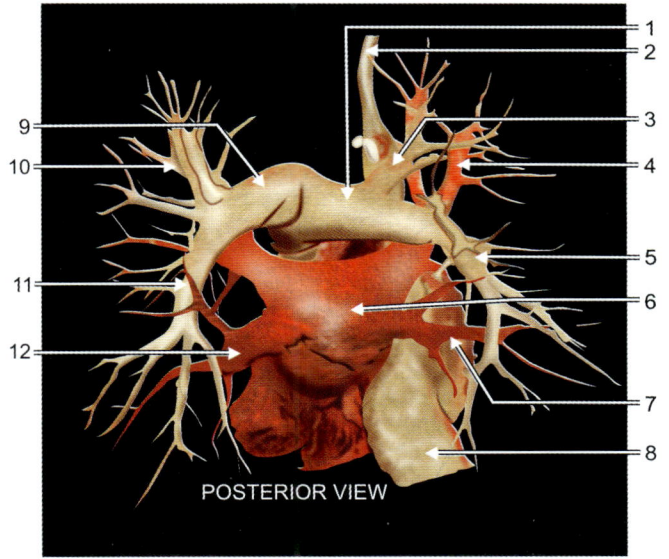

Figure 7.23

1. Right main pulmonary artery	5. Inferior pulmonary artery	9. Left main pulmonary artery
2. SVC	6. Left atrium	10. Superior pulmonary vein
3. RT superior pulmonary artery	7. Inferior pulmonary vein	11. Inferior pulmonary artery
4. Superior pulmonary vein	8. IVC	12. Inferior pulmonary vein

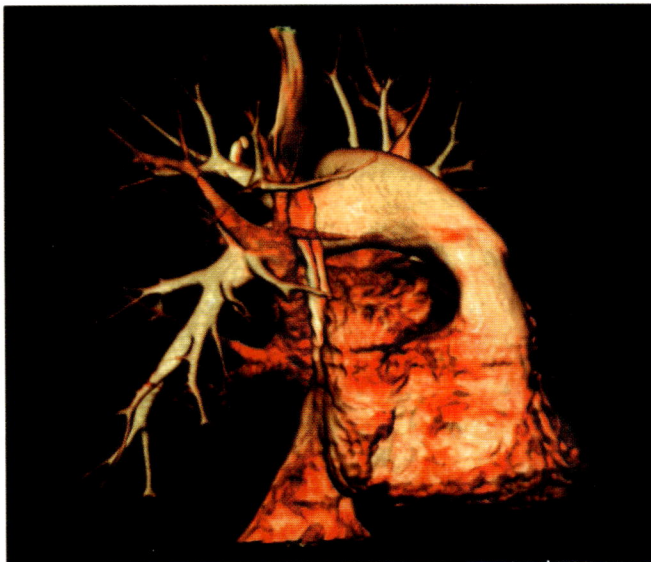

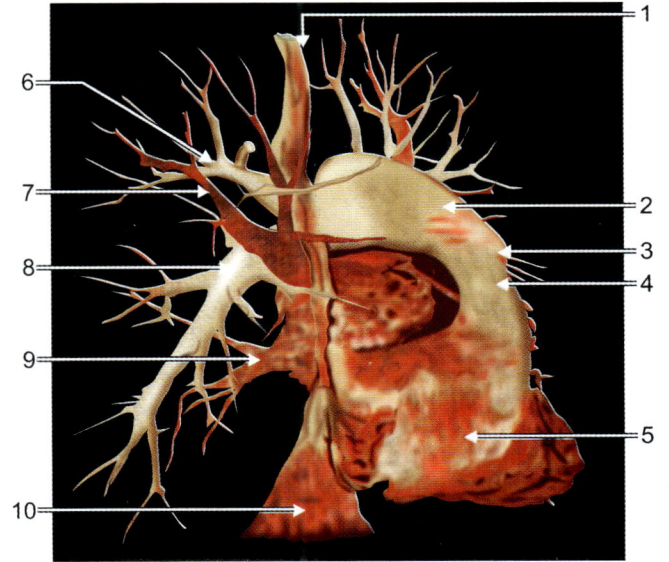

Figure 7.24

1. SVC	5. Right ventricle	9. Inferior pulmonary vein
2. Main pulmonary artery	6. Right superior pulmonary artery	10. IVC
3. Pulmonic valve	7. Right superior pulmonary vein	
4. Infundibulum	8. Inferior pulmonary artery	

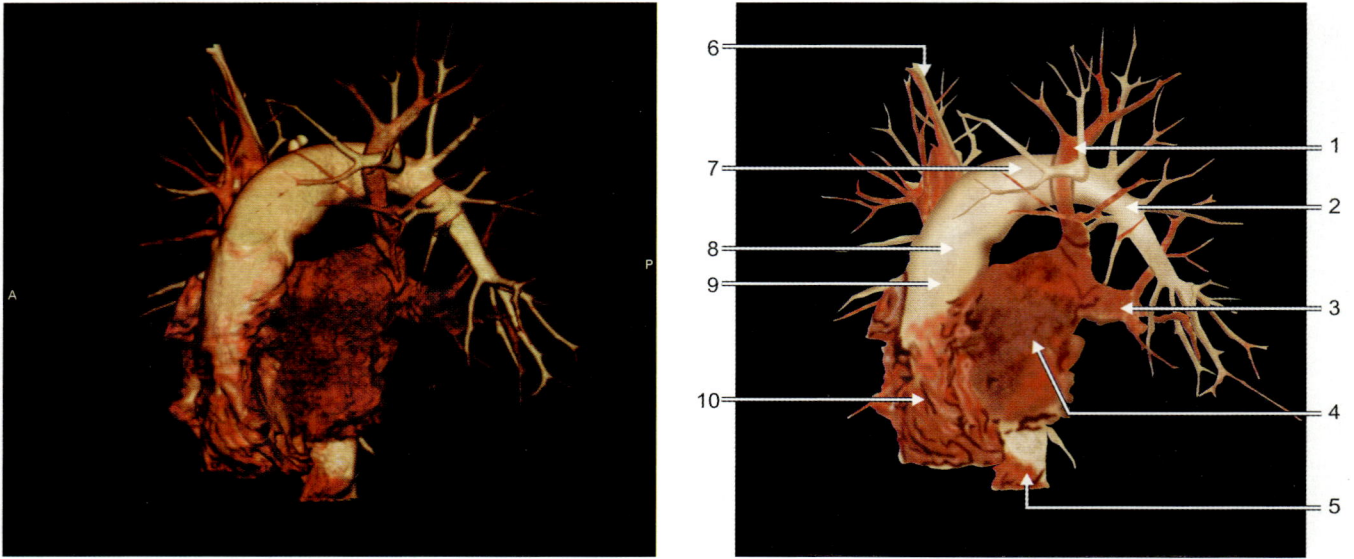

Figure 7.25

1. Left superior pulmonary vein	5. IVC	9. Infundibulum
2. Left inferior pulmonary artery	6. SVC	10. Right ventricle
3. Left inferior pulmonary vein	7. Left pulmonary artery	
4. Left atrium	8. Pulmonic valve	

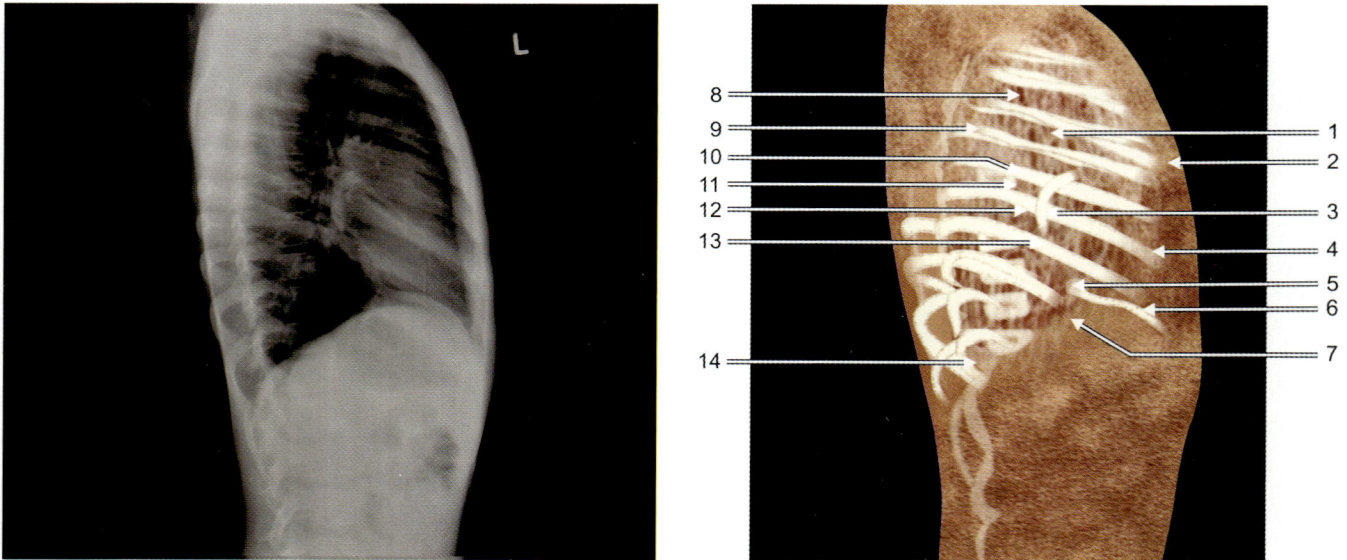

Figure 7.26

1. Arch of aorta	6. Right diaphragm	11. Left main bronchus
2. Sternum	7. Left dome of diaphragm effaced by heart anteriorly	12. Right main bronchus
3. Right pulmonary artery		13. Left atrial border
4. Anterior cardiac border formed by RV	8. Trachea	14. Posterior costophrenic recess
	9. Scapula	
5. IVC	10. Left main pulmonary artery	

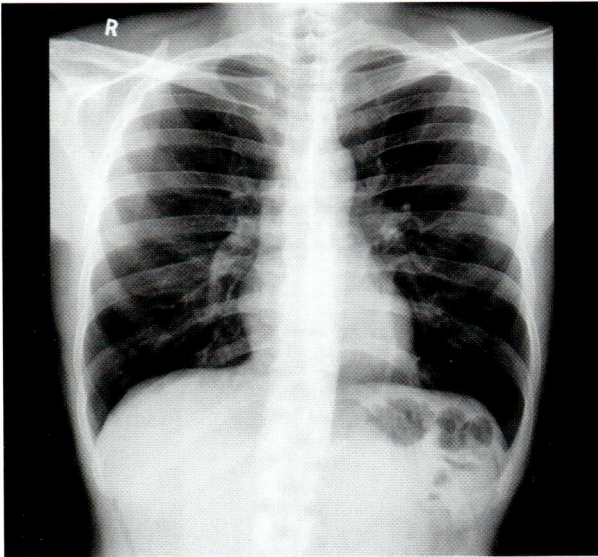

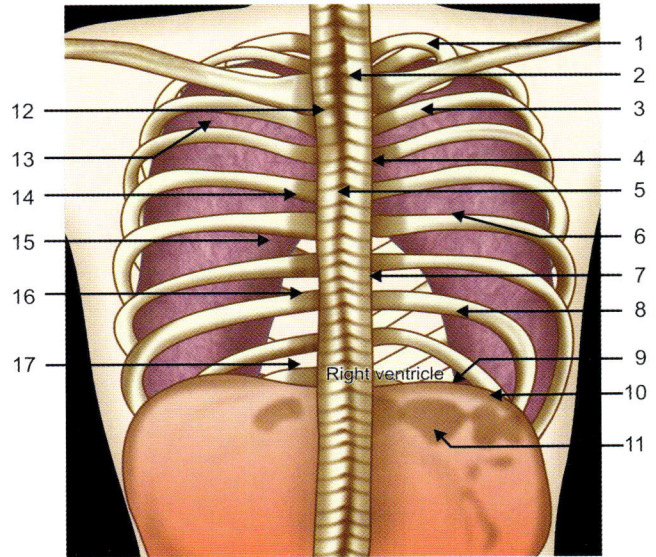

Figure 7.27

1. First rib	7. Descending aorta	13. Anterior rib
2. Spinous process	8. Left ventricle	14. Superior vena cava
3. Posterior rib	9. Cardiophrenic angle	15. Right pulmonary artery
4. Aortic knuckle	10. Left dome of diaphragm	16. Right atrium
5. Carina	11. Fundic gas bubble	17. IVC
6. Left pulmonary artery	12. Trachea	

CHAPTER 8

Abdomen

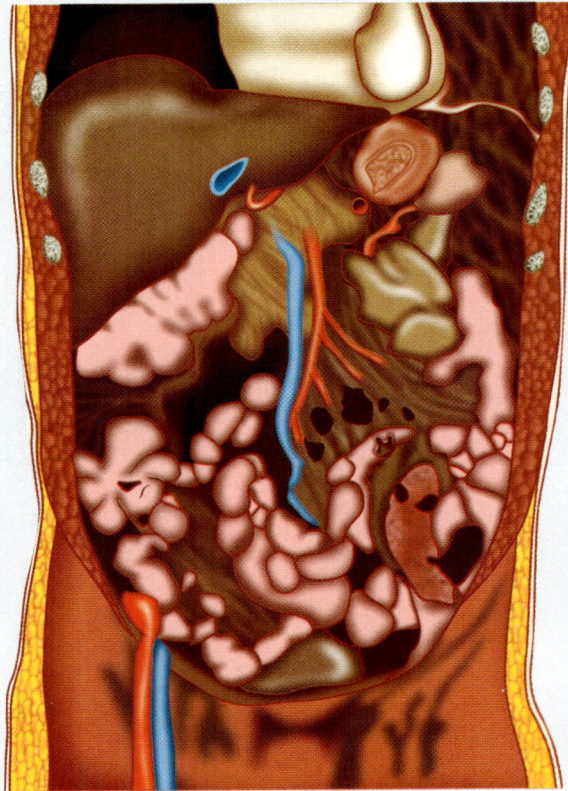

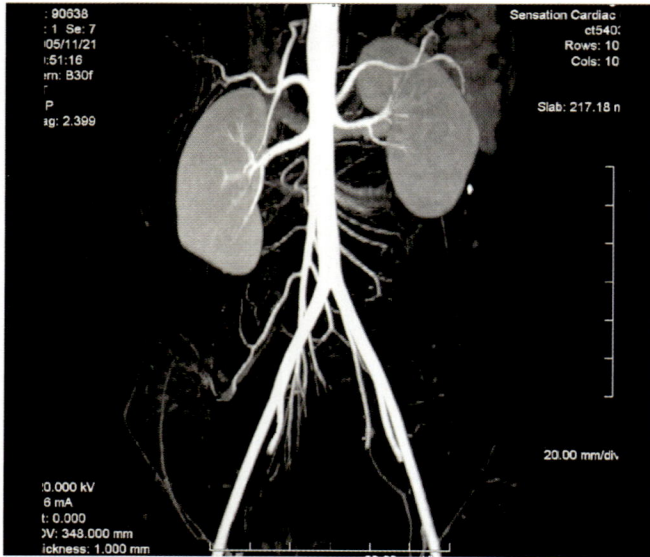
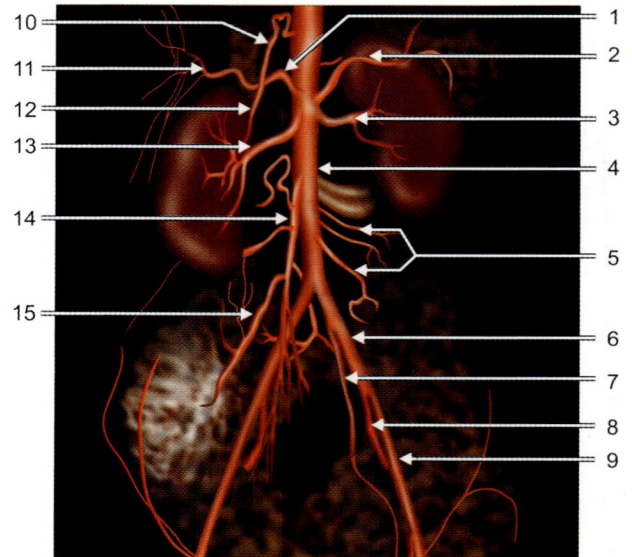

Figure 8.1

1. Hepatic artery	5. Jejunal branches of SMA	9. External iliac artery	13. Right renal artery
2. Splenic artery	6. Common iliac artery	10. Left hepatic artery	14. Superior mesenteric artery
3. Left renal artery	7. Inferior mesenteric artery	11. Right hepatic artery	
4. Aorta	8. Internal iliac artery	12. Gastroduodenal artery	15. Ileocolic artery

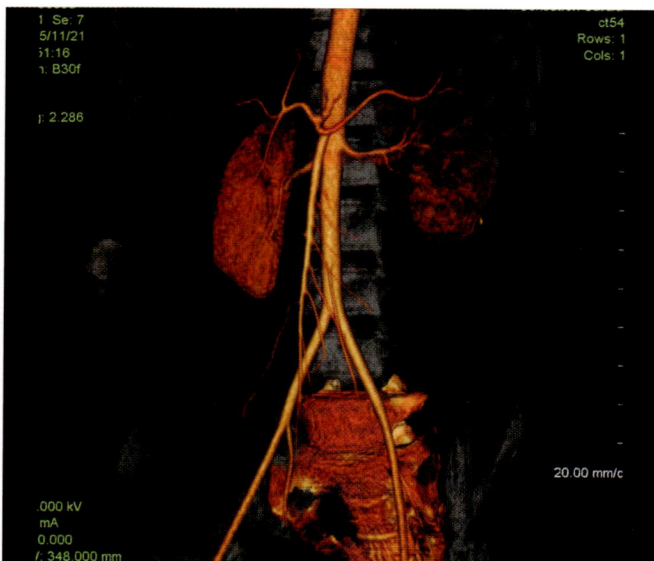
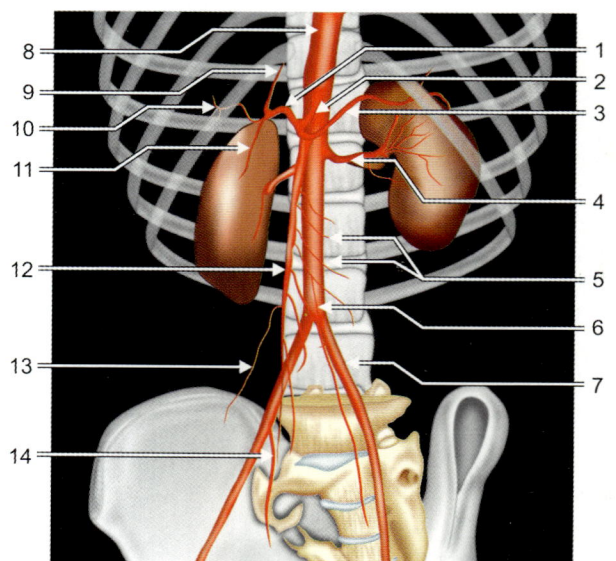

Figure 8.2

1. Hepatic artery	5. Jejunal branches	8. Aorta	12. Superior mesenteric artery
2. Celiac artery	6. Inferior mesenteric artery	9. Left hepatic artery	13. Ileocolic artery
3. Splenic artery		10. Right hepatic artery	14. Right internal iliac artery
4. Left renal artery	7. Left common iliac artery	11. Gastroduodenal artery	

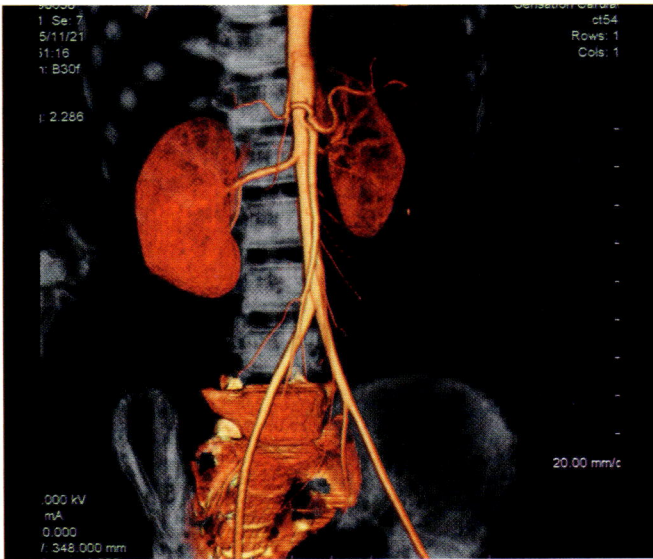

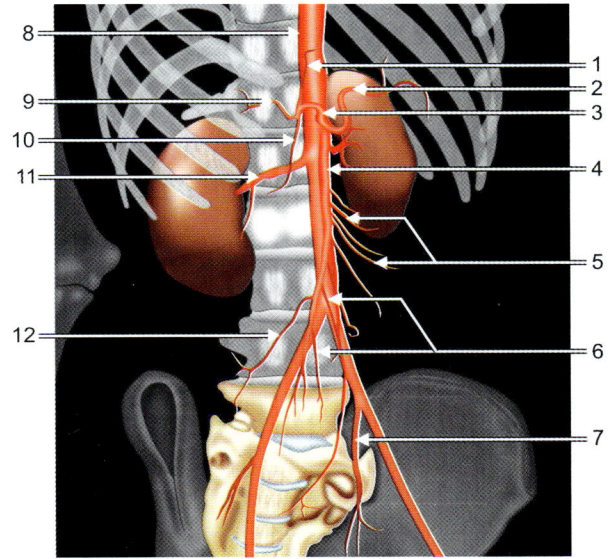

Figure 8.3

1. Left hepatic artery	5. Jejunal branches	9. Right hepatic artery
2. Splenic artery	6. Iliac branches	10. Gastroduodenal artery
3. Celiac artery	7. Left internal iliac artery	11. Right renal artery
4. Superior mesenteric artery	8. Aorta	12. Ileocolic artery

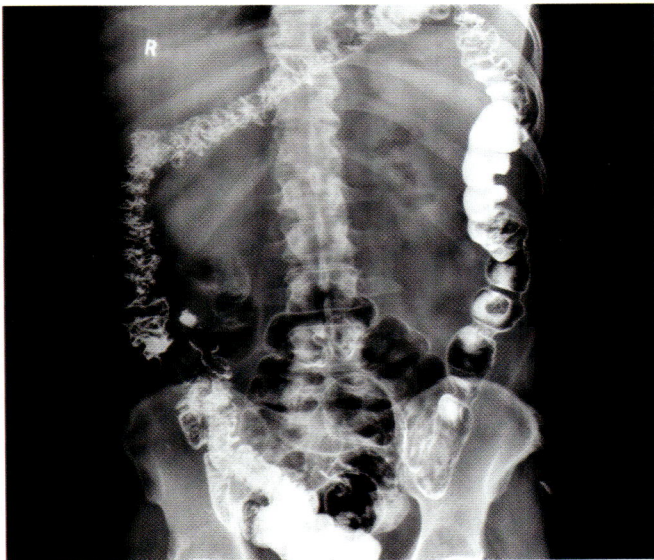

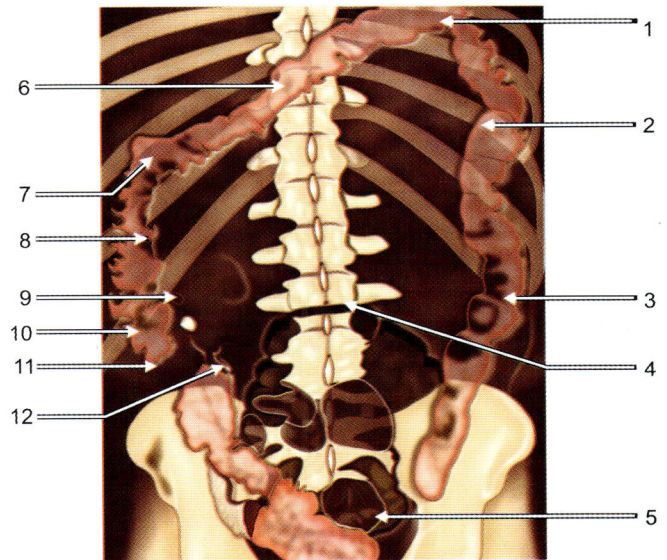

Figure 8.4

Large Intestine

1. Splenic flexure	5. Rectum	10. Caecum
2. Descending colon	6. Transverse colon	11. Appendix
3. Haustra	7. Hepatic flexure	12. Terminal ileum
4. Sigmoid colon	8. Ascending colon	
	9. IC junction	

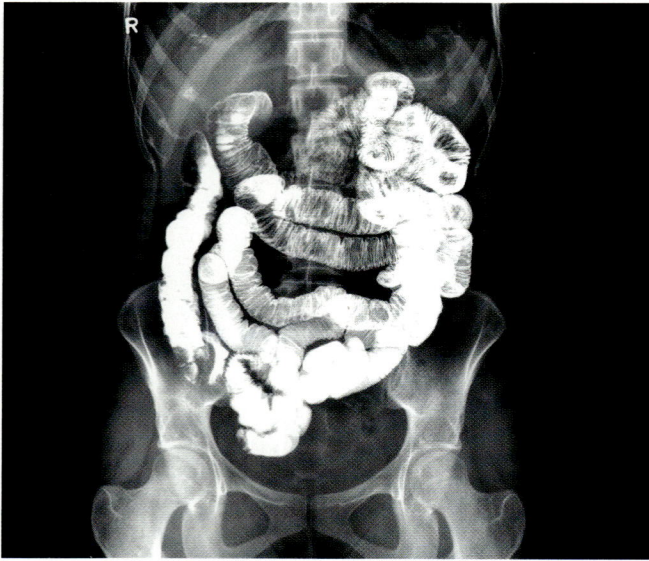

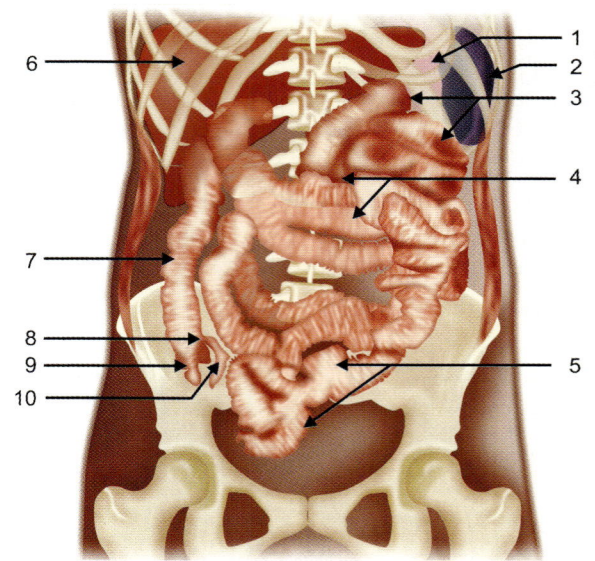

Figure 8.5

Small Intestine
1. Fundic bubble
2. Spleen
3. Jejunal loops
4. Valvulae conniventes
5. Ileal loops
6. Liver
7. Ascending colon
8. Ileocecal junction
9. Cecum
10. Terminal ileum

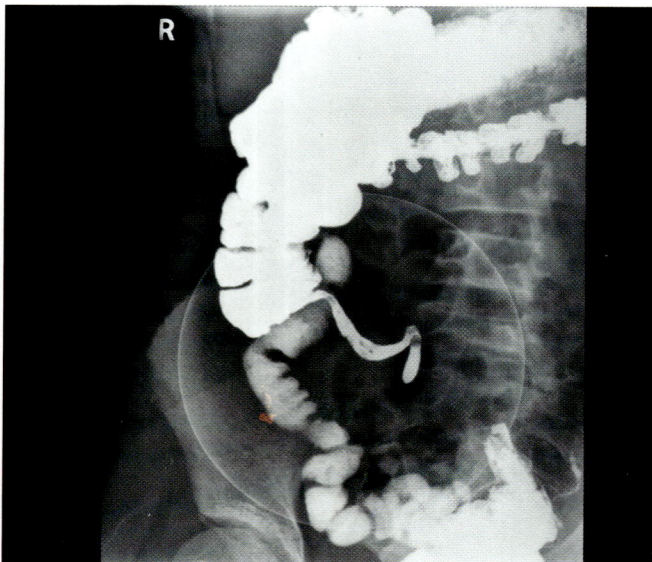

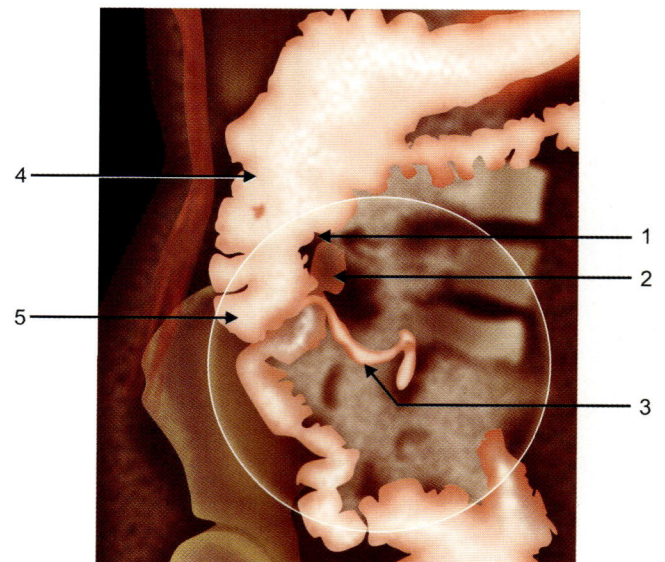

Figure 8.6

1. Ileocecal junction
2. Terminal ileum
3. Appendix
4. Ascending colon
5. Cecum

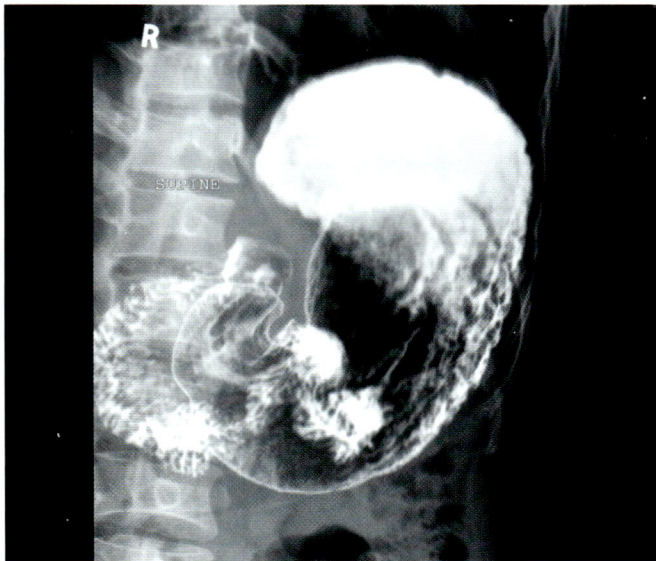

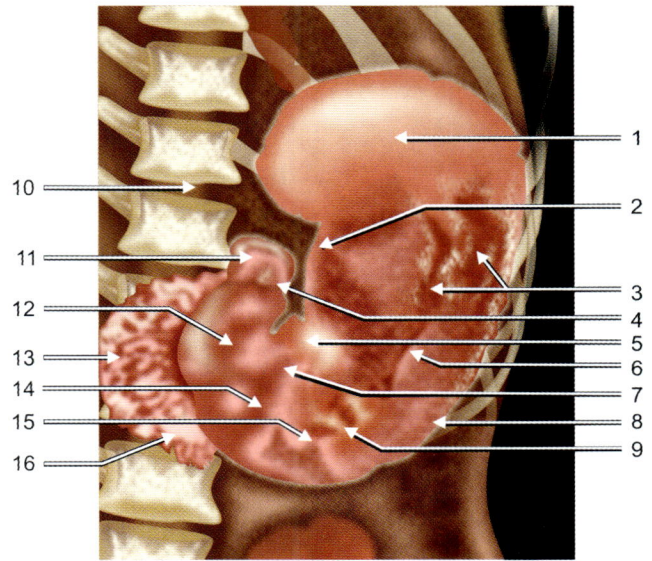

Figure 8.7

1. Fundus	7. Duodenojejunal junction	13. Duodenum, D2
2. Lesser curvature	8. Greater curvature	14. D4
3. Gastric rugae	9. Jejunum	15. Antrum
4. Pyloric canal	10. Disk space	16. Duodenum, D3
5. Incisura angularis, stomach	11. Duodenal cap (D1)	
6. Stomach, body	12. Pyloric antrum	

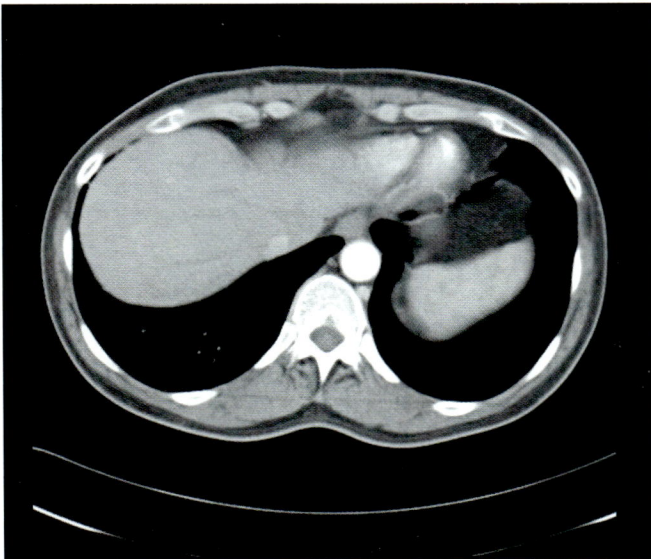

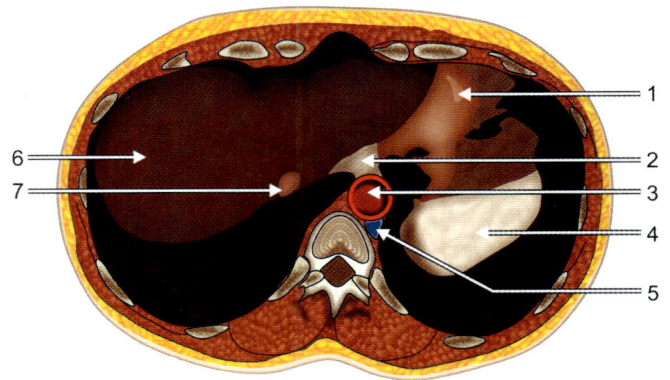

Figure 8.8

1. Heart	5. Azygos vein
2. Esophagus	6. Liver
3. Aorta	7. IVC
4. Spleen	

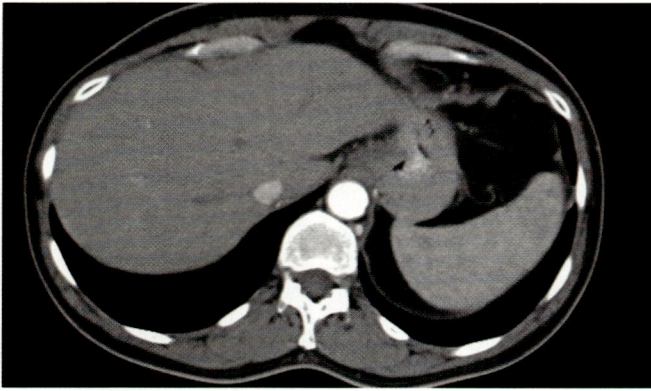

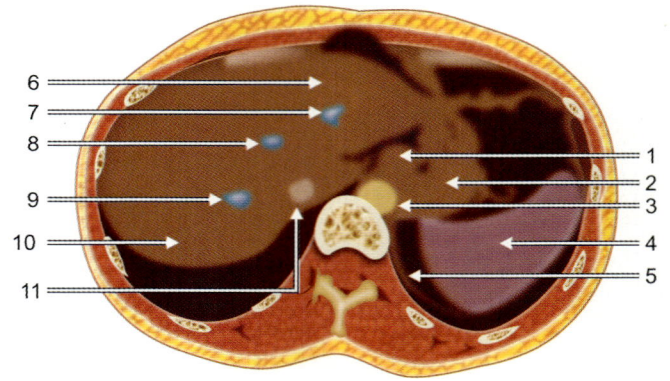

Figure 8.9

1. GE junction	7. Left hepatic vein
2. Stomach	8. Middle hepatic vein
3. Descending aorta	9. Right hepatic vein
4. Spleen	10. Liver
5. Diaphragm	11. IVC
6. Left hepatic lobe	

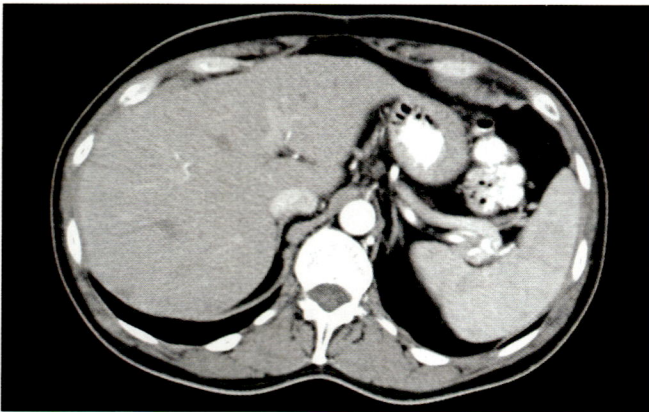

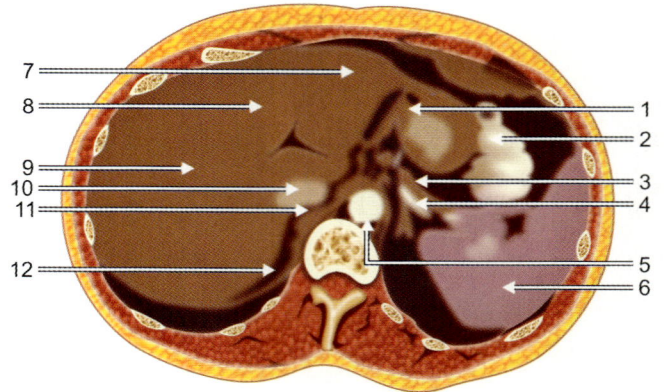

Figure 8.10

1. Stomach	7. Left lobe of liver
2. Splenic flexure of colon	8. Left portal vein
3. Splenic vein	9. Right lobe of liver
4. Splenic artery	10. IVC
5. Aorta	11. Crura of diaphragm
6. Spleen	12. Diaphragm

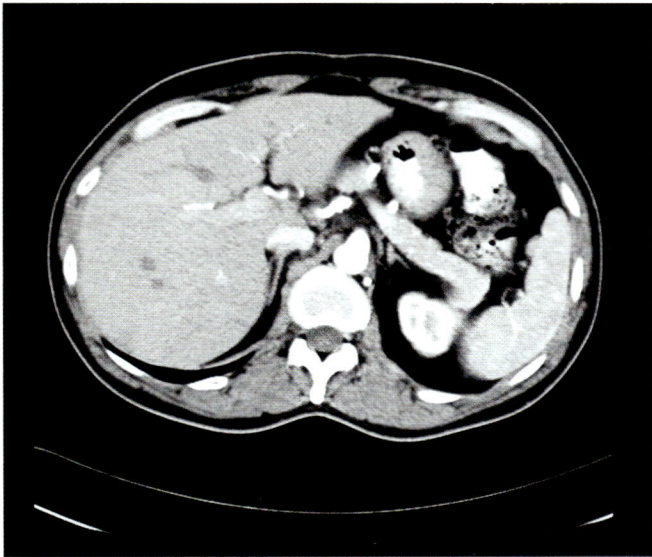

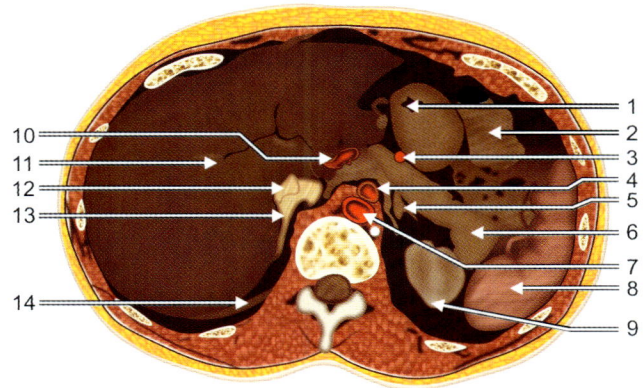

Figure 8.11

1. Stomach	6. Tail of pancreas	11. Right portal vein
2. Splenic flexure	7. Aorta	12. IVC
3. Splenic artery	8. Spleen	13. Right adrenal gland
4. Celiac trunk	9. Left kidney	14. Diaphragm
5. Left adrenal gland	10. Hepatic artery	

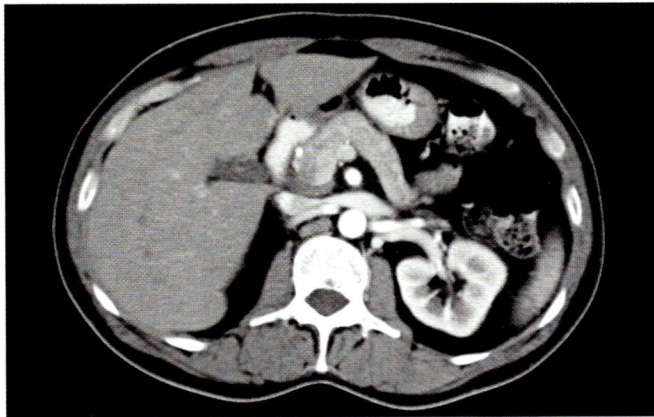

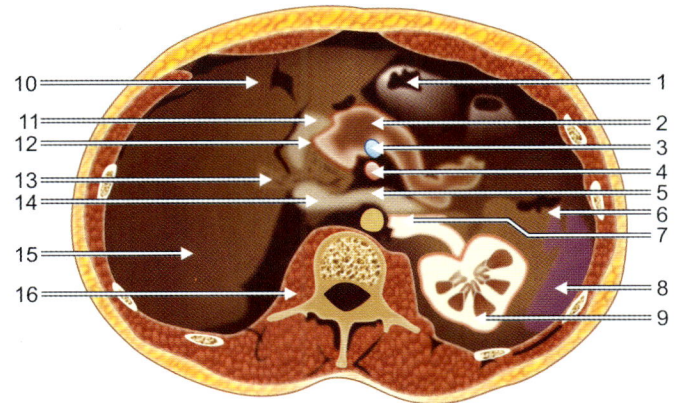

Figure 8.12

1. Stomach	7. Left renal artery	13. Gallbladder neck
2. Body of pancreas	8. Spleen	14. IVC
3. Superior mesenteric vein	9. Left kidney	15. Right lobe of liver
4. Superior mesenteric artery	10. Fissure for ligamentum venosum	16. Psoas
5. Left renal vein	11. Duodenum	
6. Descending colon	12. Gastroduodenal artery	

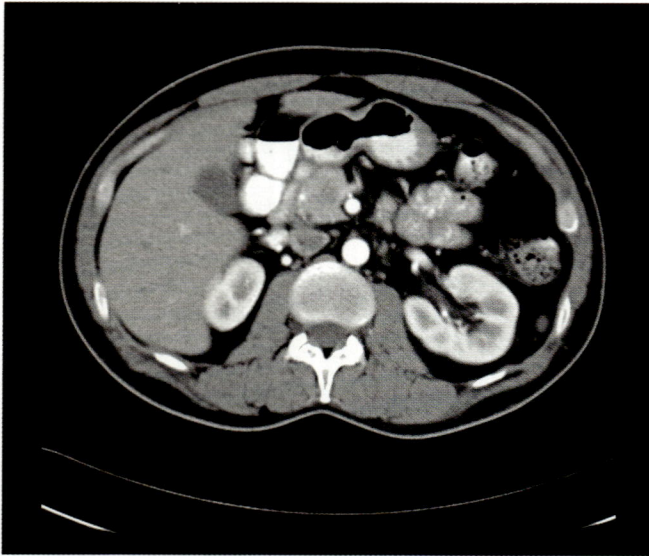

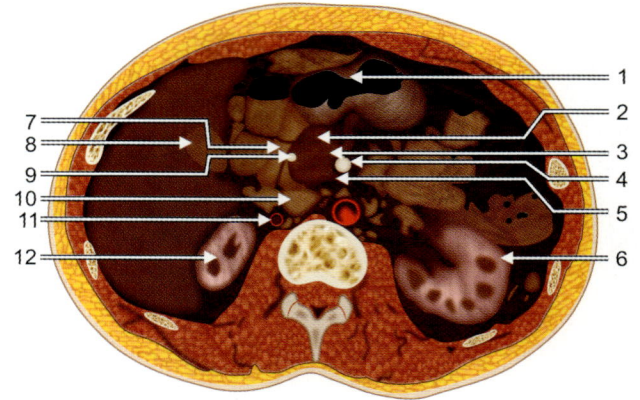

Figure 8.13

1. Stomach	5. Uncinate process, pancreas	9. Gastroduodenal artery
2. Head of pancreas	6. Left kidney	10. IVC
3. SMV	7. Duodenum	11. Right renal artery
4. SMA	8. Gallbladder	12. Right kidney

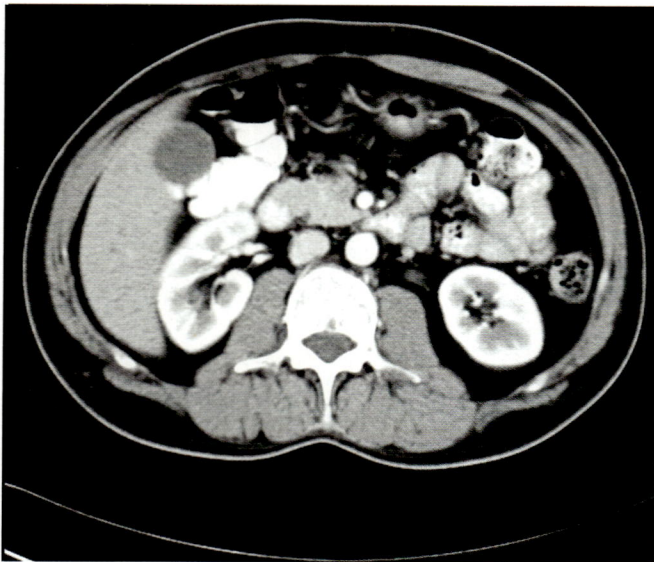

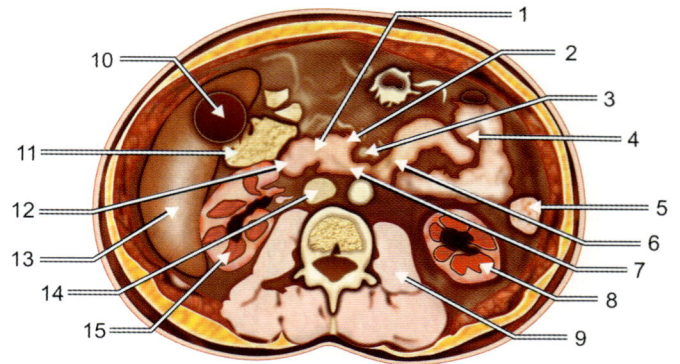

Figure 8.14

1. Head of pancreas	6. Duodenojejunal flexure	11. Hepatic flexure
2. SMV	7. Uncinate process	12. Duodenum
3. SMA	8. Left kidney	13. Liver
4. Jejunal loops	9. Psoas	14. IVC
5. Descending colon	10. Gallbladder	15. Right kidney

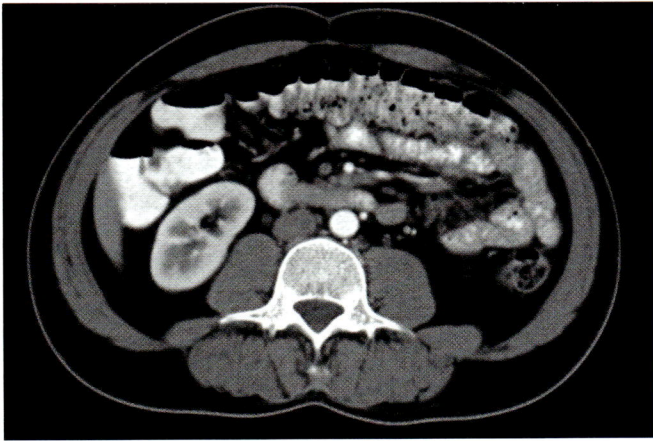

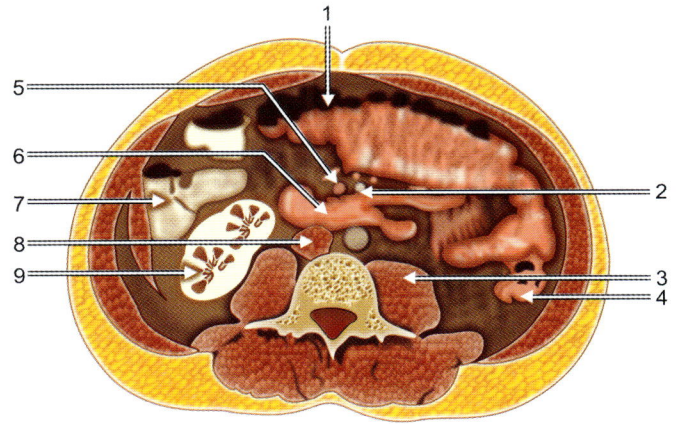

Figure 8.15

1. Transverse colon	6. Duodenum, third part
2. SMA	7. Ascending colon
3. Psoas	8. IVC
4. Descending colon	9. Right kidney
5. SMV	

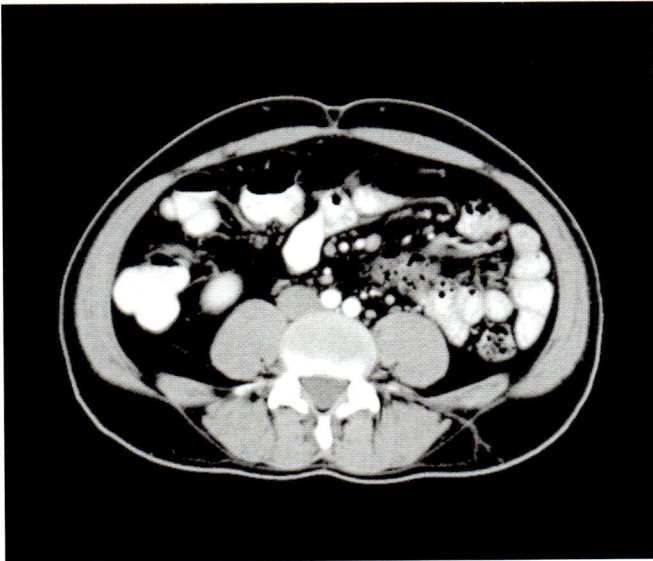

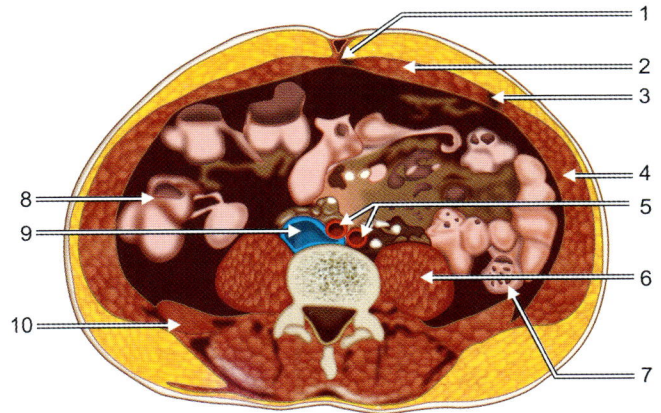

Figure 8.16

1. Linea alba	6. Psoas
2. Rectus abdominis	7. Descending colon
3. Linea semilunaris	8. Ascending colon
4. Oblique muscle	9. IVC
5. RT & LT common iliac arteries	10. Quadratus lumborum

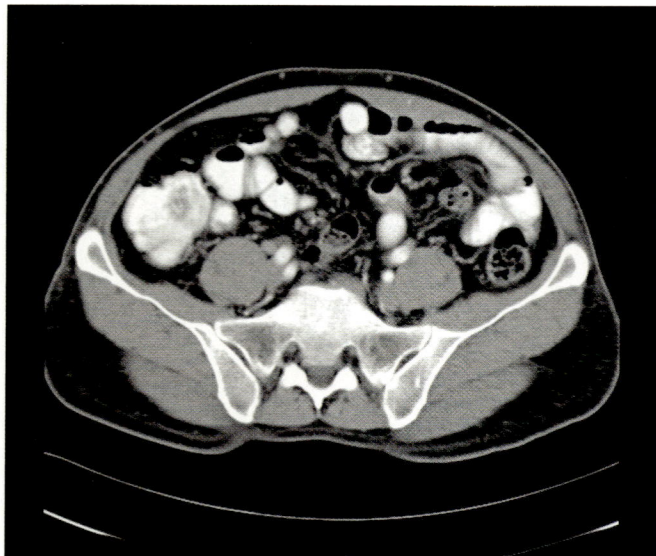
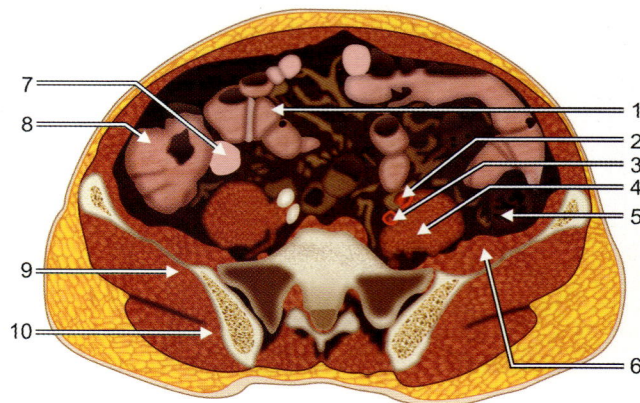

Figure 8.17

1. Iliac loops	6. Iliacus
2. Left external iliac artery	7. Terminal ileum
3. Left internal iliac artery	8. caecum
4. Psoas	9. Gluteus medius
5. Descending colon	10. Gluteus maximus

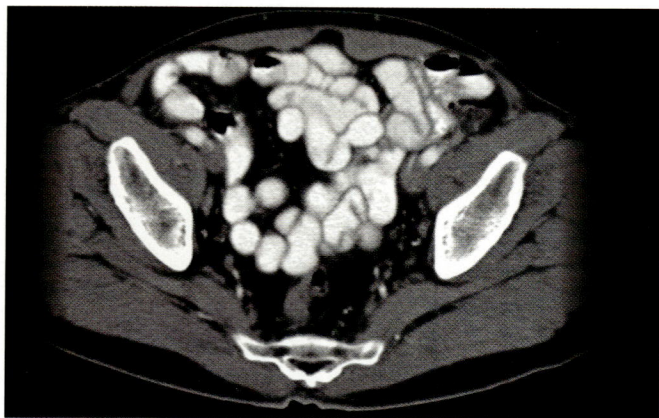
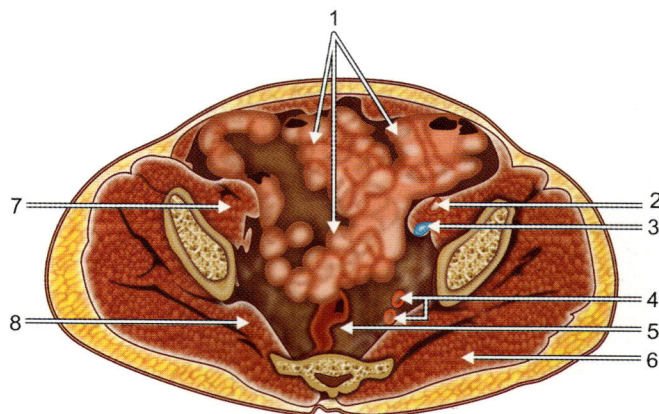

Figure 8.18

1. Ileal loops	5. Rectum
2. External iliac artery	6. Gluteus maximus
3. External iliac vein	7. Iliopsoas
4. Internal iliac branches	8. Piriformis muscle

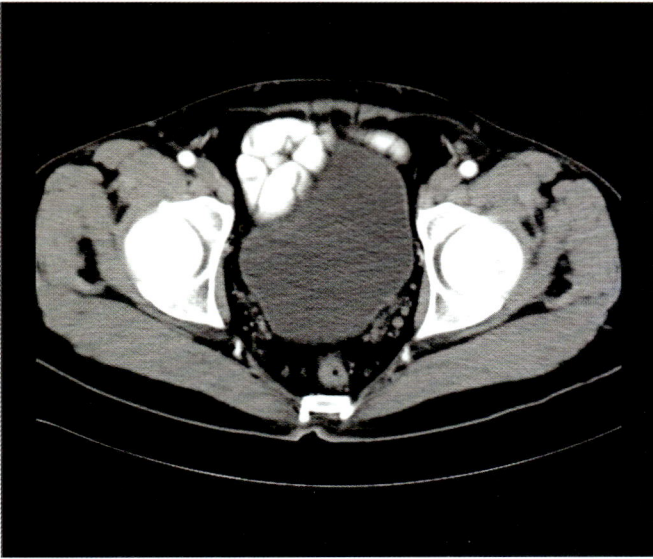

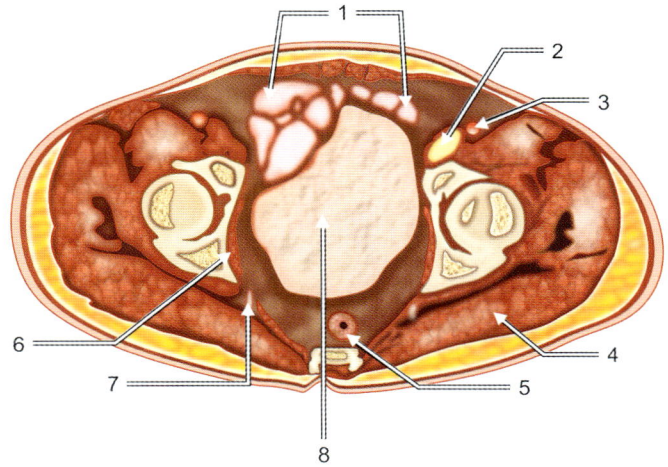

Figure 8.19

1. Iliac loops	5. Rectum
2. Femoral vein	6. Obturator internus
3. Femoral artery	7. Inferior gluteal artery
4. Gluteus maximus	8. Urinary bladder

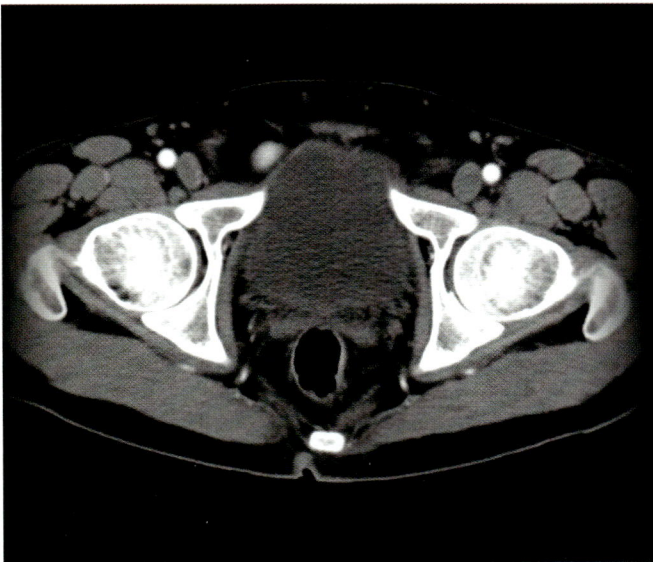

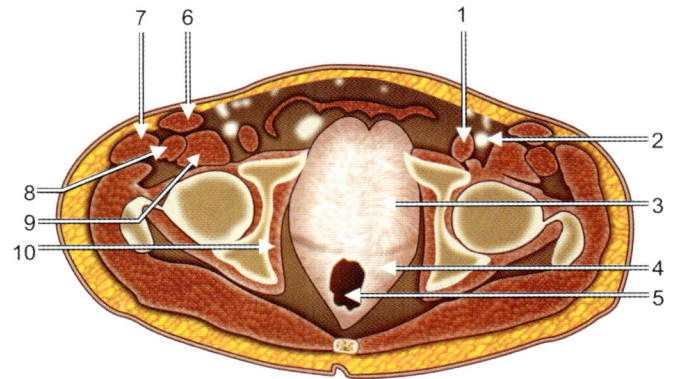

Figure 8.20

1. Femoral vein	5. Rectum	9. Iliopsoas
2. Femoral artery	6. Sartorius	10. Obturator internus
3. Urinary bladder	7. Tensor fascia lata muscle	
4. Seminal vesicle	8. Rectus femoris	

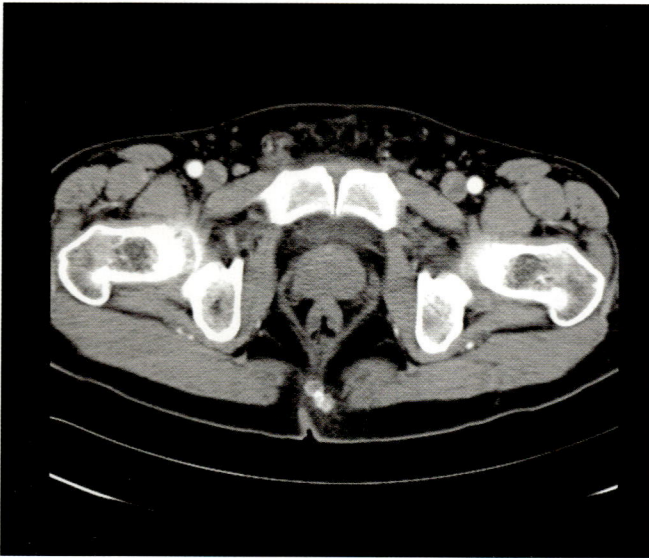

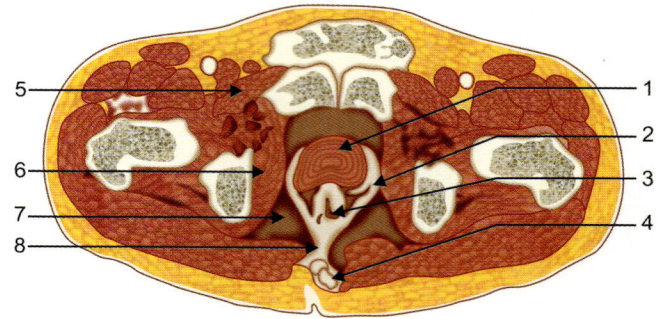

Figure 8.21

1. Prostate gland	5. Pectineus muscle
2. Levator ani muscle	6. Obturator internus
3. Anal canal	7. Ischiorectal fossa
4. Coccyx	8. Coccygeus

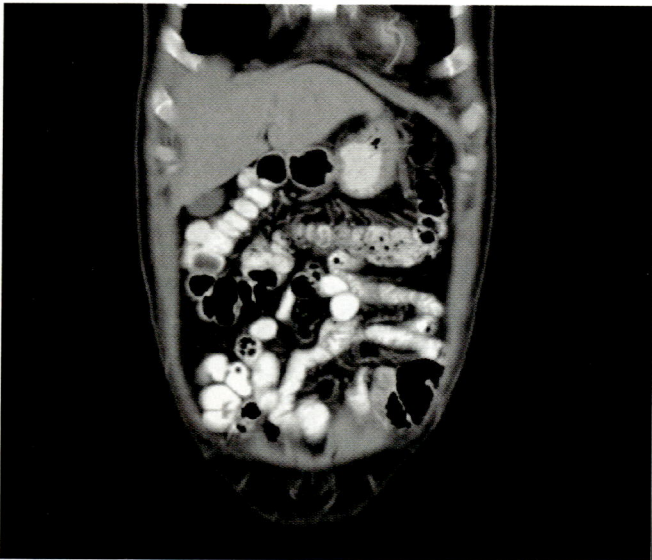

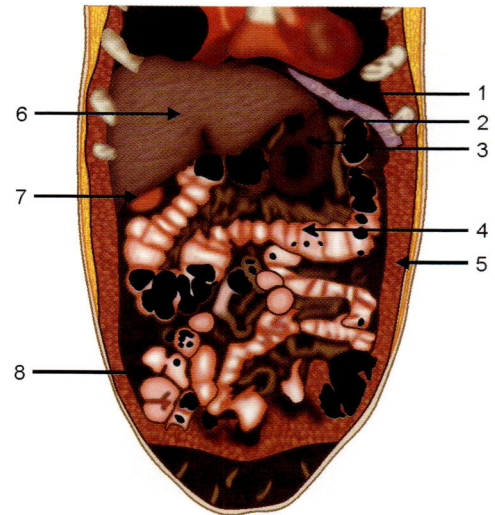

Figure 8.22

1. Diaphragm	5. Abdominal wall
2. Splenic flexure	6. Liver
3. Stomach	7. Gallbladder
4. Transverse colon	8. Ileal loops

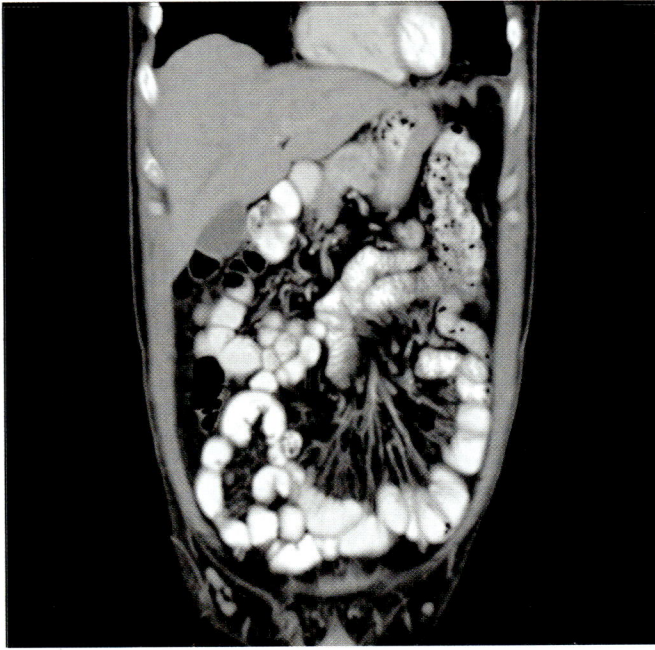

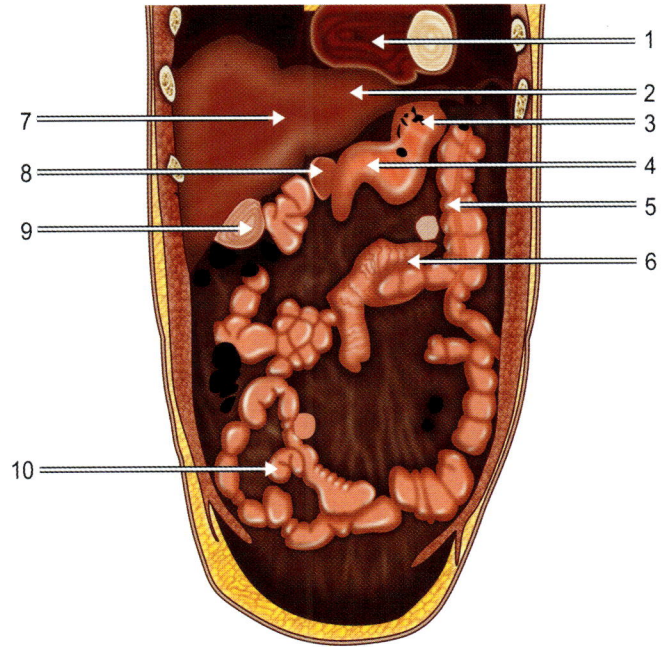

Figure 8.23

1. Heart	5. Transverse colon	9. Gallbladder
2. Liver, left lobe	6. Jejunal loops	10. Ileal loops
3. Stomach	7. Liver, right lobe	
4. Pancreas, body	8. Duodenum	

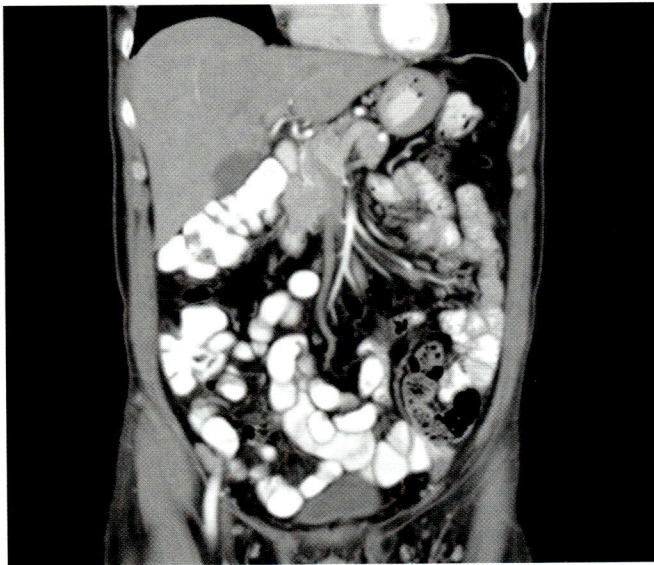

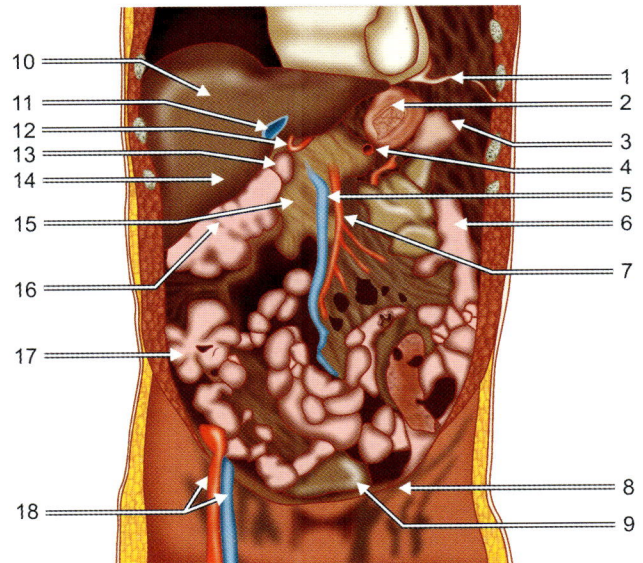

Figure 8.24

1. Diaphragm	7. SMA	13. Duodenum
2. Stomach	8. Inguinal ligament	14. Gallbladder
3. Splenic flexure	9. Urinary bladder	15. Pancreas, head
4. Splenic artery	10. Liver	16. Hepatic flexure
5. SMV	11. Portal vein	17. Caecum
6. Jejunal loops	12. Hepatic artery	18. Femoral vessels

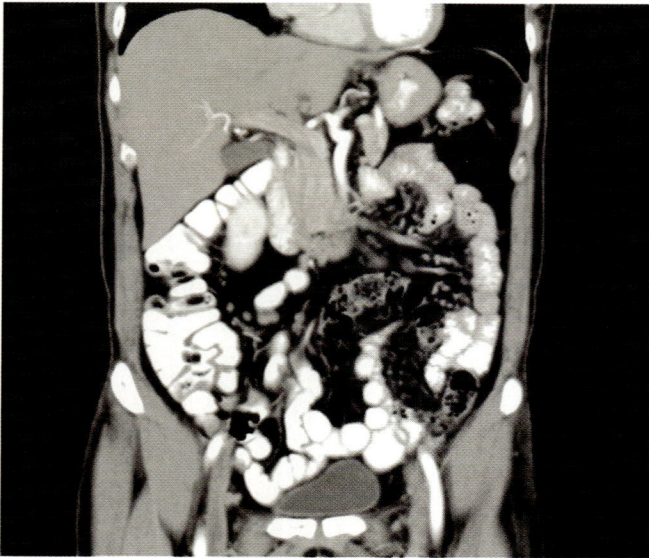

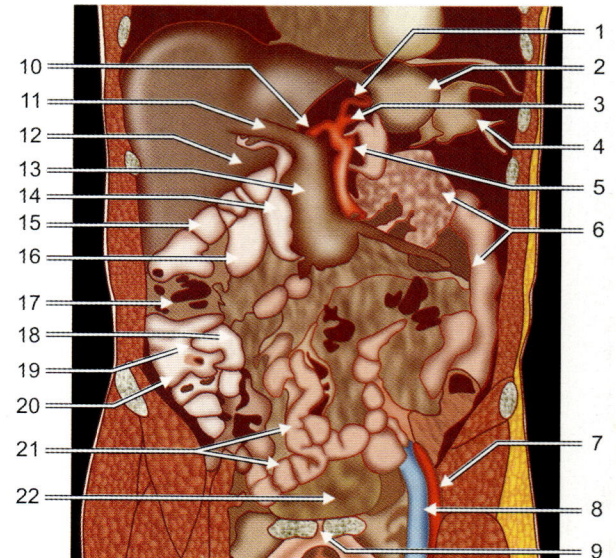

Figure 8.25

1. Left gastric artery	7. Femoral artery	13. Pancreas	19. Ileocecal valve
2. Stomach, fundus	8. Femoral vein	14. Duodenum	20. Caecum
3. Splenic artery	9. Pubic symphysis	15. Hepatic flexure	21. Ileal loops
4. Splenic flexure	10. Hepatic artery	16. Right kidney	22. Urinary bladder
5. Coeliac artery	11. Portal vein	17. Ascending colon	
6. Jejunal loops	12. Gallbladder	18. Terminal ileum	

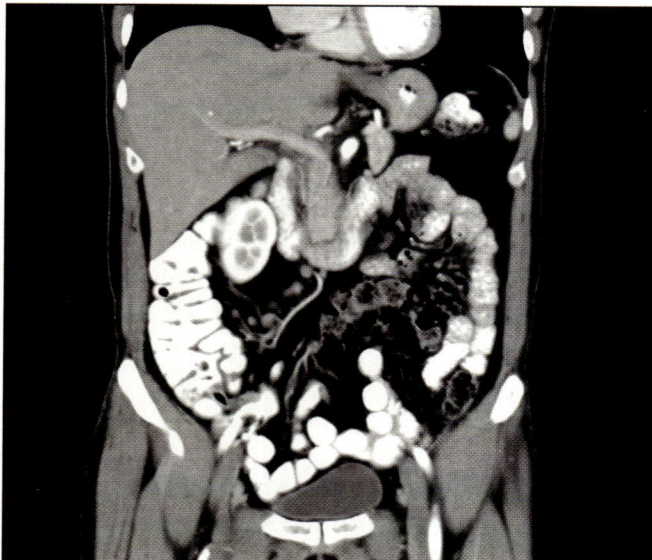

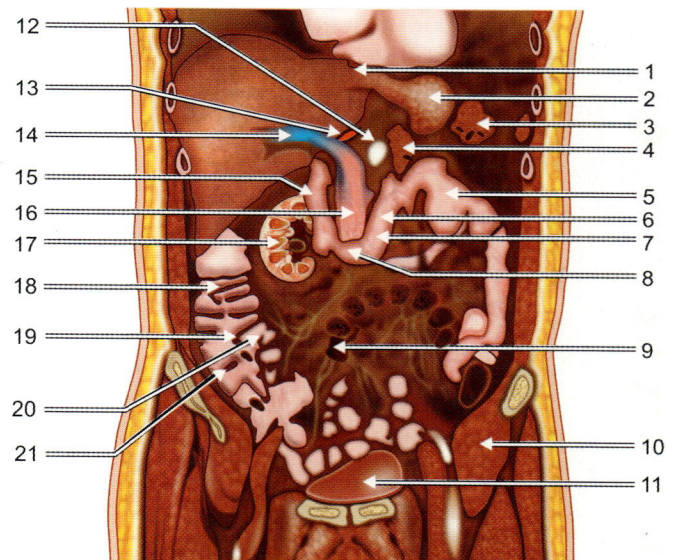

Figure 8.26

1. Gastroesophageal junction	6. Duodeno-jejunal flexure	12. Celiac	18. Ascending colon
2. Stomach	7. Duodenum, D4	13. Hepatic artery	19. IC valve
3. Splenic flexure	8. Duodenum, D3	14. Portal vein	20. Terminal ileum
4. Pancreas, body	9. Iliocolic artery	15. Duodenum, D2	21. Caecum
5. Jejunal loops	10. Iliopsoas	16. Pancreas, head	
	11. Urinary bladder	17. Right kidney	

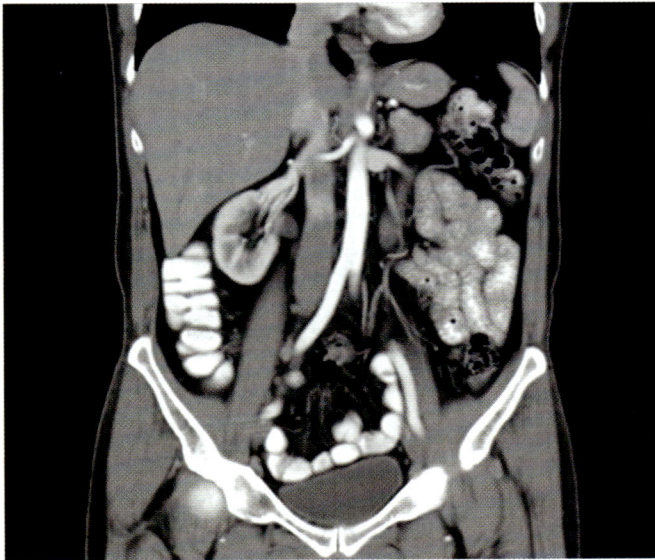

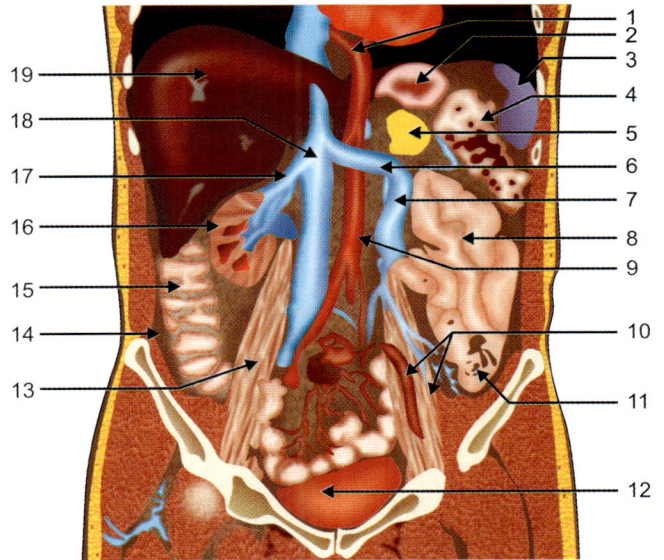

Figure 8.27

1. Esophagus	6. Left renal vein	11. Descending colon	16. Right kidney
2. Stomach	7. Inferior mesenteric vein	12. Urinary bladder	17. Right renal vein
3. Spleen	8. Jejunal loops	13. Psoas	18. IVC
4. Splenic flexure	9. Aorta	14. Paracolic gutter	19. Liver
5. Pancreas	10. External iliac vessels	15. Ascending colon	

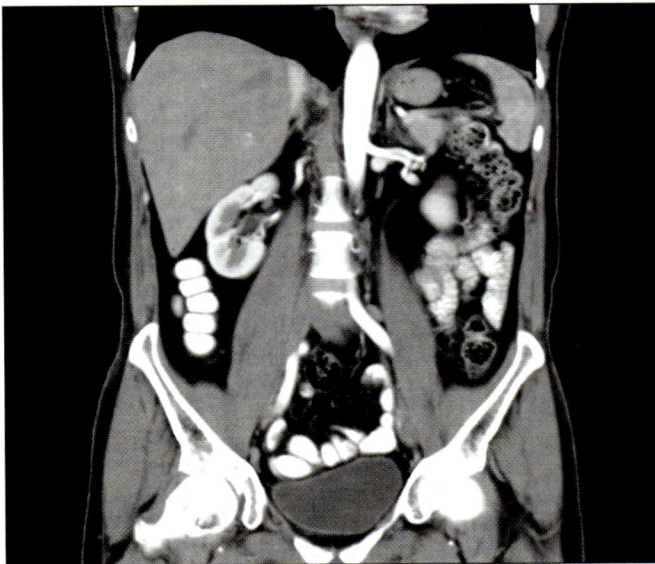

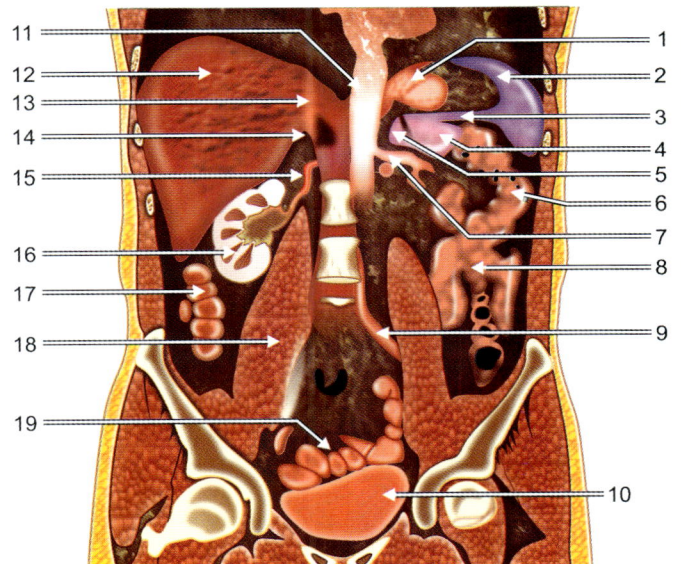

Figure 8.28

1. Stomach	6. Descending colon	10. Urinary bladder	15. Right renal artery
2. Spleen	7. Left renal artery	11. Aorta	16. Right kidney
3. Splenic vein	8. Jejunal loops	12. Liver	17. Ascending colon
4. Pancreas, tail	9. Left common iliac artery	13. IVC	18. Psoas
5. Left adrenal gland		14. Right adrenal gland	19. Ileal loops

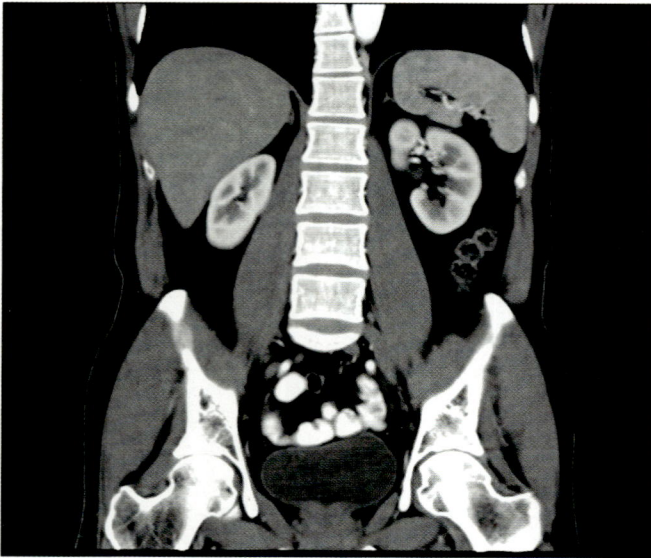

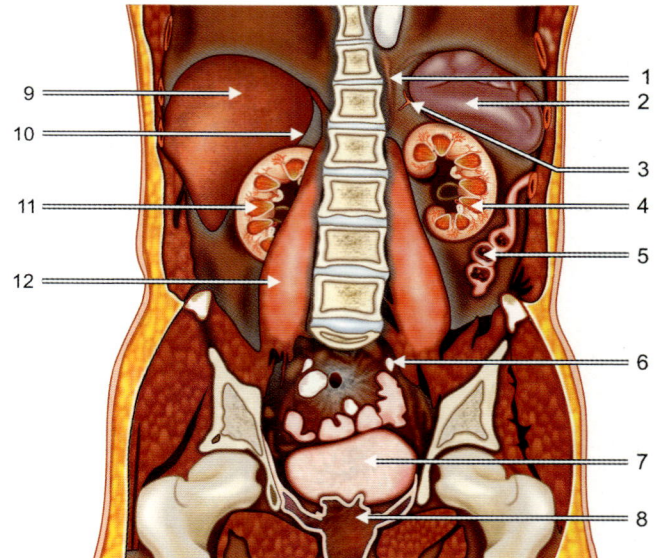

Figure 8.29

1. Crus, diaphragm	5. Descending colon	9. Liver
2. Spleen	6. Internal iliac artery	10. Right adrenal gland
3. Left adrenal gland	7. Urinary bladder	11. Right kidney
4. Left kidney	8. Prostate	12. Psoas

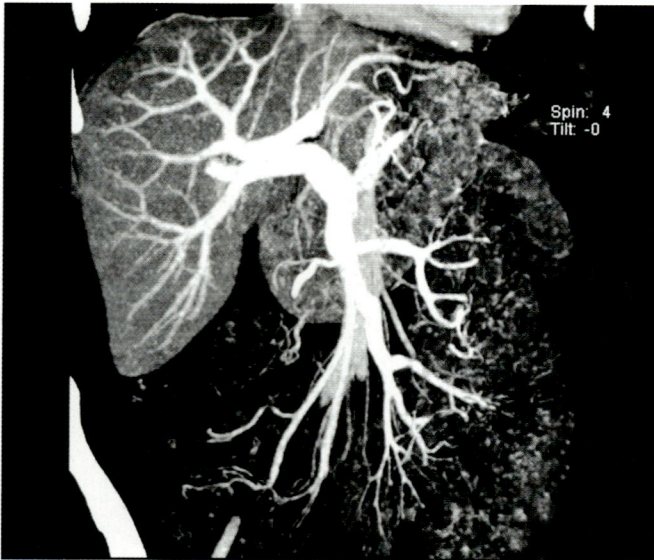

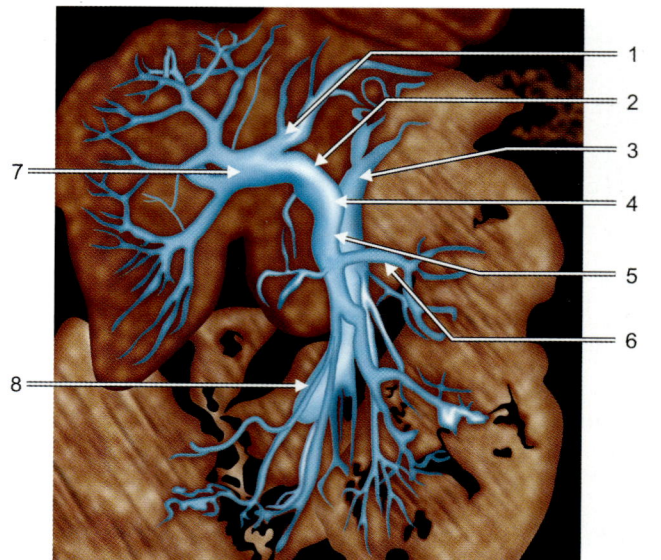

Figure 8.30

1. Left portal vein	5. Superior mesenteric vein
2. Portal vein	6. Jejunal vein
3. Splenic vein	7. Right portal vein
4. Portal confluence	8. Ileocolic veins

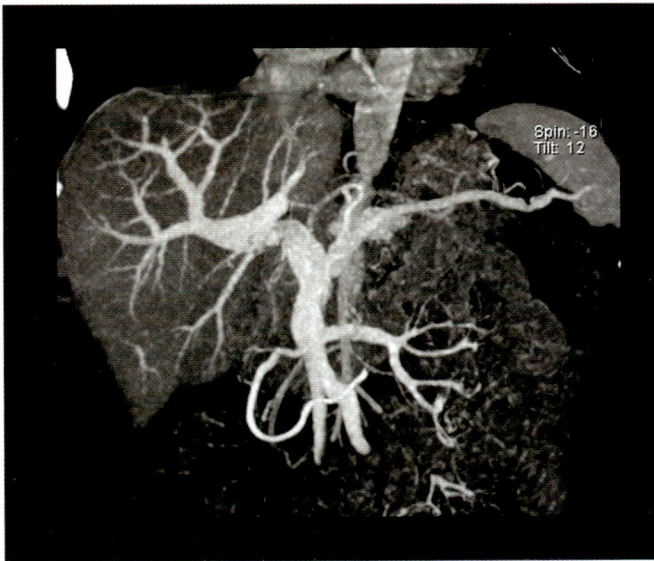

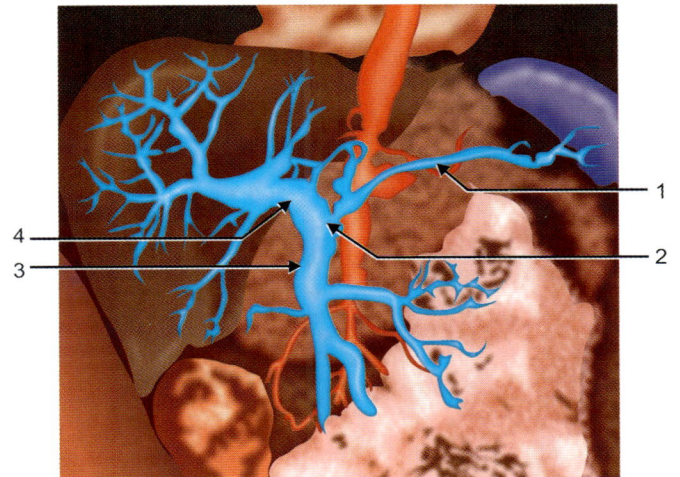

Figure 8.31

1. Splenic vein
2. Portal confluence
3. Portal vein
4. Superior mesenteric vein

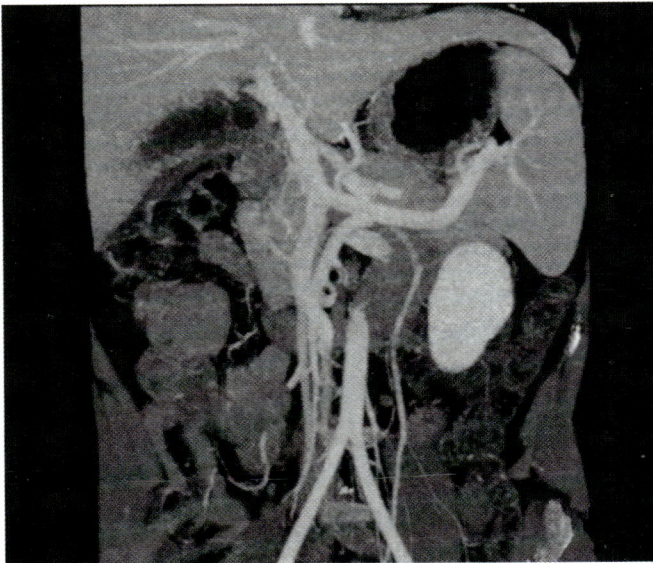

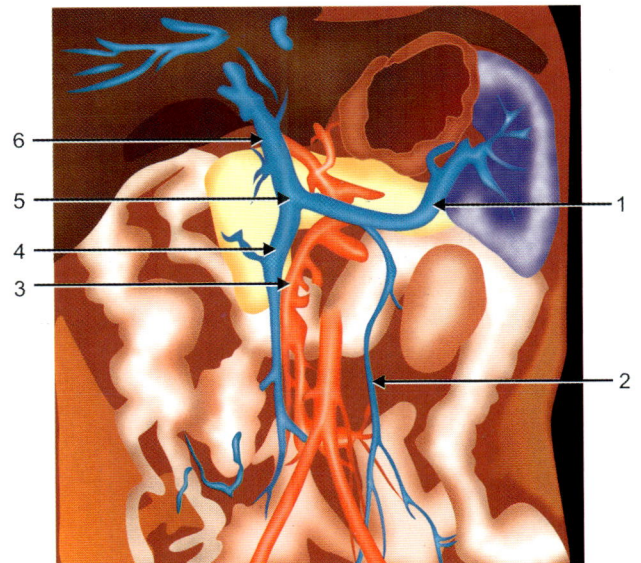

Figure 8.32

1. Splenic vein
2. Inferior mesenteric vein
3. Portal vein
4. Portal confluence
5. Superior mesenteric vein
6. Superior mesenteric artery

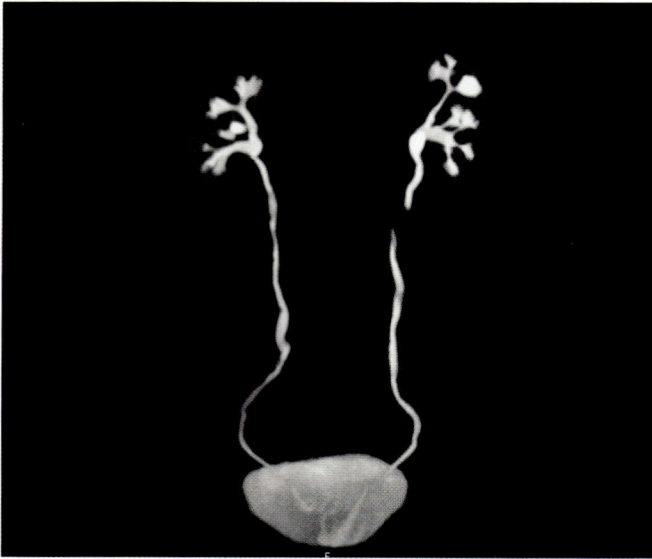

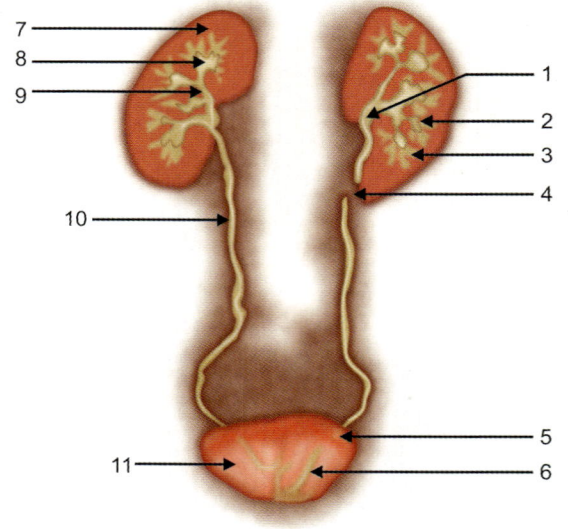

TRUNK

Figure 8.33

1. Renal pelvis	5. UV junction	9. Major calyx
2. Papilla	6. Ureteric jet	10. Ureter
3. Pyramid	7. Renal cortex	11. Urinary bladder
4. Vascular impression	8. Minor calyx	

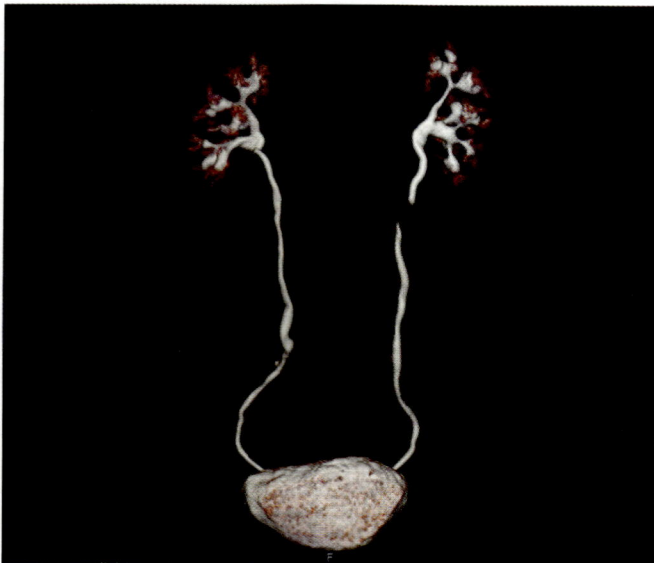

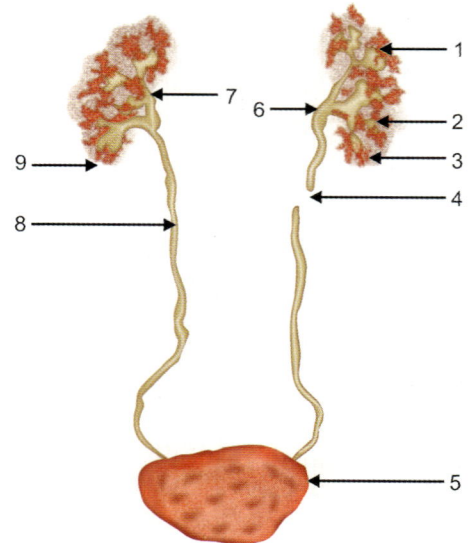

Figure 8.34

1. Papilla	4. Vascular impression	7. Major calyx
2. Minor calyx	5. Urinary bladder	8. Renal cortex
3. Medullary pyramid	6. Pelvis	9. Ureter

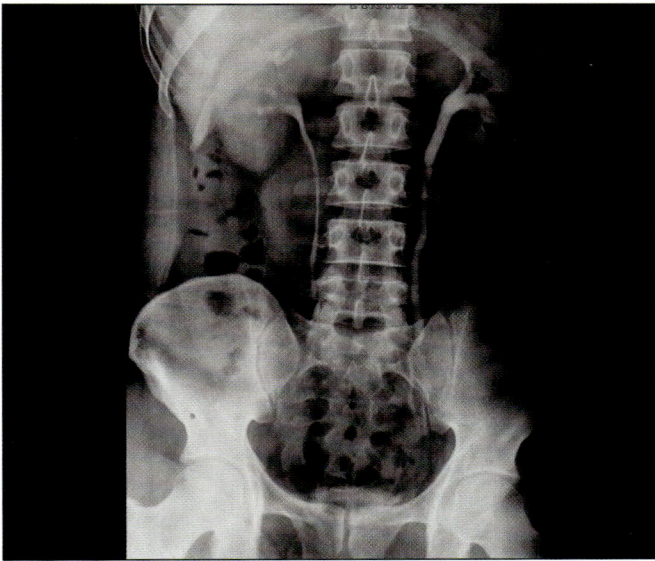

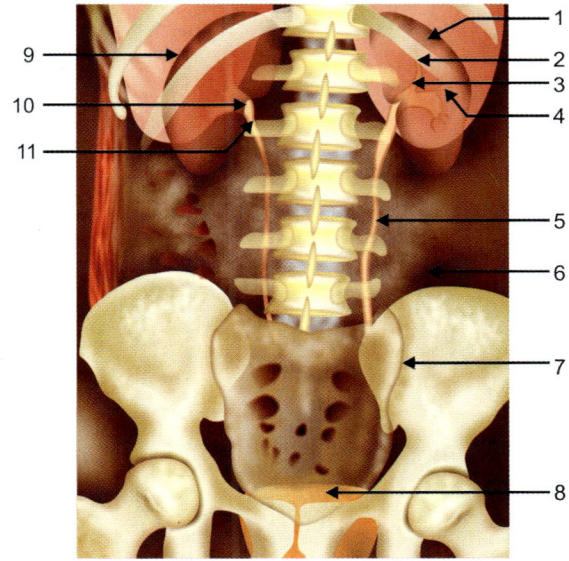

Figure 8.35

Intravenous Urogram (IVU)
1. Left kidney
2. Minor calyx
3. Major calyx
4. Papilla
5. Ureter
6. Psoas shadow
7. Sacroiliac joint
8. Bladder
9. Right kidney
10. Pelvis
11. Pelviureteric junction

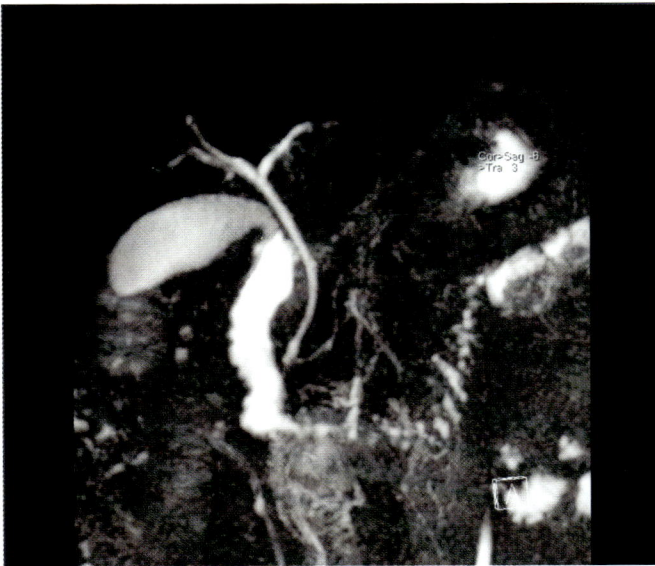

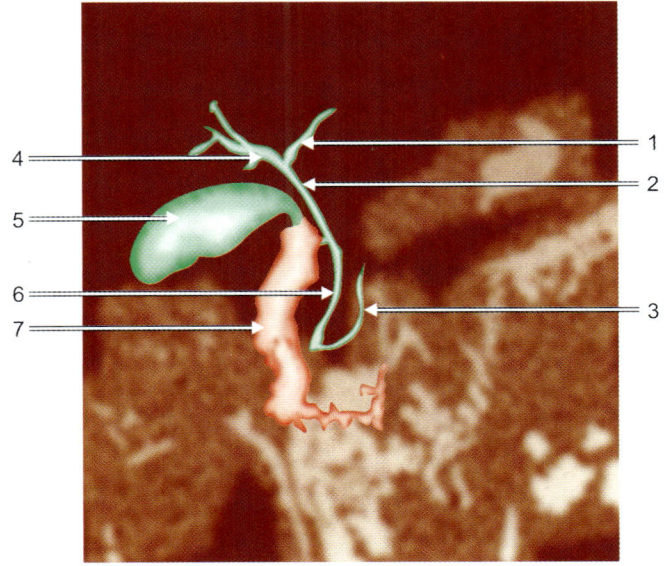

Figure 8.36

MRCP
1. Left hepatic duct
2. Common hepatic duct
3. Pancreatic duct
4. Right hepatic duct
5. Gallbladder
6. Common bile duct
7. Duodenum

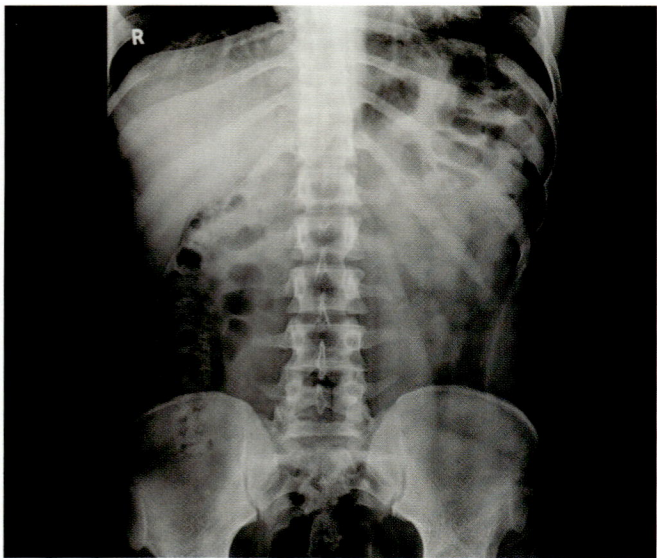

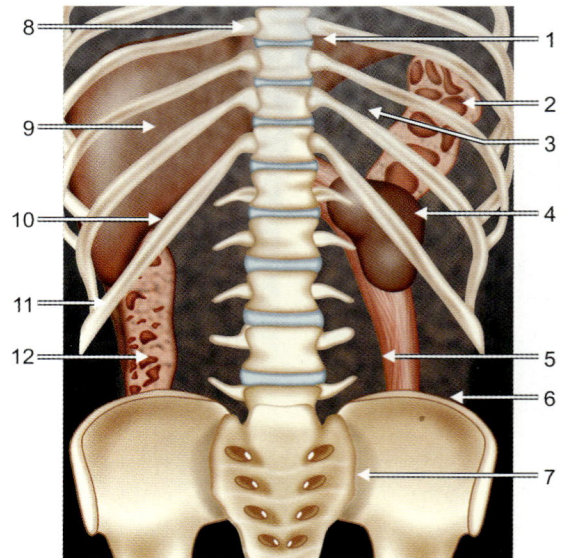

Figure 8.37

1. Descending aorta	7. Left sacroiliac joint
2. Splenic flexure	8. IVC
3. Fundic bubble	9. Liver
4. Left kidney	10. Hepatic flexure
5. Left psoas muscle	11. Fat stripe
6. Iliac crest	12. Ascending colon

CHAPTER 9

Pelvis

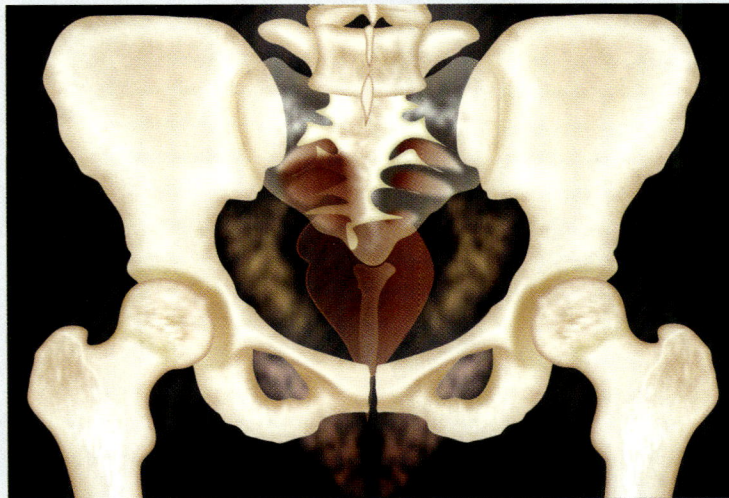

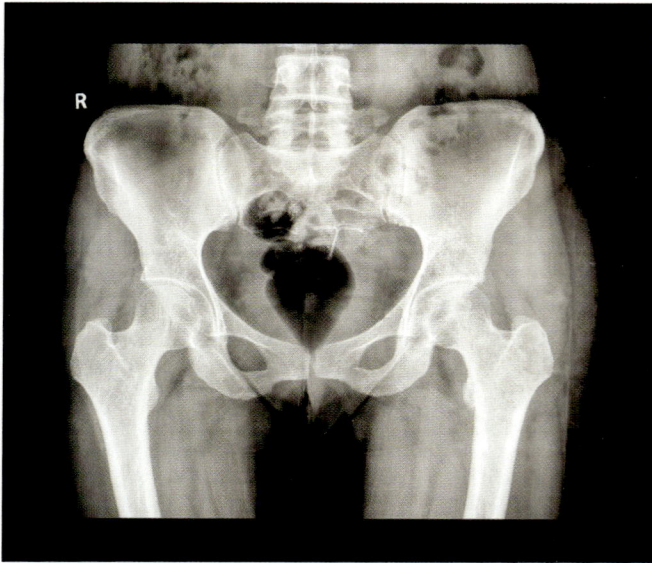

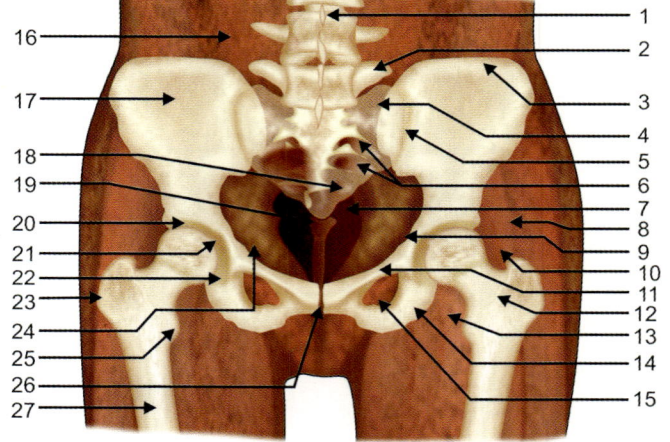

Figure 9.1

1. Spinous process	10. Supracapsular fat plane	19. Coccyx
2. L5 transverse process	11. Superior pubic ramus	20. Superior compartment of hip joint
3. Iliac crest	12. Intertrochanteric line	21. Axial compartment of hip joint
4. Sacral ala	13. Psoas fat plane	22. Medial compartment of hip joint
5. Sacroiliac joint	14. Ischial tuberosity	23. Greater trochanter
6. Sacral foramina	15. Obturator foramen	24. Obturator internus fat plane
7. Rectal gas shadow	16. Psoas	25. Lesser trochanter
8. Gluteus medius fat plane	17. Iliac bone	26. Pubic symphysis
9. Ischial spine	18. Copper-T	27. Femur

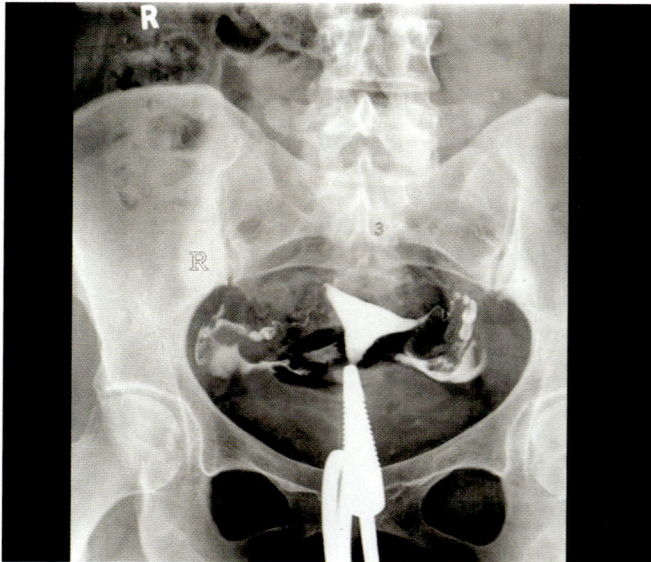

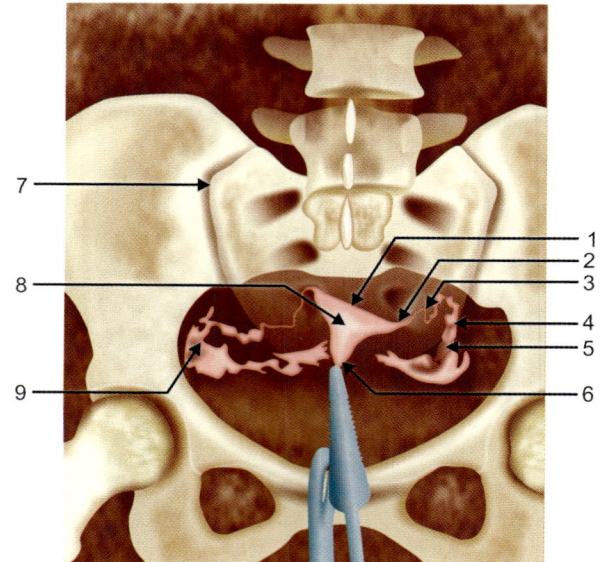

Figure 9.2

1. Fundus of uterus	4. Ampullary part	7. Sacroiliac joint
2. Cornu of uterus	5. Infundibulum	8. Body of uterus
3. Isthmus of fallopian tube	6. Cervix	9. Free spill of contrast in the pelvis

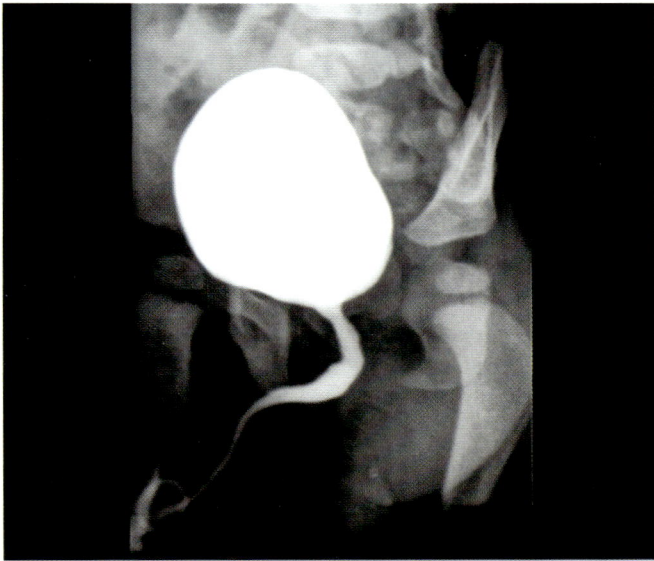

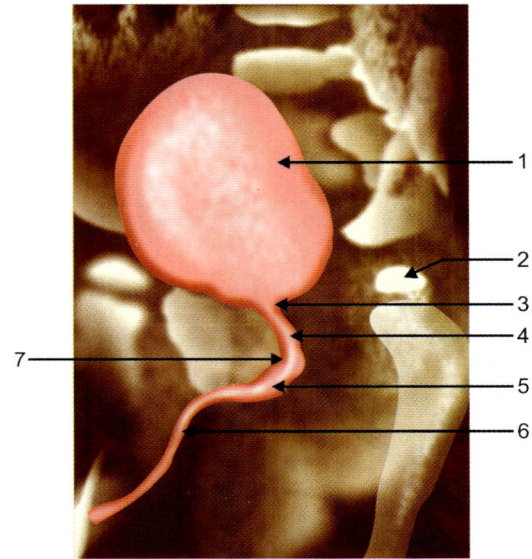

Figure 9.3

1. Urinary bladder	5. Bulbous urethra
2. Femur head	6. Penile (anterior) urethra
3. Bladder neck	7. Membranous urethra
4. Prostatic urethra	

FEMALE PELVIS

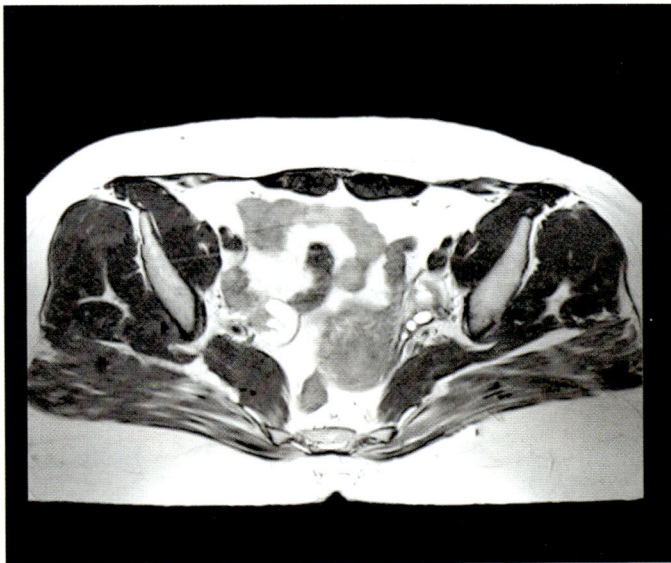

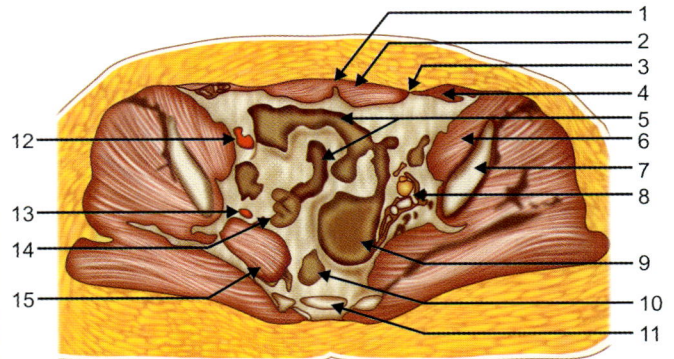

Figure 9.4

1. Linea alba	6. Iliopsoas muscle	11. Sacrum
2. Rectus abdominis muscle	7. Hip bone	12. External iliac vessels
3. Linea semilunaris	8. Left ovary	13. Internal iliac branches
4. Oblique muscles	9. Uterine fundus	14. Right ovary with follicles
5. Bowel loops	10. Rectosigmoid	15. Piriformis

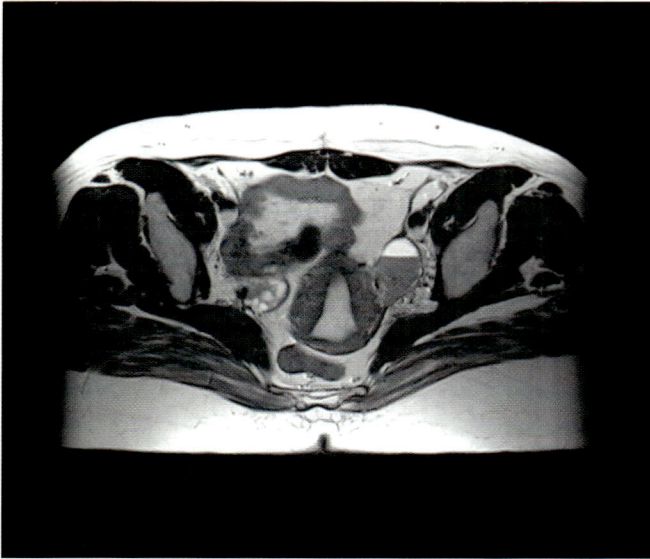

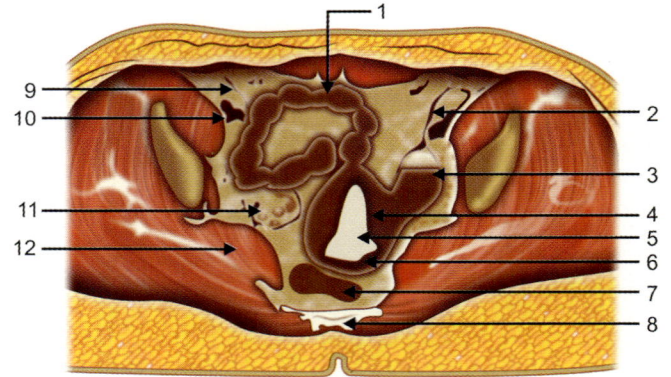

Figure 9.5

1. Bowel loops	7. Rectum
2. Round ligament	8. Sacrum
3. Left ovarian cyst with fluid level	9. Right round ligament
4. Junctional zone	10. External iliac vessels
5. Uterine cavity	11. Right ovary
6. Uterine fundus	12. Piriformis

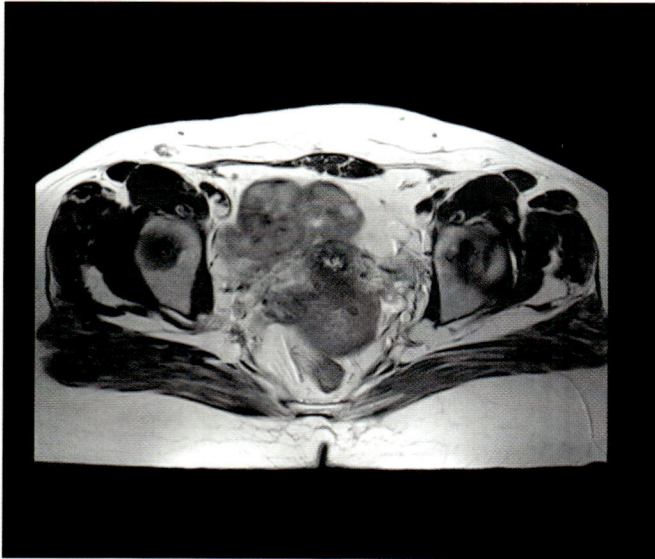

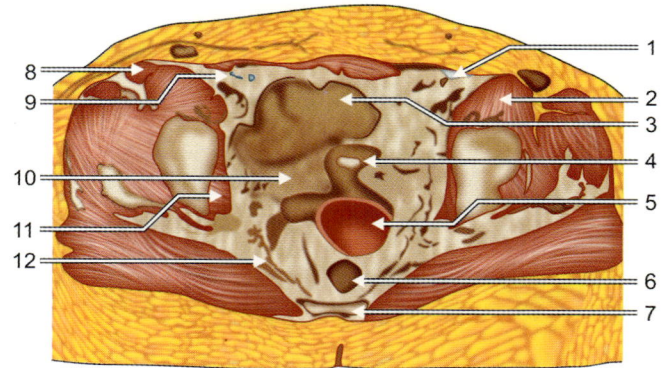

Figure 9.6

1. Round ligament	7. Sacrum
2. Iliopsoas	8. Sartorius
3. Bowel loops	9. Round ligament
4. Cervix	10. Parametrium
5. Uterus	11. Obturator internus
6. Rectum	12. Uterosacral ligament

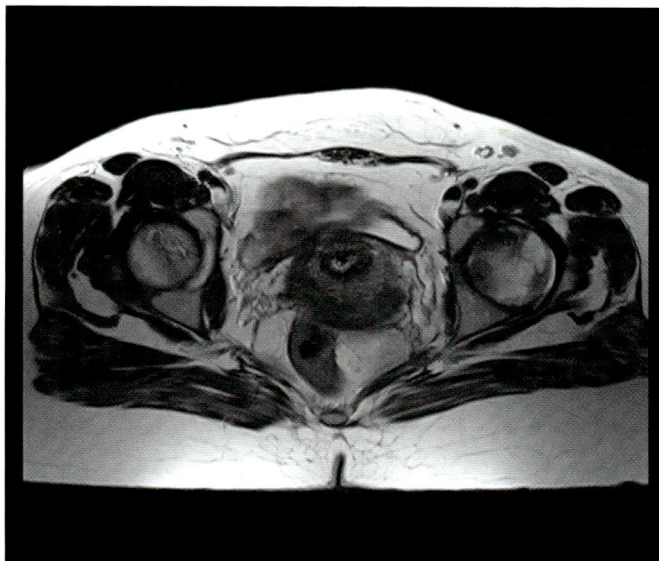

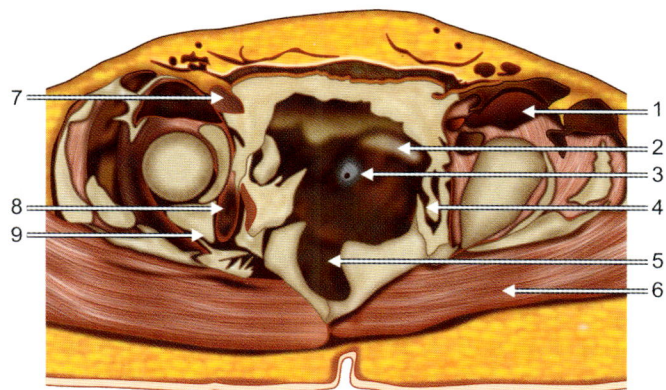

Figure 9.7

1. Iliopsoas	6. Gluteus maximus
2. Urinary bladder	7. External iliac vessels
3. Cervical canal	8. Obturator internus
4. Venous plexus	9. Ischium
5. Rectum	

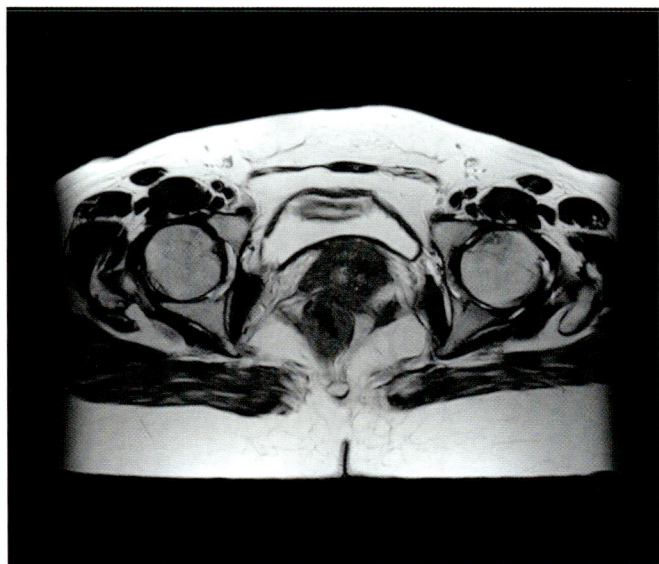

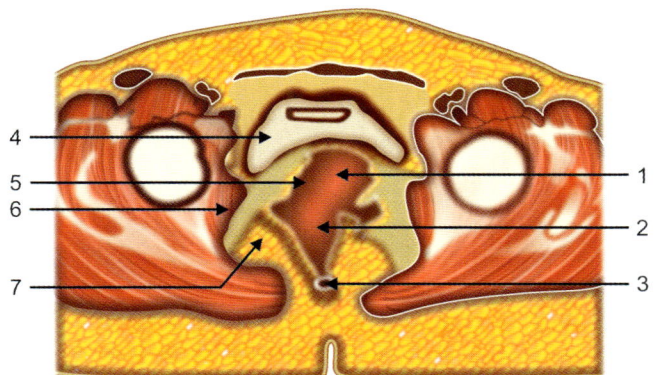

Figure 9.8

1. External OS, cervix	5. Vaginal fornix
2. Rectum	6. Obturator internus
3. Coccyx	7. Levator ani muscle
4. Urinary bladder	

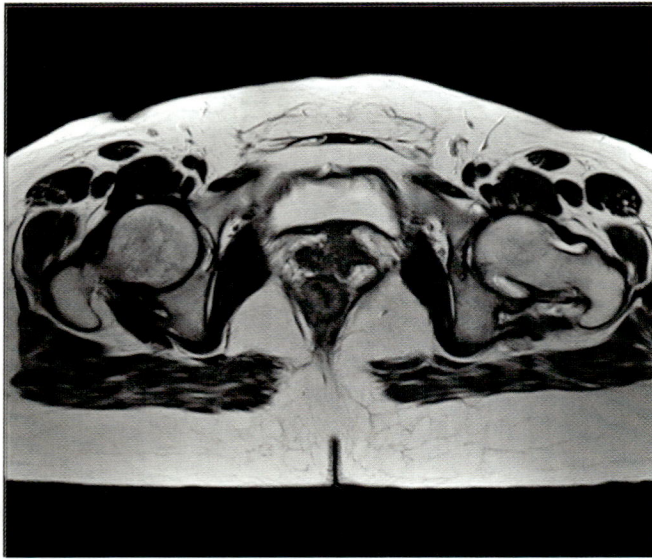

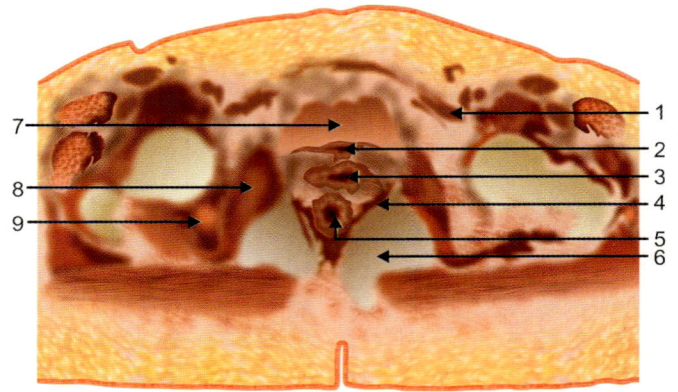

Figure 9.9

1. Pectineus muscle	6. Ischioanal fossa
2. Urethra	7. Urinary bladder
3. Vagina, fornix	8. Obturator internus
4. Levator ani muscle	9. Ischium
5. Anal canal	

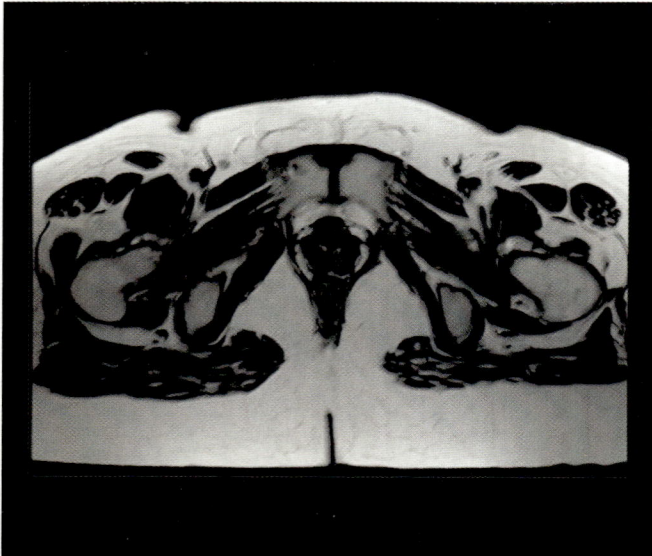

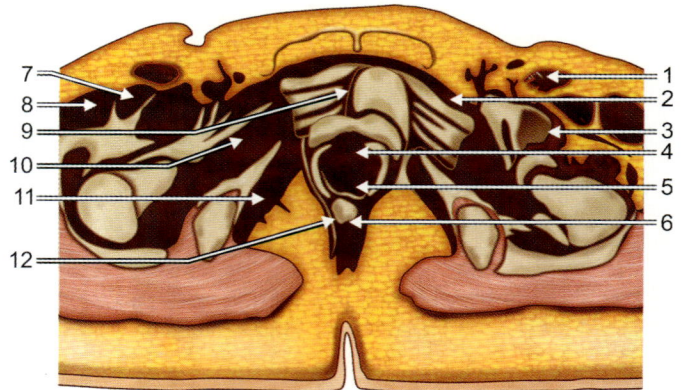

Figure 9.10

1. Sartorius	7. Rectus femoris muscle
2. Pectineus muscle	8. Tensor fascia lata muscle
3. Iliopsoas	9. Pubic symphysis
4. Urethra	10. Obturator externus
5. Vagina	11. Obturator internus
6. Anal canal	12. Levator ani

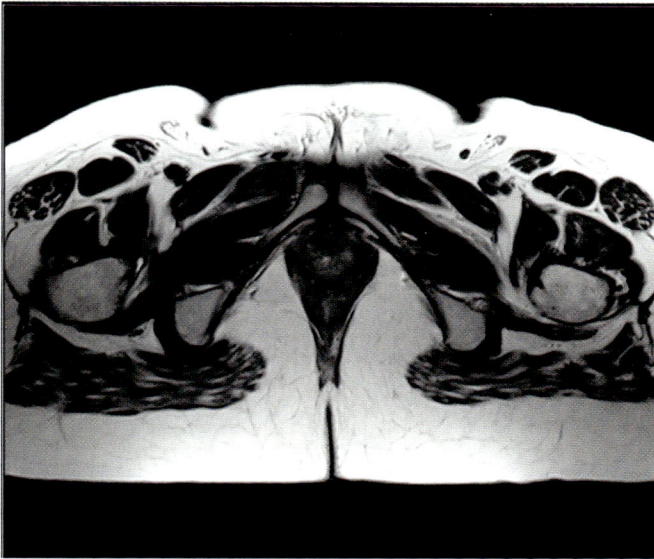

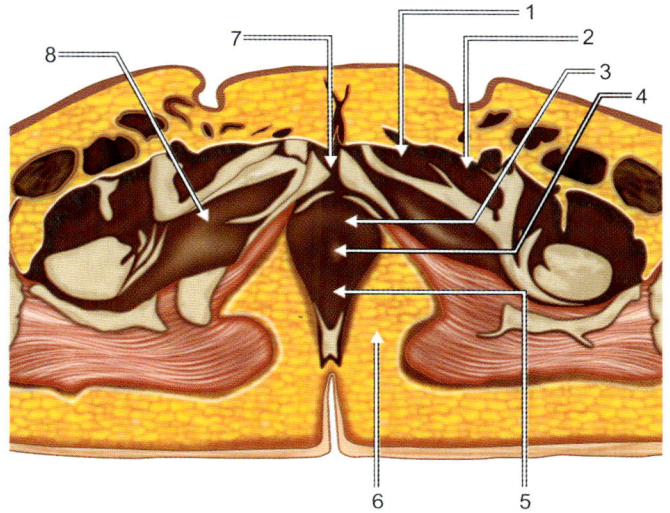

Figure 9.11

1. Adductor brevis	5. Anus
2. Pectineus	6. Ischioanal fossa
3. Urethra	7. Pubic symphysis
4. Vagina	8. Obturator externus

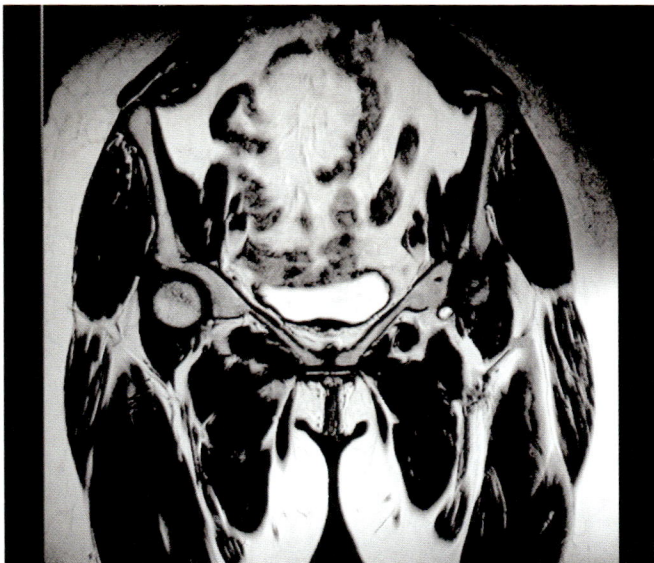

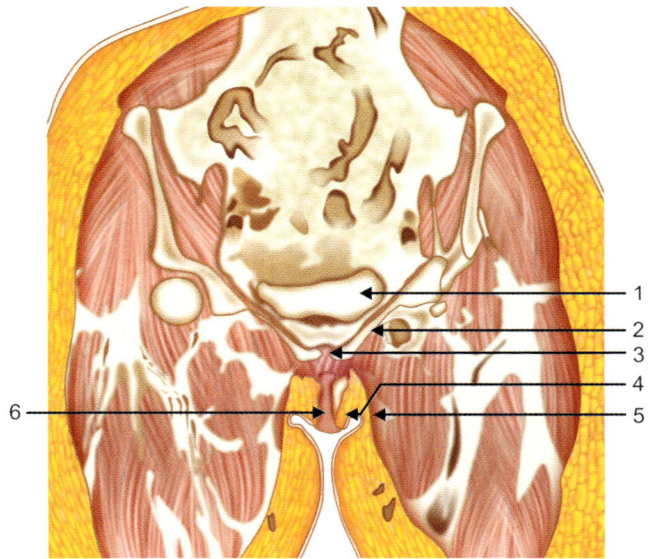

Figure 9.12

1. Urinary bladder	4. Labium majora
2. Superior pubic ramus	5. Gracilis muscle
3. Pubic symphysis	6. Clitoris

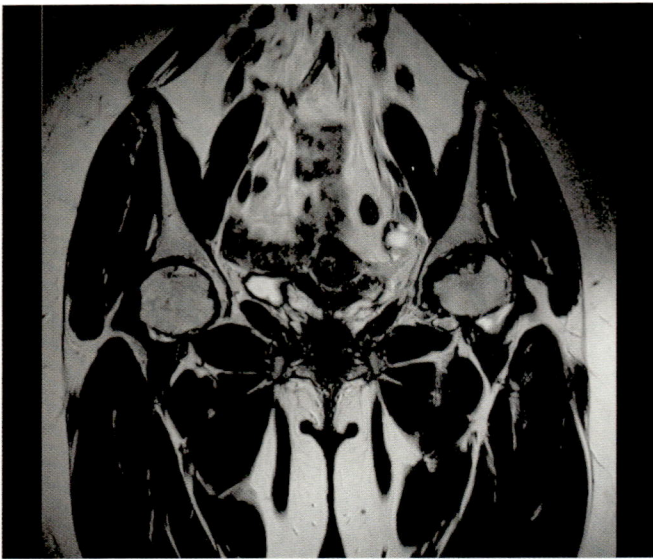

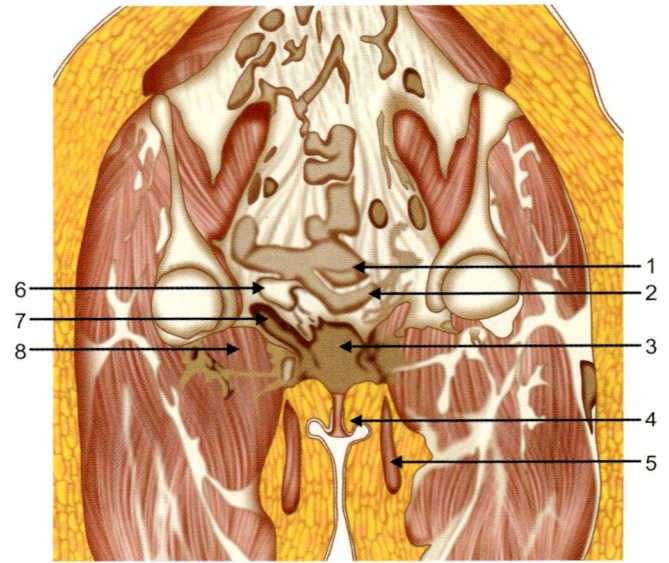

Figure 9.13

1. Part of uterus	5. Gracilis
2. Vagina, fornix	6. Urinary bladder
3. Urethra	7. Obturator internus
4. Labium majora	8. Obturator externus

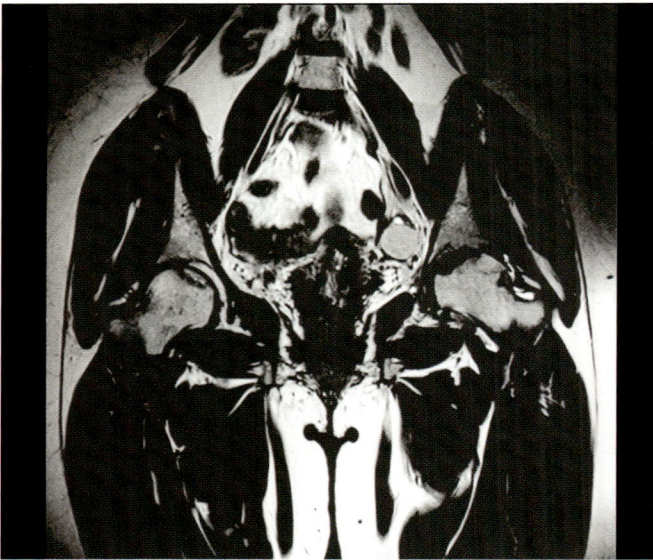

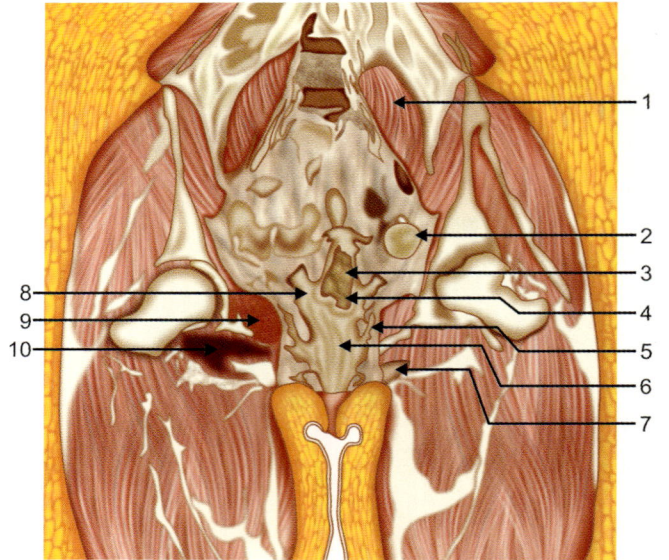

Figure 9.14

1. Psoas	6. Vagina
2. Cyst in left ovary	7. Ischiopubic ramus
3. Cervical canal	8. Vaginal fornix
4. External os	9. Obturator internus
5. Levator ani muscle	10. Obturator externus

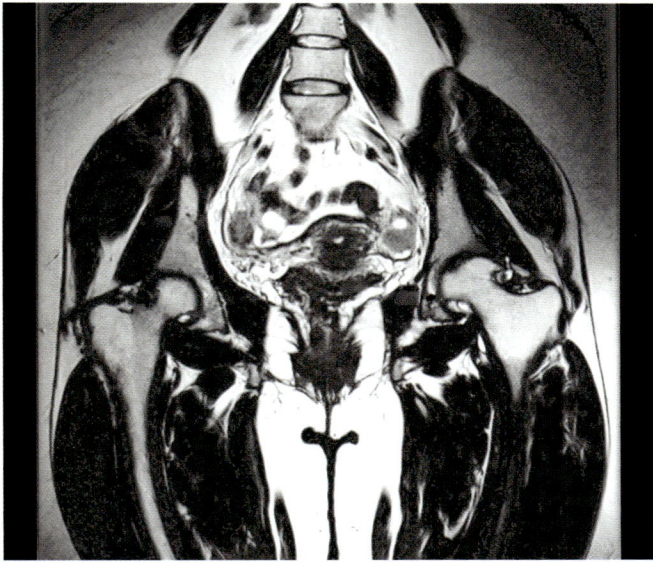
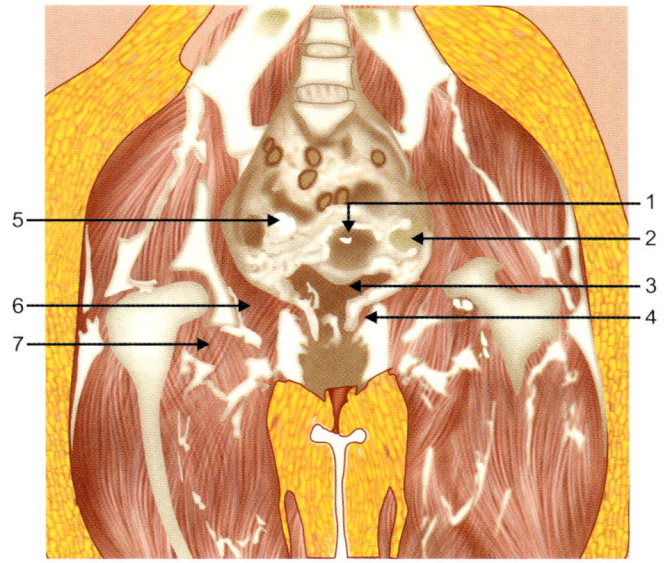

Figure 9.15

1. Uterus	5. Right ovary
2. Left ovary	6. Obturator internus
3. Posterior fornix, vagina	7. Obturator externus
4. Levator ani muscle	

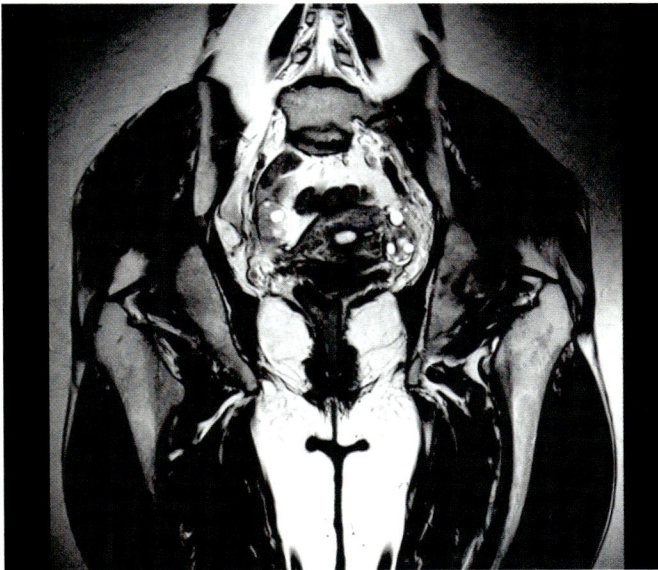
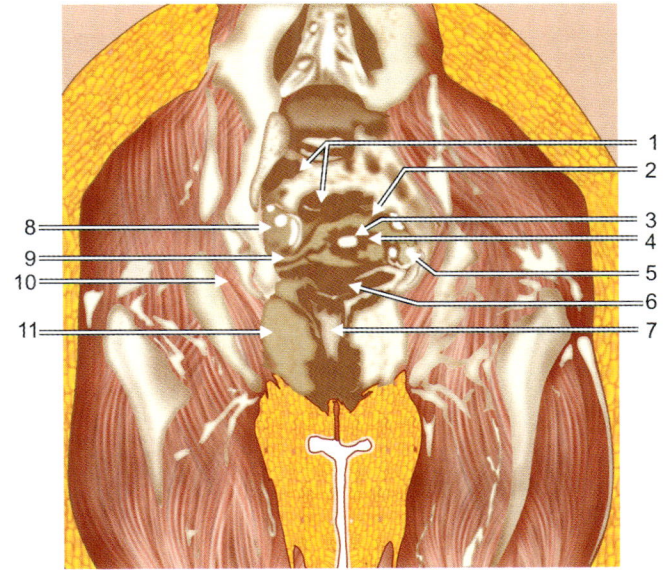

Figure 9.16

1. Bowel loops	7. Anal canal
2. Uterus	8. Right ovary
3. Endometrial cavity	9. Fallopian tube
4. Junctional zone	10. Obturator internus
5. Left ovary	11. Ischioanal fossa
6. Posterior fornix, vagina	

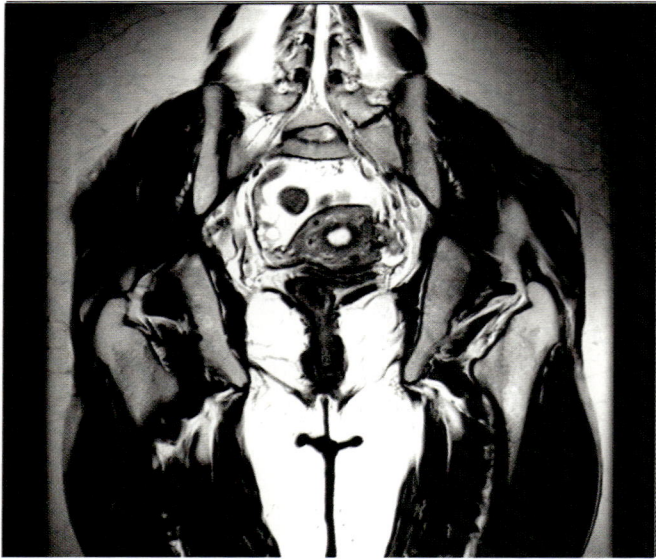
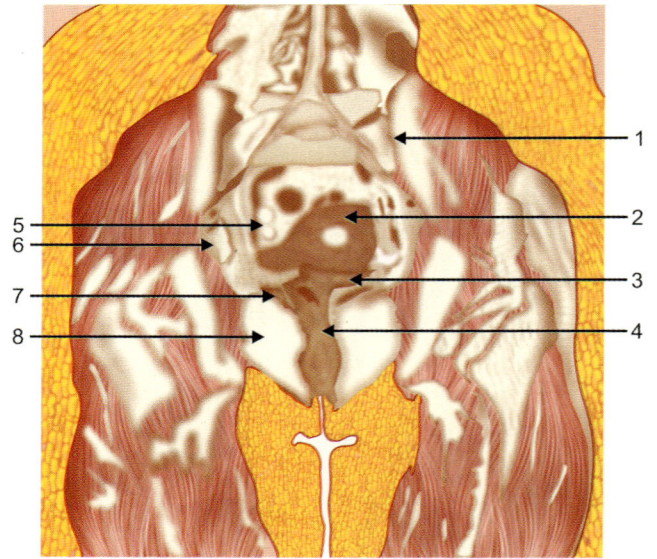

Figure 9.17

1. SI joint	5. Right ovary
2. Uterus	6. Sciatic nerve
3. Posterior fornix, vagina	7. Levator ani muscle
4. Anal canal	8. Ischioanal fossa

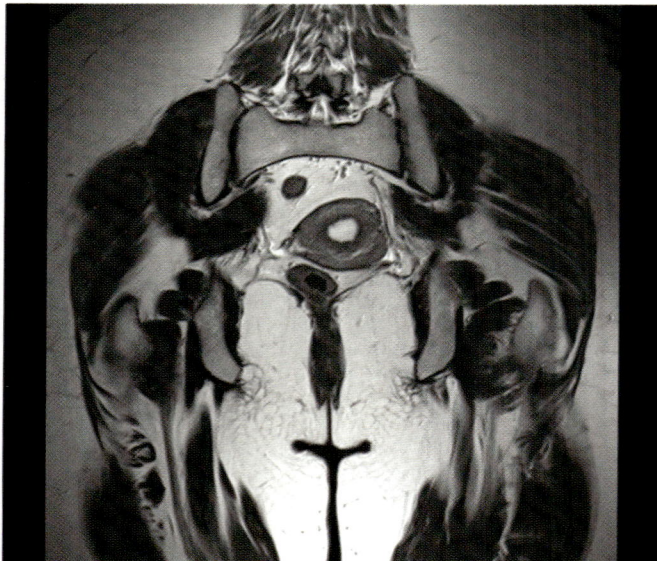
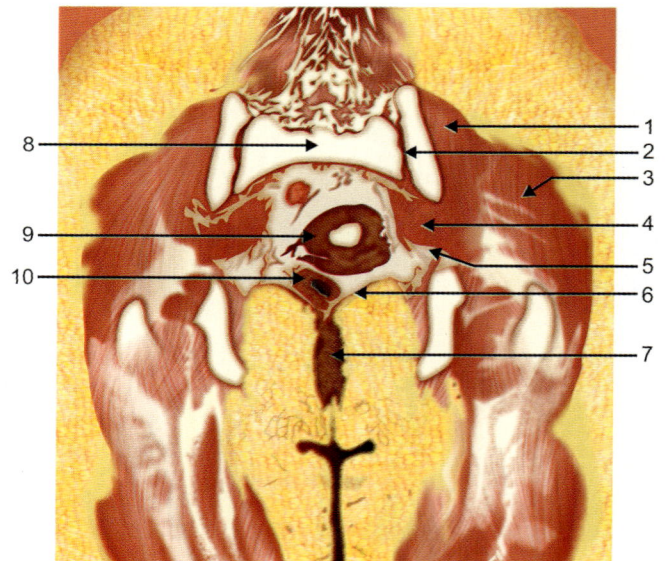

Figure 9.18

1. Gluteus medius	6. Levator ani muscle
2. SI joint	7. Anal canal
3. Gluteus maximus	8. Sacrum
4. Piriformis	9. Uterus
5. Sciatic nerve	10. Rectum

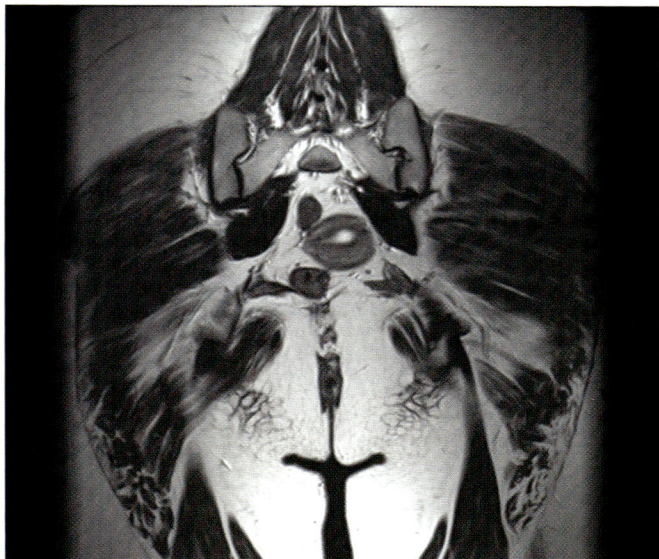
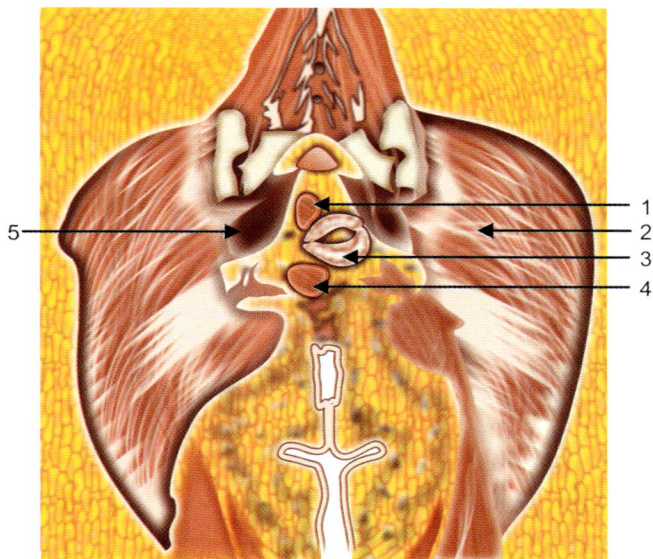

Figure 9.19

1. Rectum	4. Rectum
2. Gluteus maximus	5. Piriformis
3. Uterus, fundus	

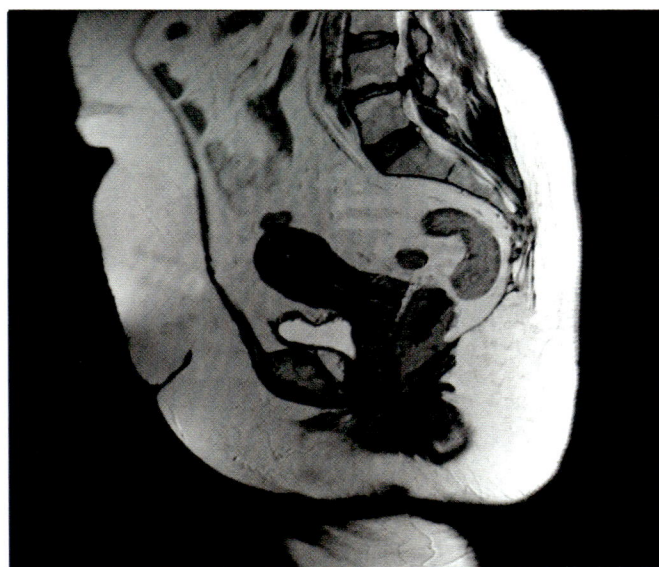
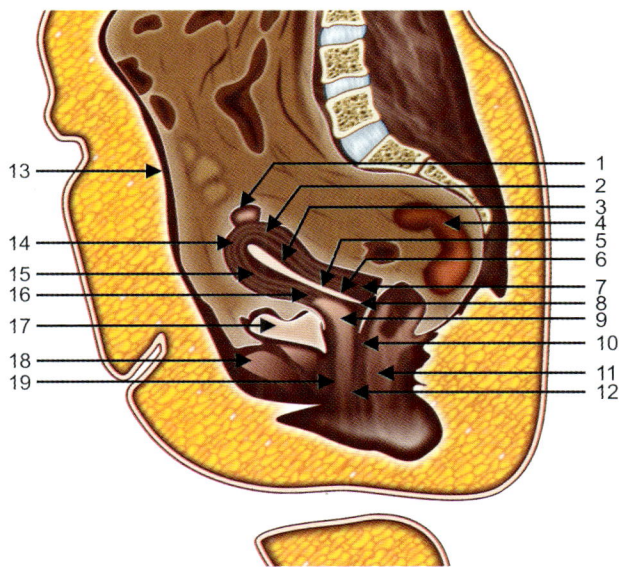

Figure 9.20

1. Bowel loop	8. External os, cervix	15. Body of uterus
2. Myometrium	9. Anterior fornix, vagina	16. Cervix
3. Endometrium	10. Rectovaginal pouch	17. Urinary bladder
4. Rectum	11. Anal canal	18. Pubis bone
5. Internal os of cervix	12. Vagina	19. Urethra
6. Cervical canal	13. Rectus abdominis	
7. Posterior fornix of vagina	14. Fundus of uterus	

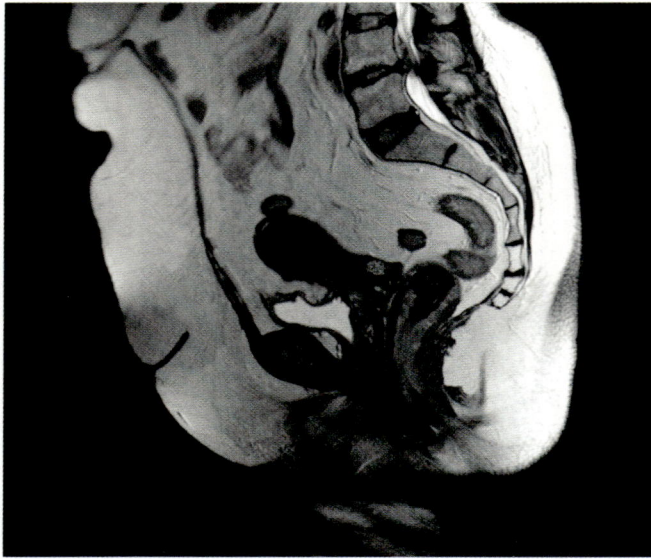

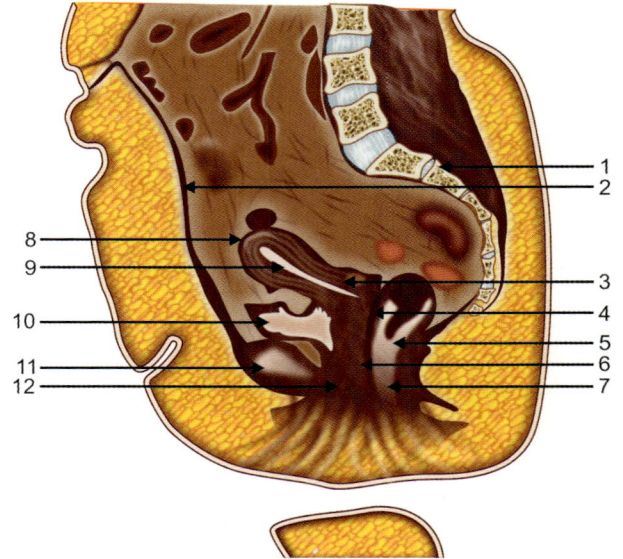

Figure 9.21

1. Sacrum	5. Rectum	9. Uterus, body
2. Rectus abdominis muscle	6. Vagina	10. Urinary bladder
3. Cervix	7. Anal canal	11. Symphysis pubis
4. Rectovaginal pouch	8. Uterus, fundus	12. Urethra

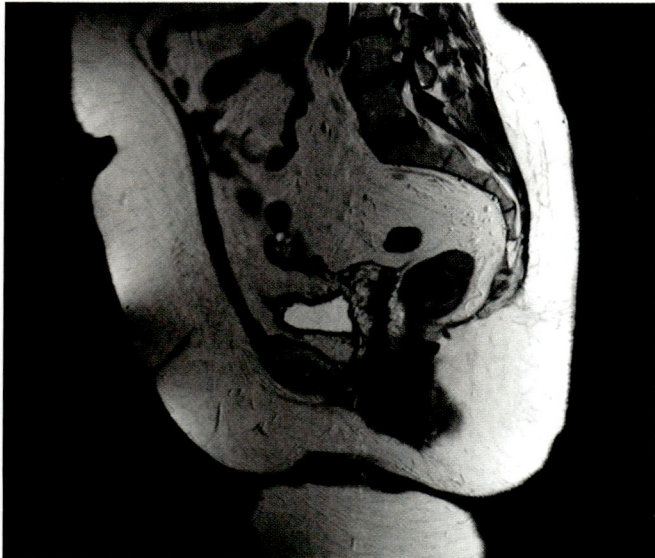

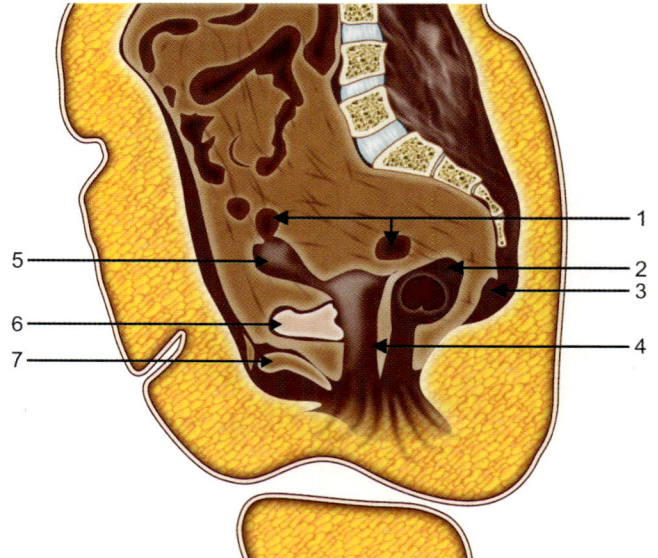

Figure 9.22

1. Bowel loops	5. Uterus, cornu
2. Rectum	6. Urinary bladder
3. Coccyx	7. Pubis bone
4. Vagina, Lateral wall	

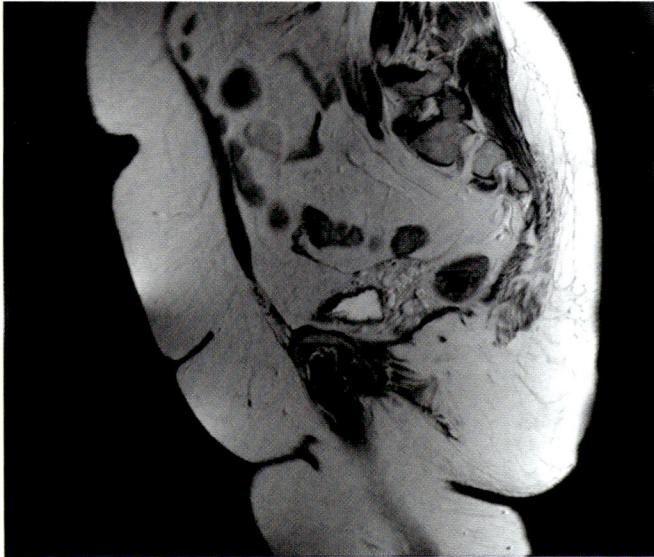

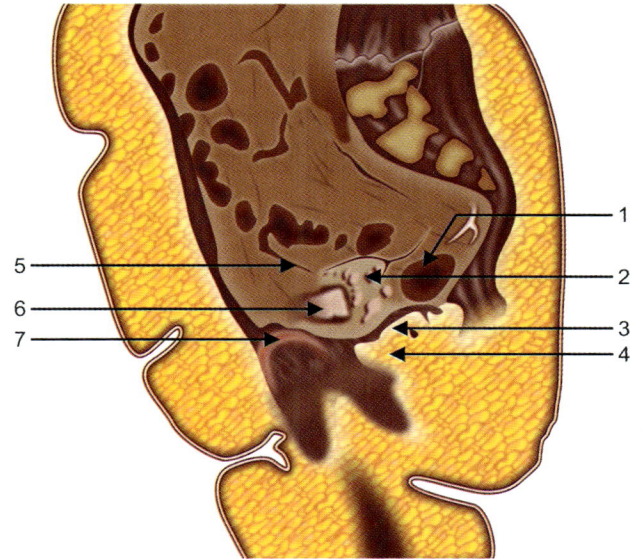

Figure 9.23

1. Rectum	5. Fallopian tube
2. Ovary	6. Bladder
3. Levator ani muscle	7. Pubis
4. Ischioanal fossa	

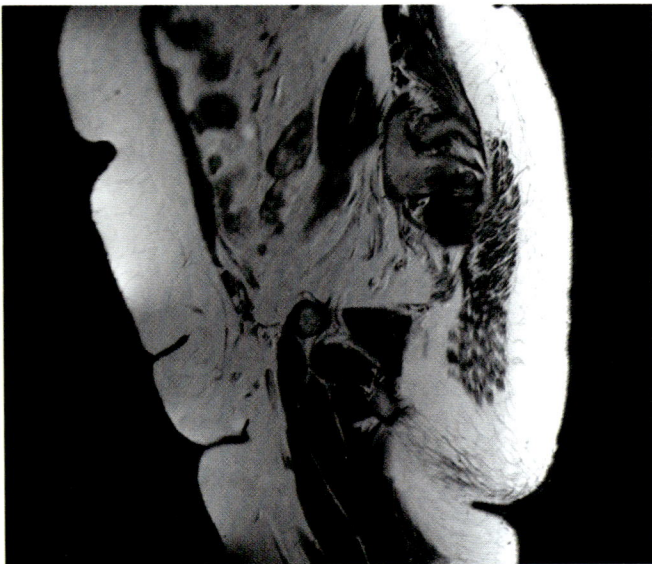

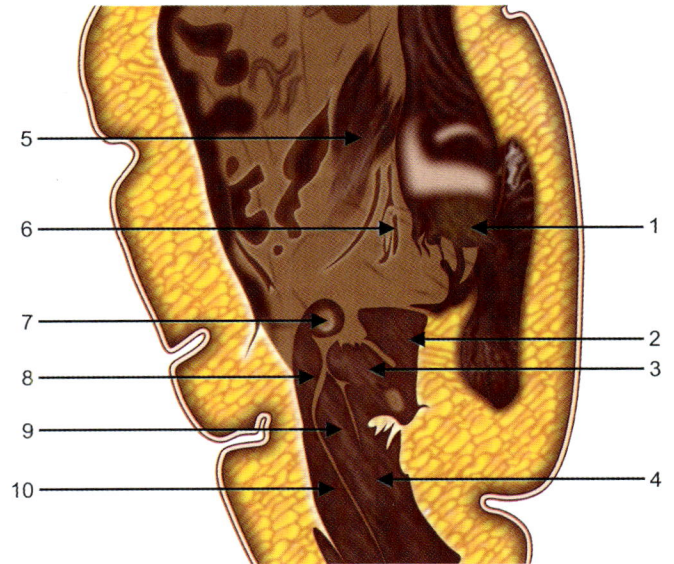

Figure 9.24

1. Piriformis muscle	5. Psoas muscle	9. Adductor brevis
2. Obturator internus muscle	6. Internal iliac vessels	10. Adductor longus
3. External obturator muscle	7. Superior pubic ramus	
4. Adductor magnus	8. Pectineus muscle	

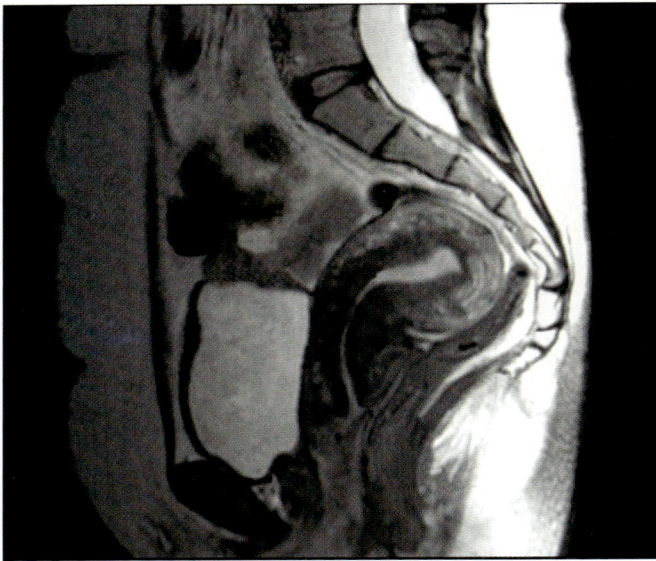
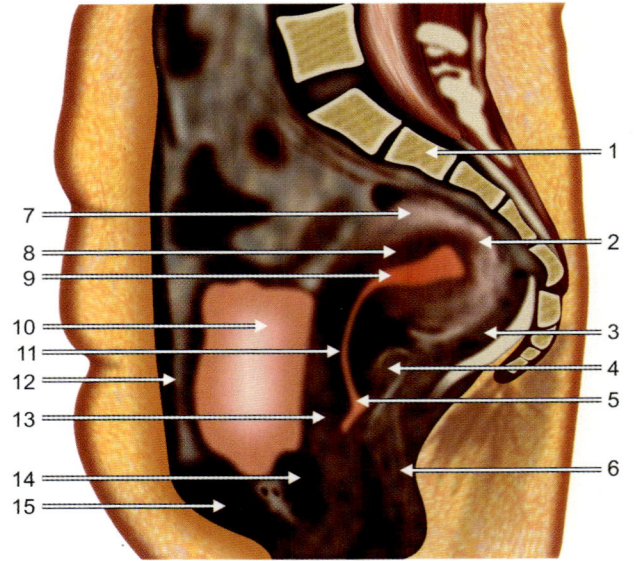

Figure 9.25

TRILAMINAR PATTERN OF UTERUS	6. Anal canal	11. Cervix
1. Sacrum	7. Outer zone: Outer myometrium	12. Rectus abdominis
2. Fundus of uterus	8. Junctional zone: Endometrium and inner myometrium	13. Anterior fornix, vagina
3. Rectum	9. Inner zone: Endometrial cavity	14. Urethra
4. Posterior fornix, vagina	10. Urinary bladder	15. Pubic symphysis
5. External os		

MALE PELVIS

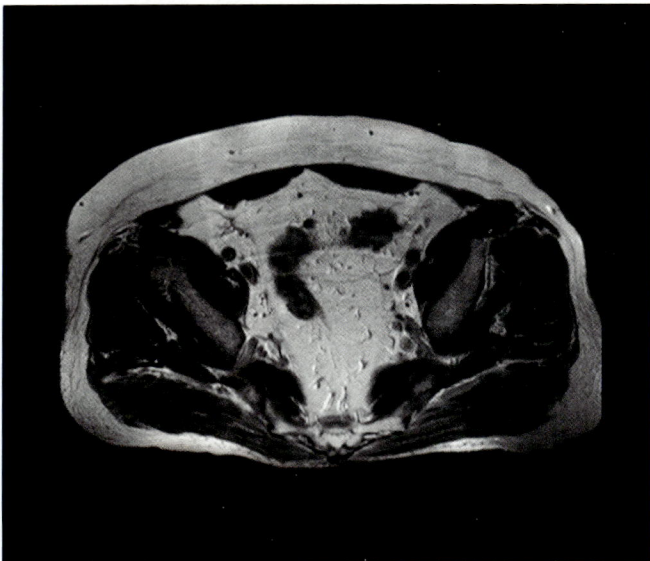
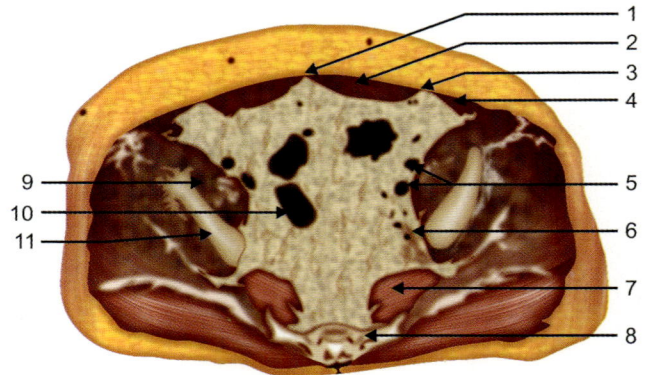

Figure 9.26

1. Linea alba	5. External iliac vessels	9. Iliopsoas muscle
2. Rectus abdominis muscle	6. Internal iliac vessels	10. Sigmoid colon
3. Linea semilunaris	7. Pyriformis muscle	11. Iliac bone
4. Oblique abdominal muscles	8. Sacrum	

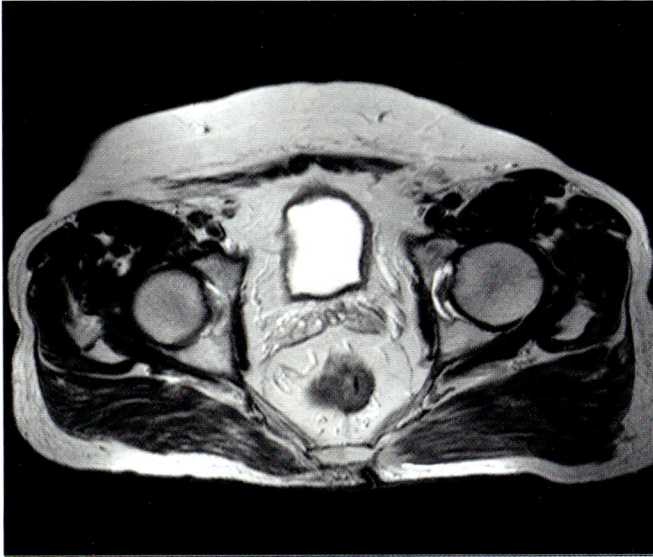

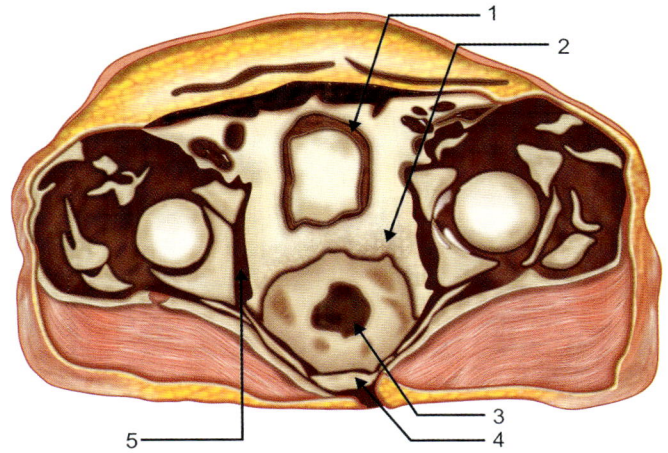

Figure 9.27

1. Urinary bladder
2. Seminal vesicle
3. Rectum
4. Sacrum
5. Obturator internus muscle

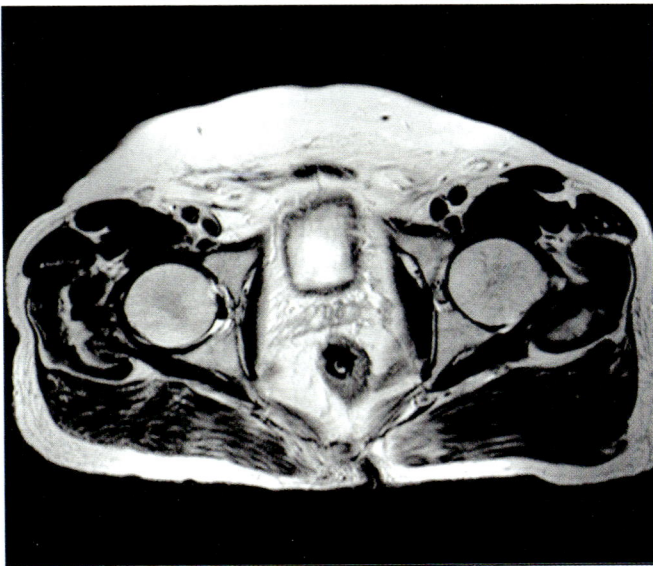

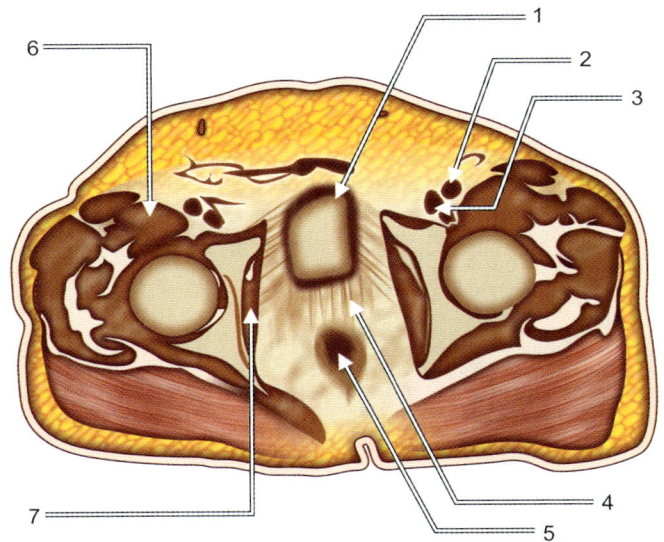

Figure 9.28

1. Urinary bladder
2. Femoral artery
3. Femoral vein
4. Seminal vesicle
5. Rectum
6. Iliopsoas muscle
7. Obturator internus muscle

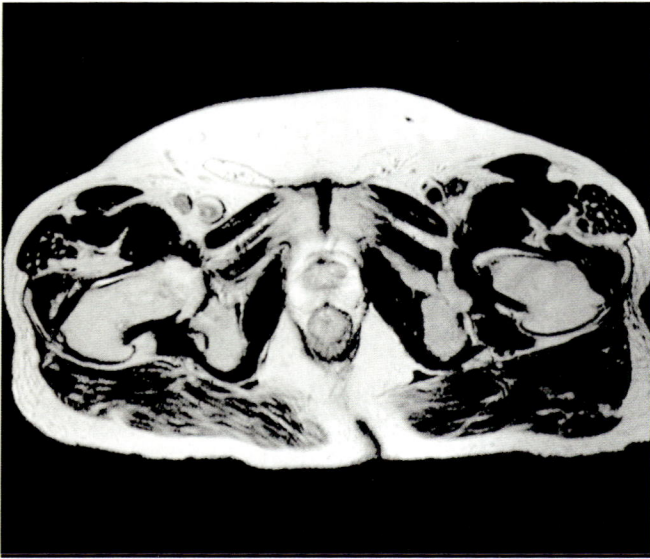

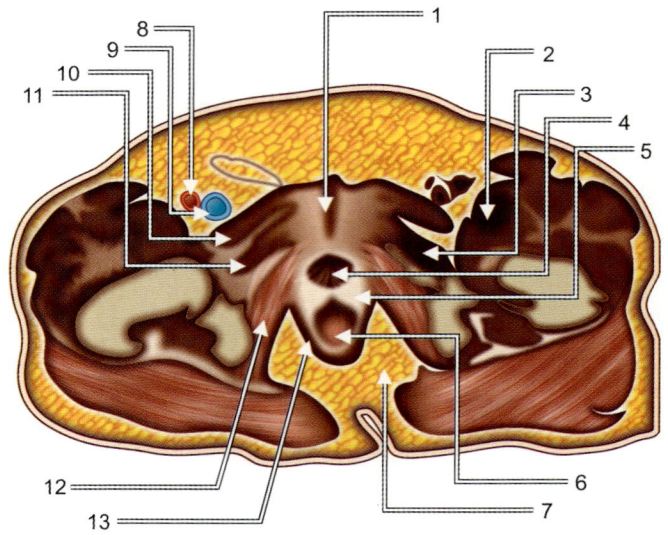

Figure 9.29

1. Pubic symphysis	6. Anal canal	11. Obturator externus
2. Iliopsoas muscle	7. Fat in ischiorectal fossa	12. Obturator internus muscle
3. Obturator externus	8. Femoral artery	13. Levator ani muscle
4. Prostate-central (fibromuscular) zone	9. Femoral vein	
5. Prostate peripheral zone	10. Pectineus muscle	

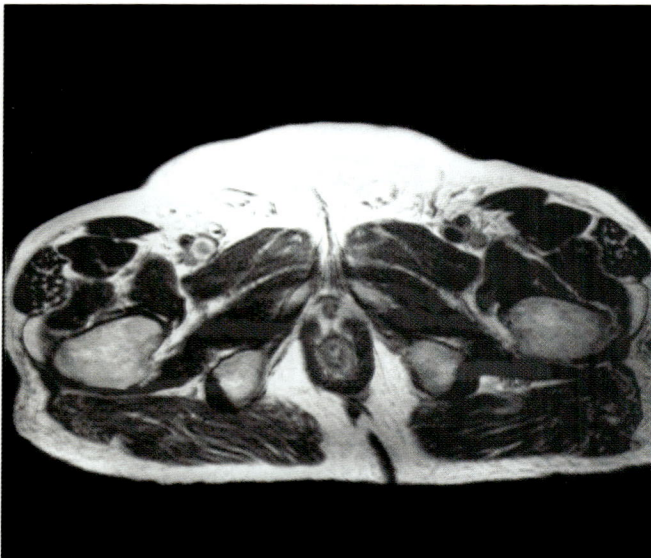

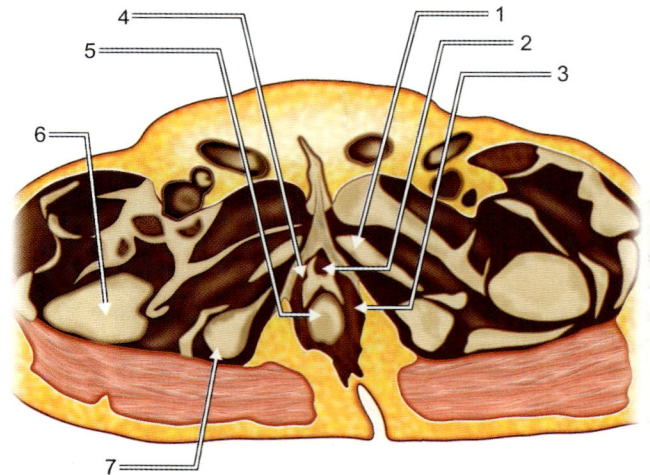

Figure 9.30

1. Pubic ramus	5. Anus
2. Urethra, membranous segment	6. Femur
3. Levator ani muscle	7. Ischial tuberosity
4. Urogenital diaphragm	

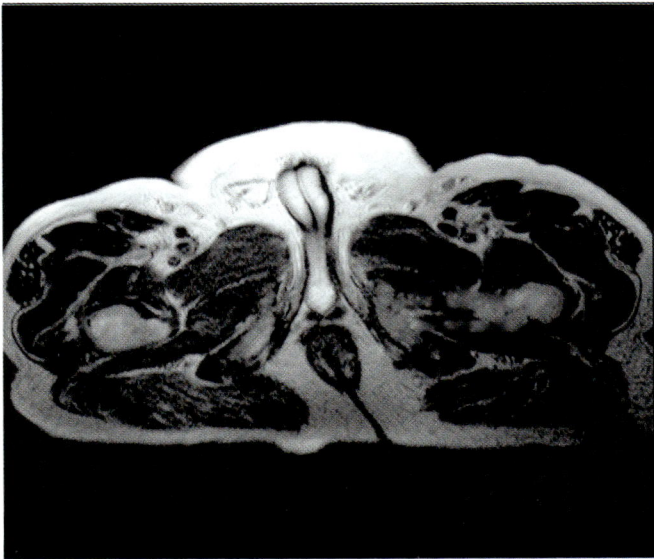

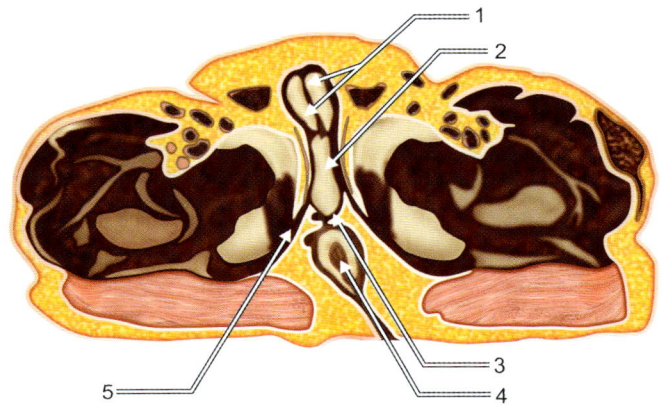

Figure 9.31

1. Corpora cavernosa, penis
2. Corpus spongiosum, penis
3. Bulbospongiosus muscle
4. Anus
5. Ischiocavernosus muscle

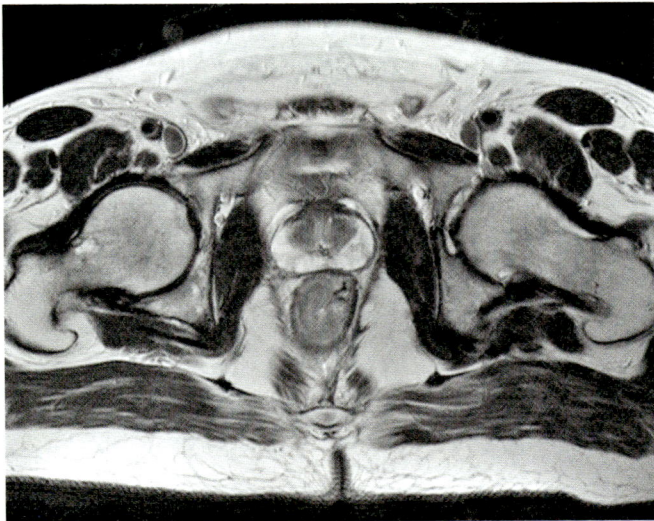

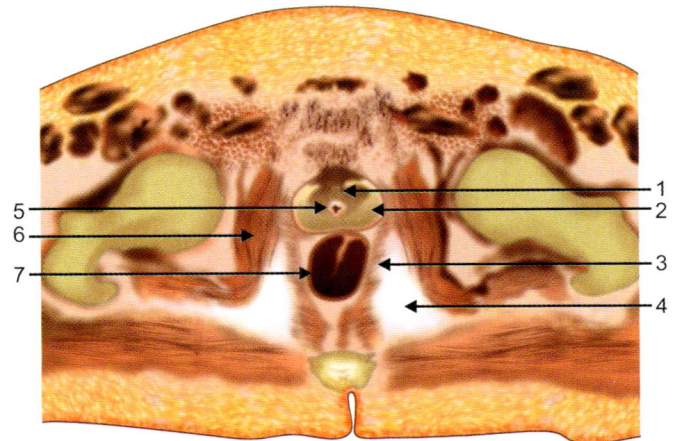

Figure 9.32

1. Prostate-central zone
2. Prostate-peripheral zone
3. Levator ani muscle
4. Ischiorectal fossa
5. Prostatic urethra
6. Obturator internus
7. Rectum

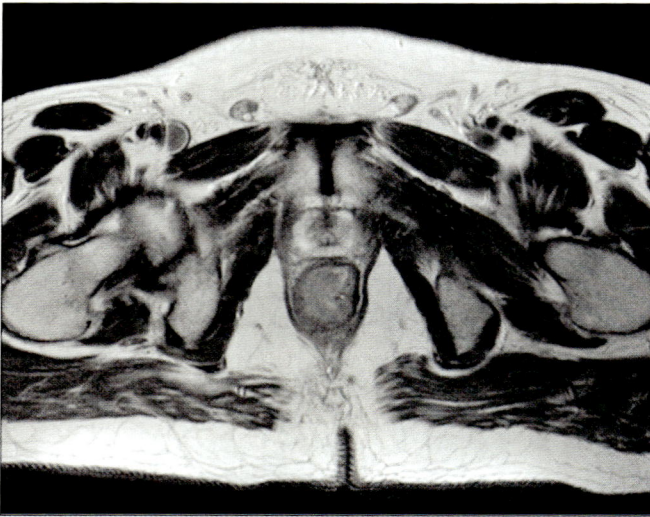

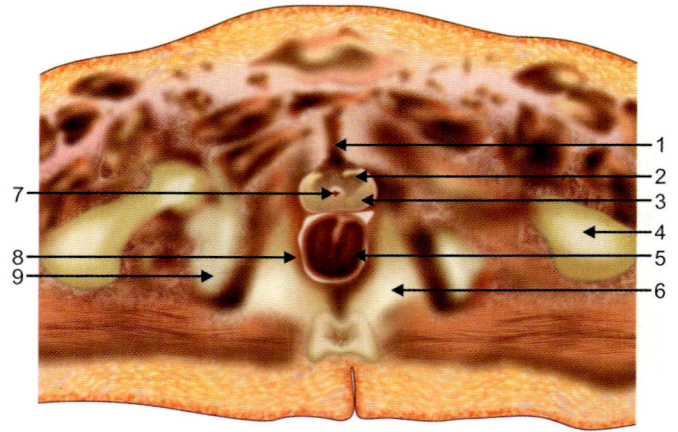

Figure 9.33

1. Pubic symphysis	6. Ischiorectal fossa
2. Central zone	7. Urethra
3. Peripheral zone	8. Levator ani muscle
4. Femur	9. Ischial tuberosity
5. Anal canal	

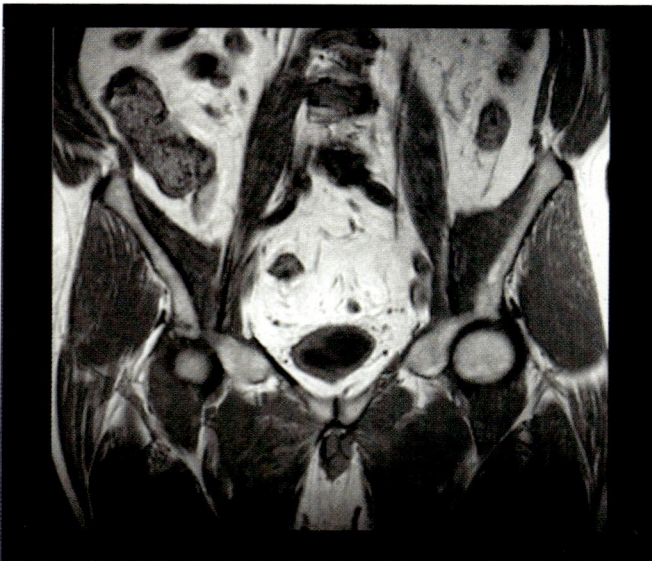

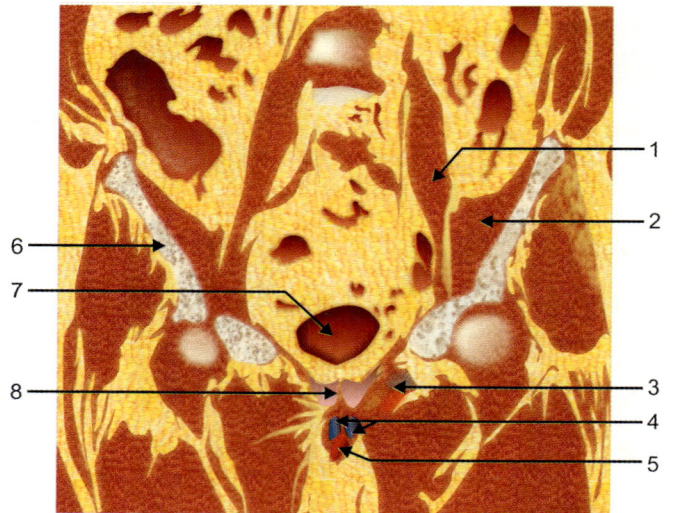

Figure 9.34

1. Psoas	5. Corpus spongiosum
2. Iliacus	6. Ilium
3. Obturator externus	7. Urinary bladder
4. Corpora cavernosa	8. Pubic symphysis

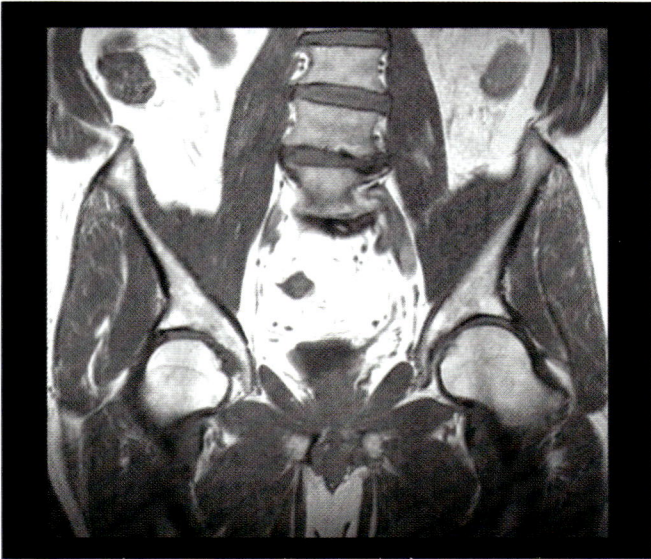
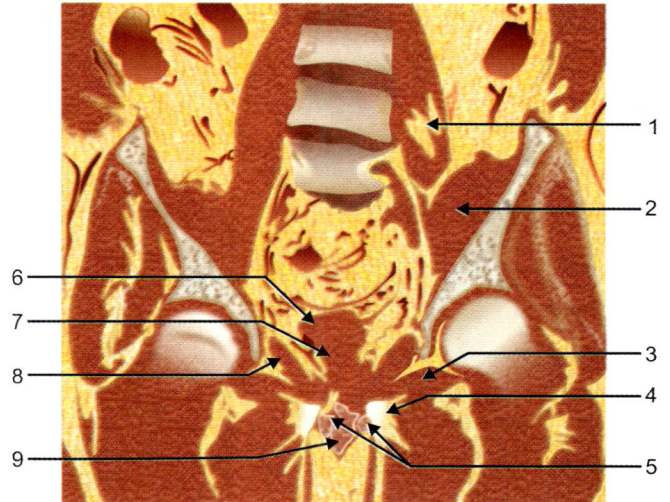

Figure 9.35

1. Psoas	6. Urinary bladder
2. Iliacus	7. Prostate
3. Obturator externus	8. Obturator internus
4. Pubic ramus	9. Corpus spongiosum
5. Corpora cavernosa	

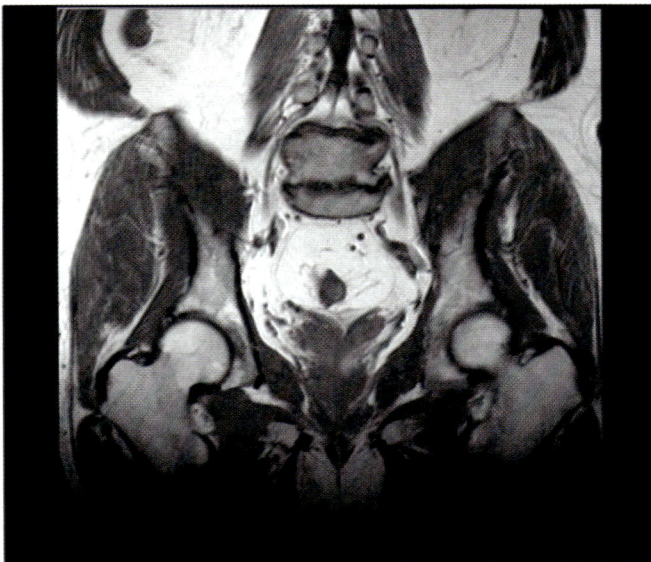
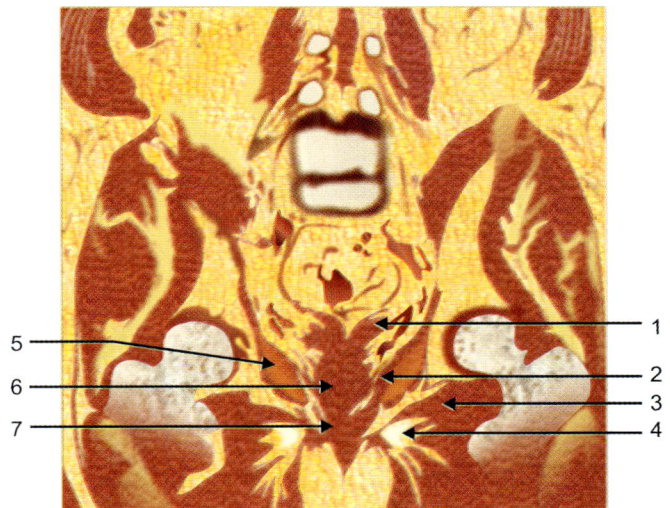

Figure 9.36

1. Seminal vesicle	5. Obturator internus
2. Levator ani muscle	6. Prostate gland
3. Obturator externus	7. Urogenital diaphragm
4. Pubic ramus	

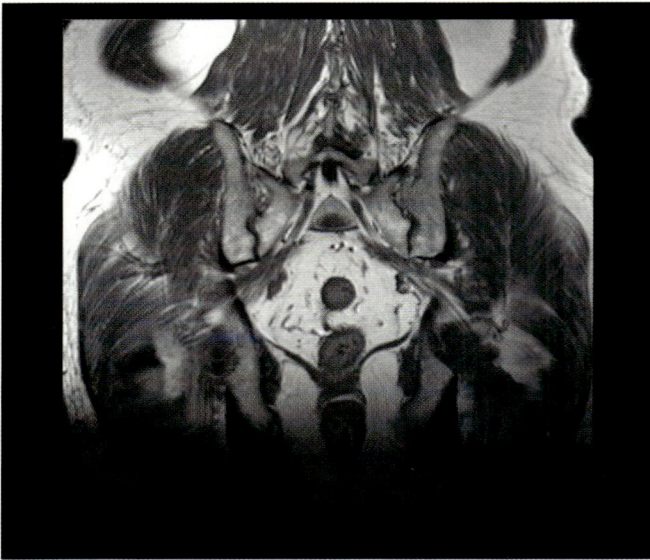

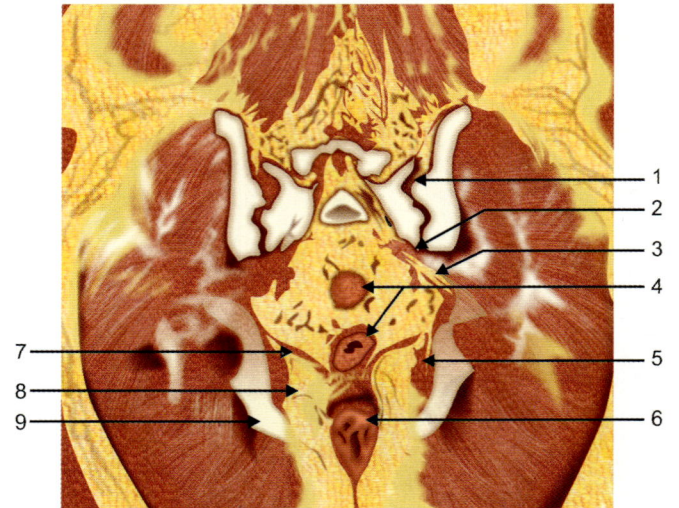

Figure 9.37

1. SI joint	6. Anal canal
2. Piriformis muscle	7. Levator ani muscle
3. Lumbosacral plexus	8. Ischiorectal fossa
4. Rectum	9. Ischium
5. Obturator internus muscle	

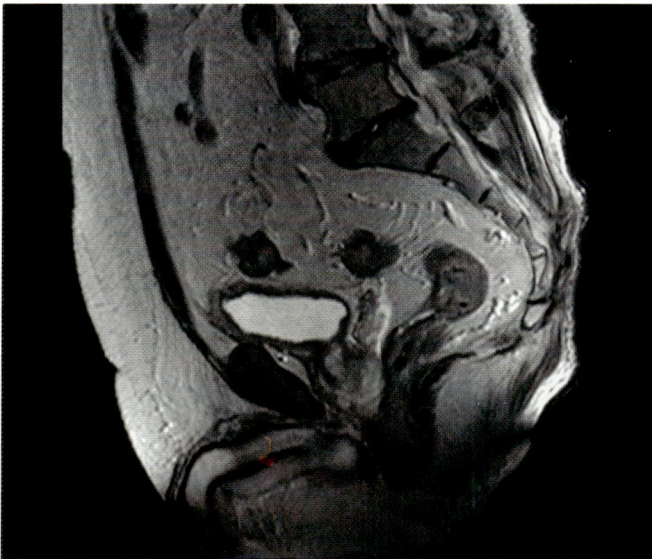

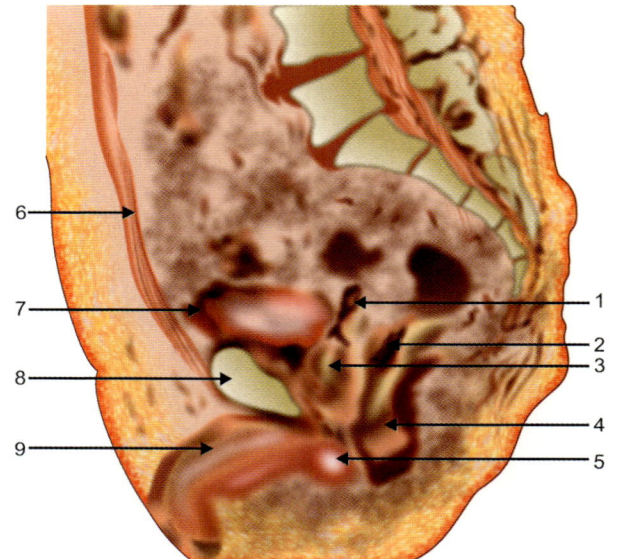

Figure 9.38

1. Seminal vesicle	6. Rectus abdominis
2. Rectum	7. Urinary bladder
3. Prostate	8. Pubic bone
4. Anal canal	9. Corpus cavernosum
5. Bulb of penis	

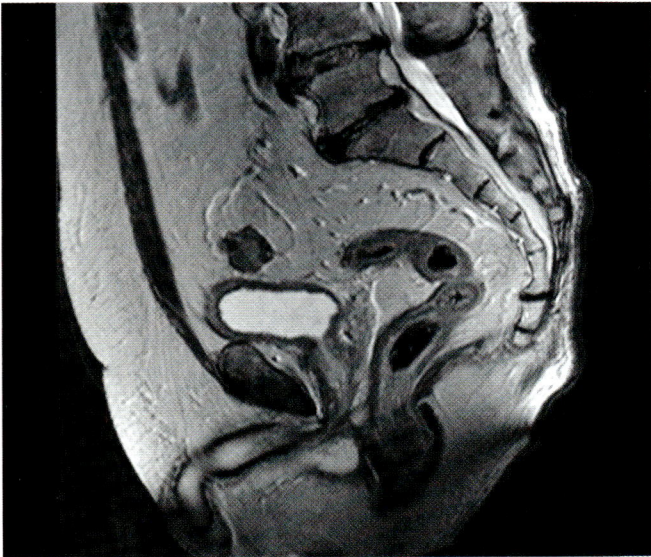

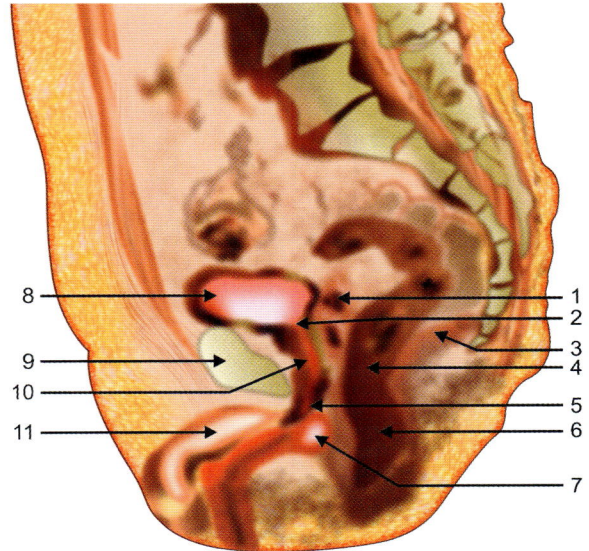

Figure 9.39

1. Seminal vesicle	5. Urogenital diaphragm	9. Pubis bone
2. Bladder neck	6. Anal canal	10. Prostatic urethra
3. Levator ani muscle	7. Bulb of penis	11. Penis
4. Rectum	8. Urinary bladder	

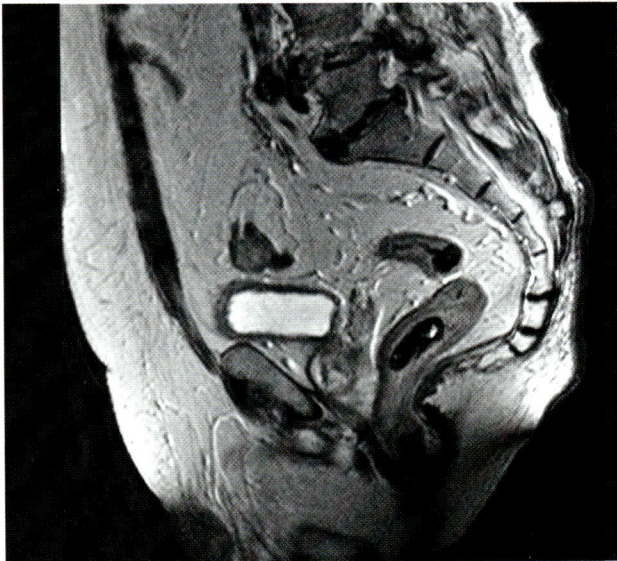

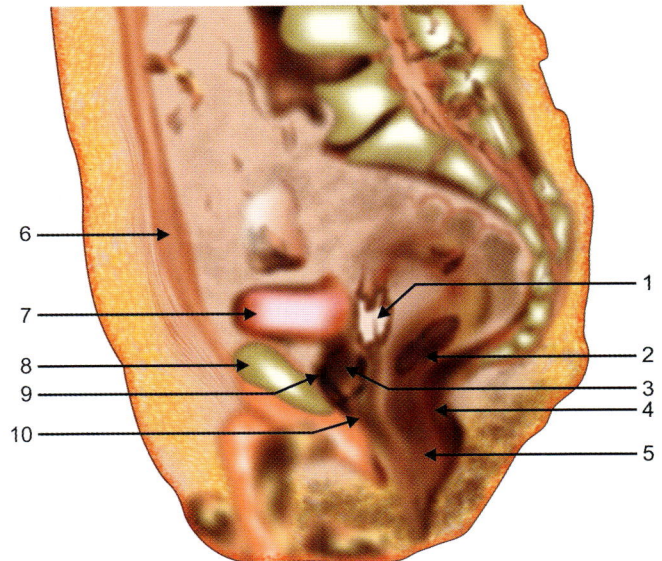

Figure 9.40

1. Seminal vesicle	6. Rectus abdominis muscle
2. Rectum	7. Urinary bladder
3. Prostate, central zone	8. Pubic ramus
4. Levator ani & coccygeus muscle	9. Prostate, peripheral zone
5. Anal canal	10. Obturator internus

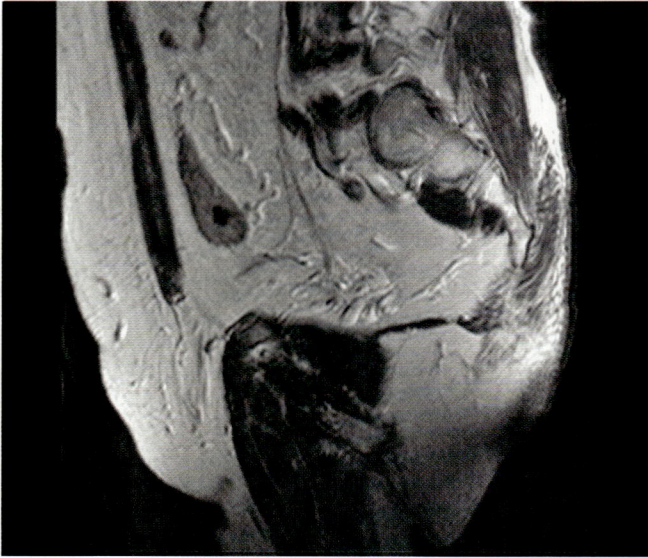

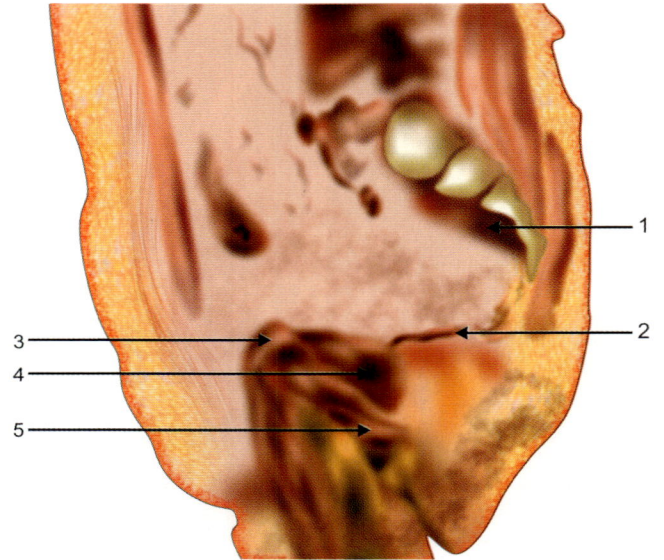

Figure 9.41

1. Pyriformis
2. Levator ani muscle
3. Pubic ramus
4. Obturator internus
5. Ischium

Section 4

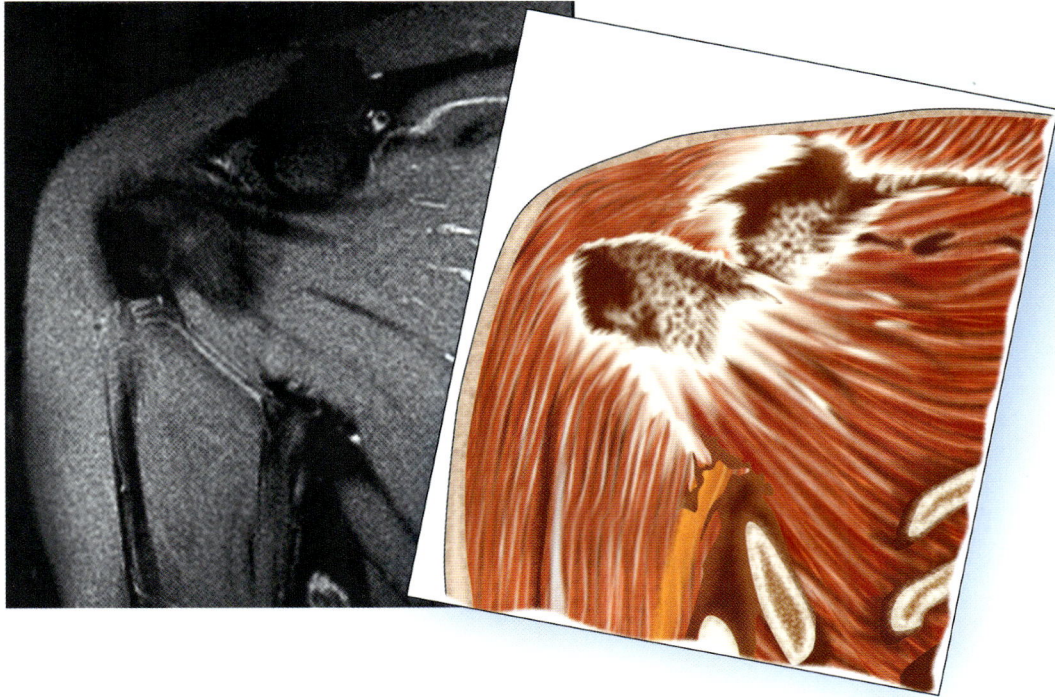

Upper Extremity

- Shoulder
- Arm and Forearm
- Elbow
- Wrist
- Upper Extremity Vessels

CHAPTER 10

Shoulder

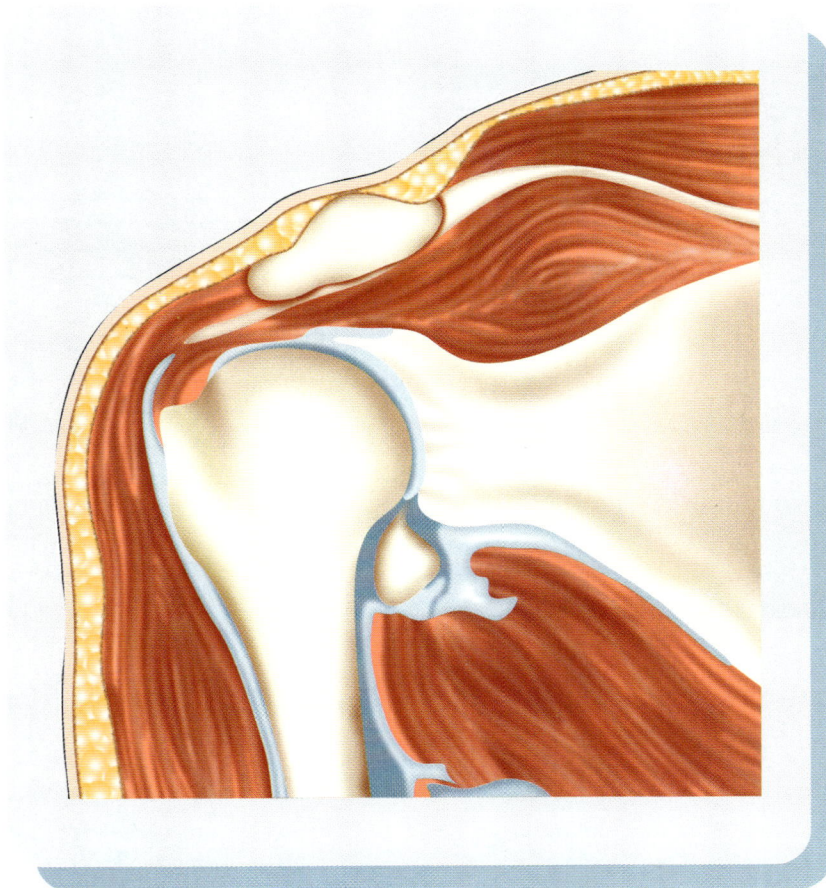

X-RAYS

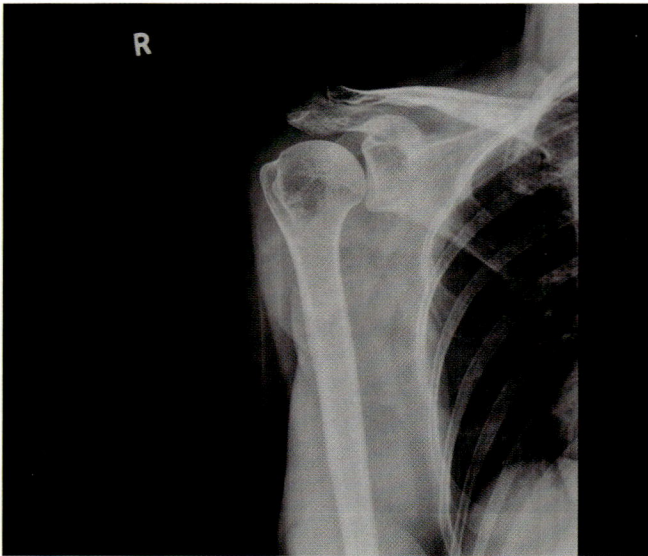
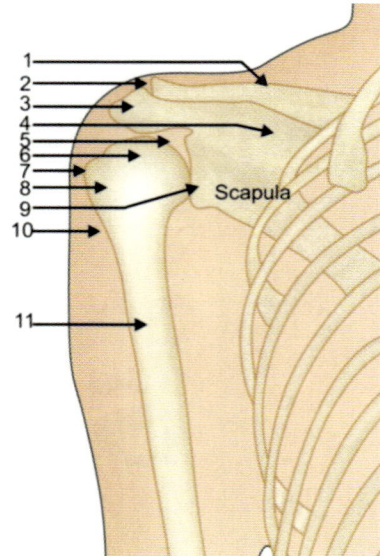

Figure 10.1

1. Clavicle	5. Coracoid process	9. Glenoid fassa
2. Acromio-clavicular joint	6. Humerus, head	10. Surgical neck
3. Acromion process	7. Greater tuberosity	11. Humerus shaft
4. Scapula spine	8. Lesser tuberosity	

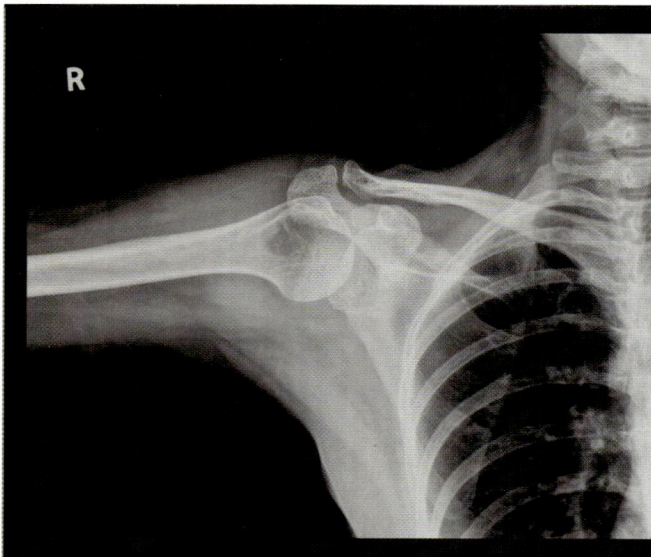
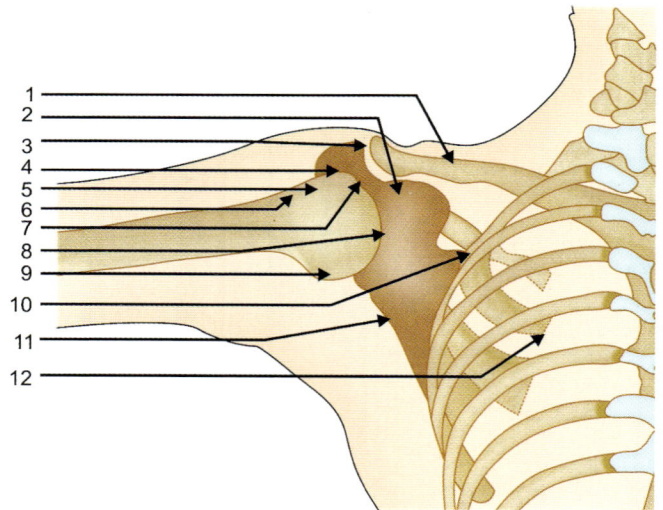

Figure 10.2

1. Clavicle	7. Acromion process
2. Coracoid process	8. Glenoid fassa
3. Acromio-clavicular joint	9. Humerus, head
4. Greater tuberosity	10. Scapular spine
5. Lesser tuberosity	11. Scapula, lateral border
6. Intertubercular sulcus	12. Scapula, medial border

MR ARTHROGRAM SHOULDER JOINT: CORONAL IMAGES—ANTERIOR TO POSTERIOR

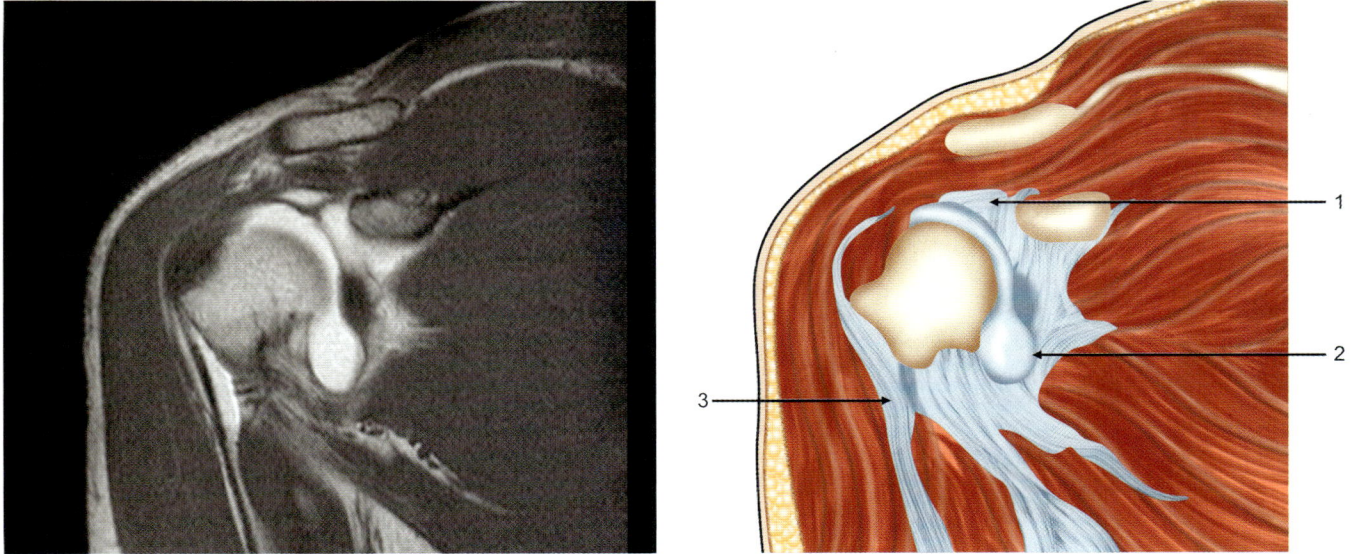

Figure 10.3

1. Superior glenohumeral ligament
2. Inferior glenohumeral ligament
3. Biceps tendon, long head

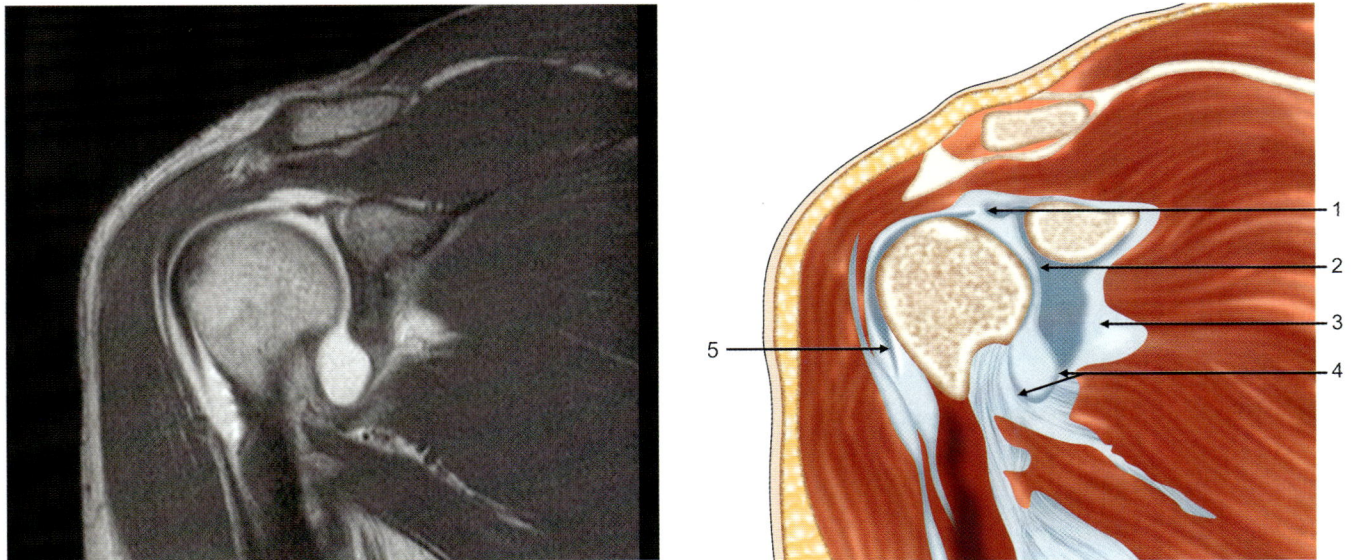

Figure 10.4

1. Biceps labral complex
2. Labrum
3. Subscapularis bursa
4. Inferior glenohumeral ligament
5. Biceps tendon, long head

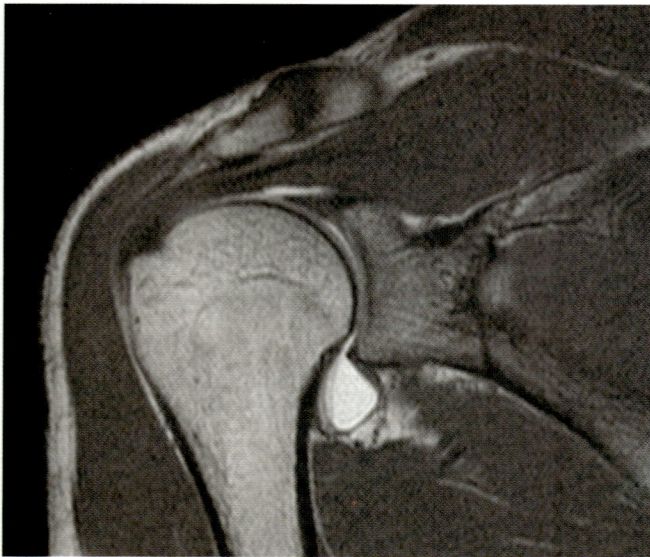

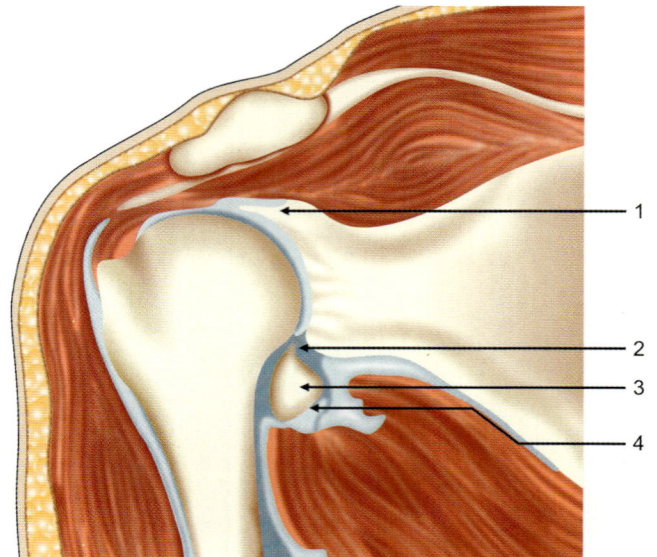

Figure 10.5

1. Superior labrum
2. Inferior labrum
3. Axillary pouch
4. Inferior glenohumeral ligament

MR ARTHROGRAM SHOULDER JOINT: SAGITTAL IMAGES—MEDIAL TO LATERAL

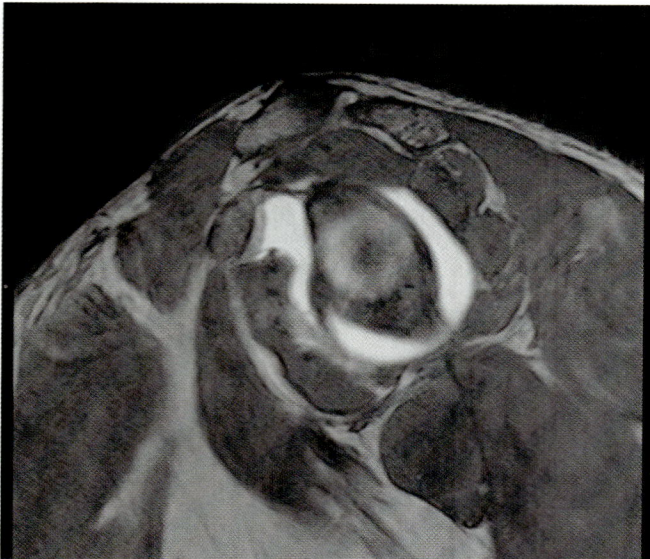

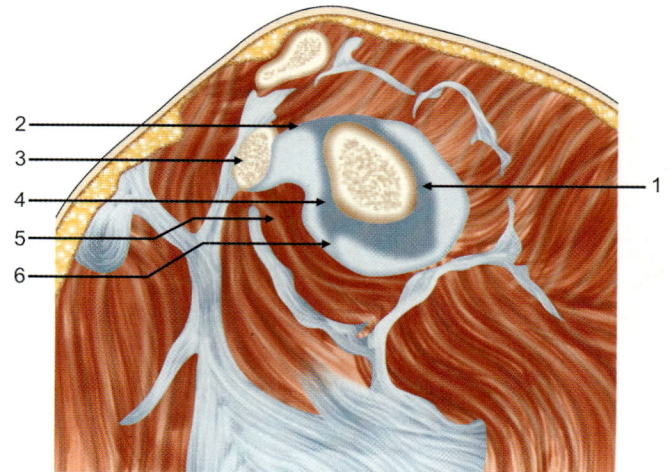

Figure 10.6

1. Posterior labrum
2. Superior glenohumeral ligament
3. Coracoid process
4. Anterior labrum
5. Subscapularis
6. Middle glenohumeral ligament

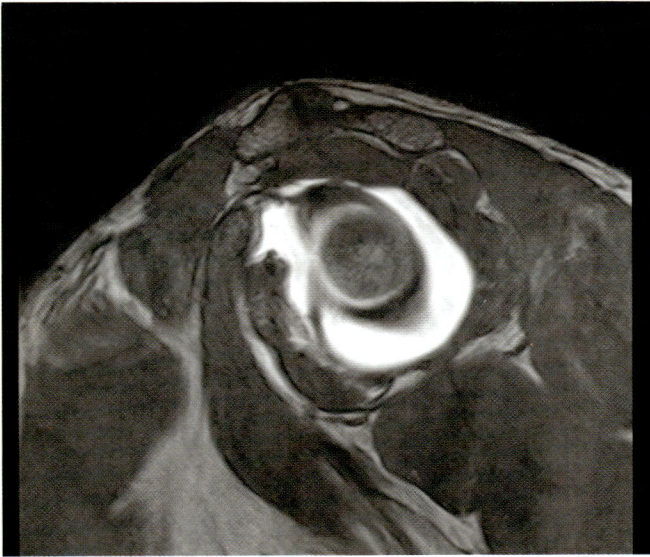

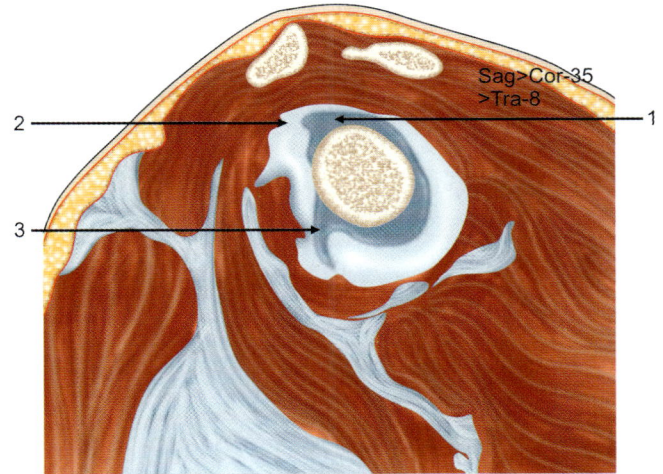

Figure 10.7

1. Biceps labral complex
2. Superior glenohumeral ligament
3. Middle glenohumeral ligament

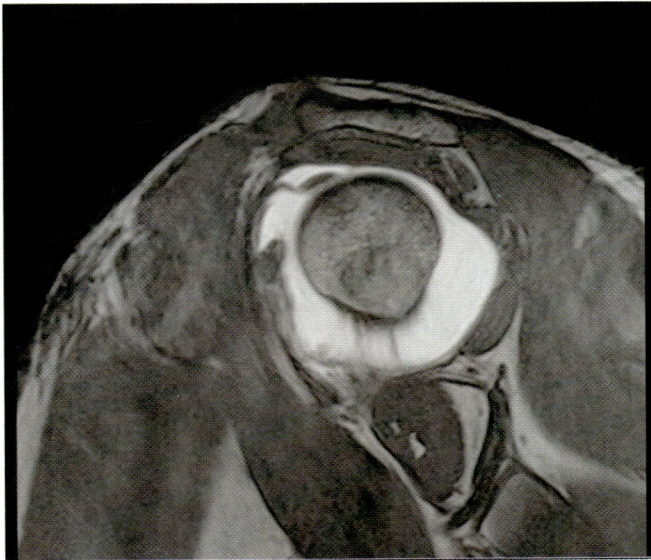

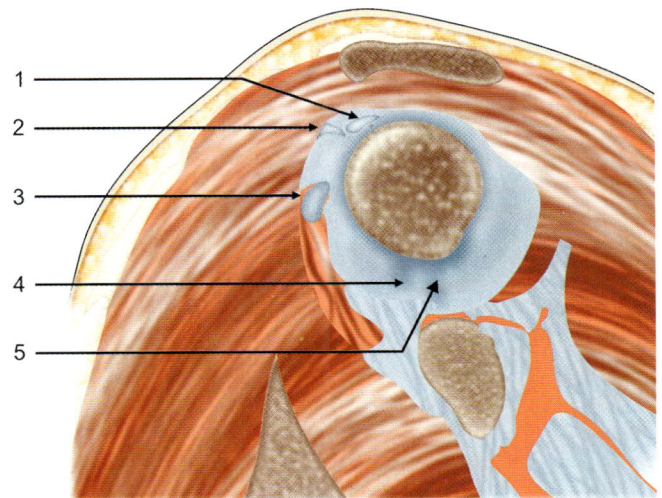

Figure 10.8

1. Biceps tendon
2. Superior glenohumeral ligament
3. Subscapularis tendon
4. Inferior glenohumeral ligament, anterior band
5. Inferior glenohumeral ligament, posterior band

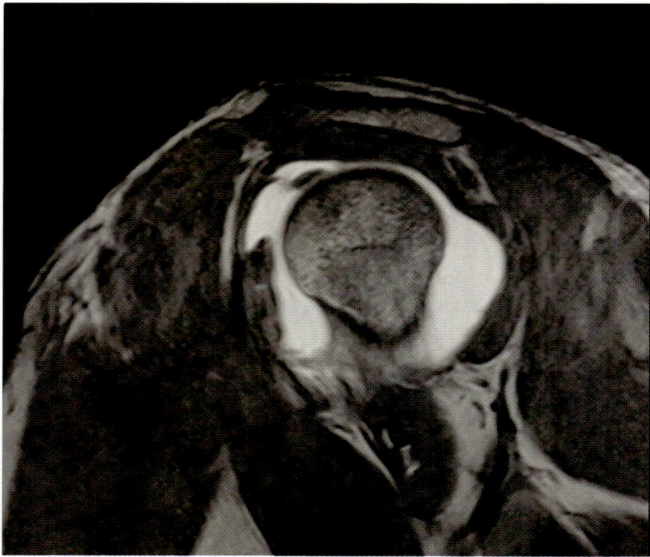

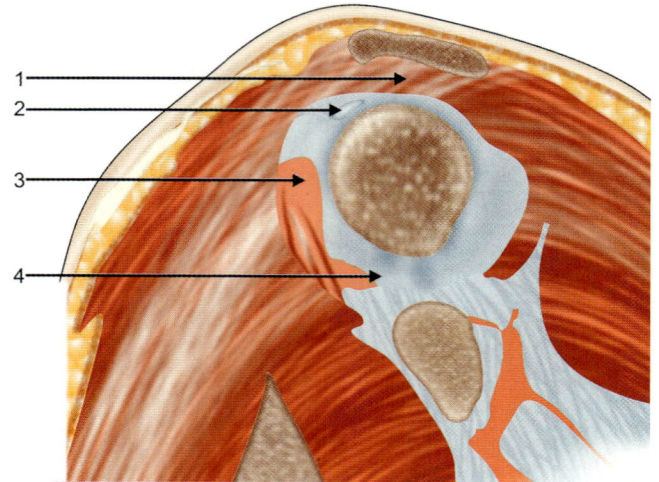

Figure 10.9

1. Supraspinatus tendon
2. Biceps tendon
3. Subscapularis tendon
4. Inferior glenohumeral ligament, axillary band

MR SHOULDER JOINT: AXIAL IMAGES—SUPERIOR TO INFERIOR

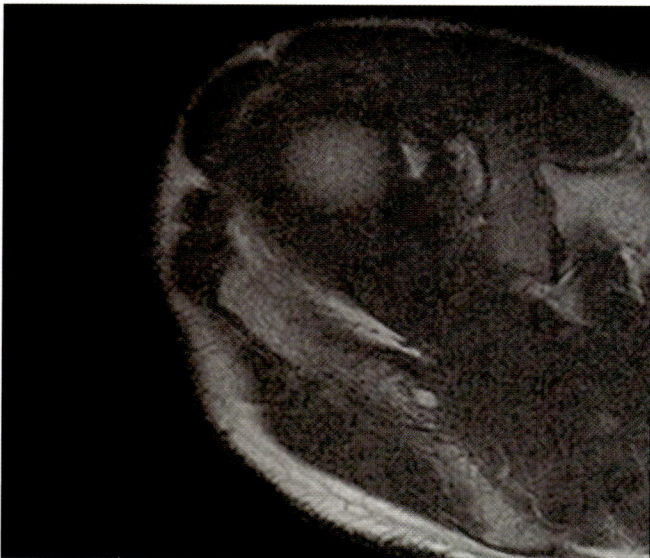

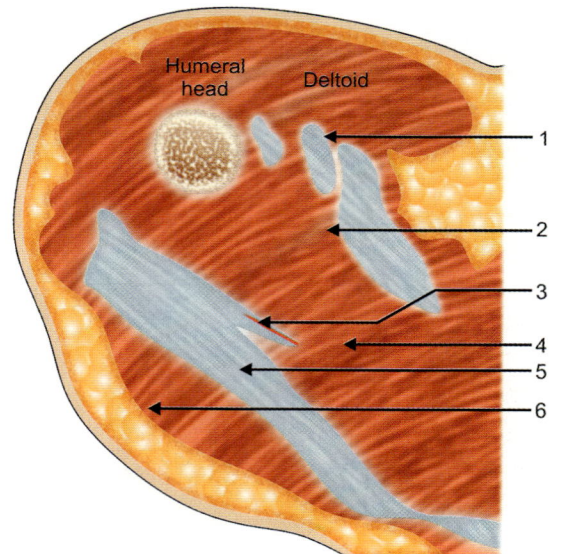

Figure 10.10

1. Coracoid process
2. Supraglenoid tuberosity
3. Suprascapular artery
4. Supraspinatus
5. Scapular spine
6. Deltoid

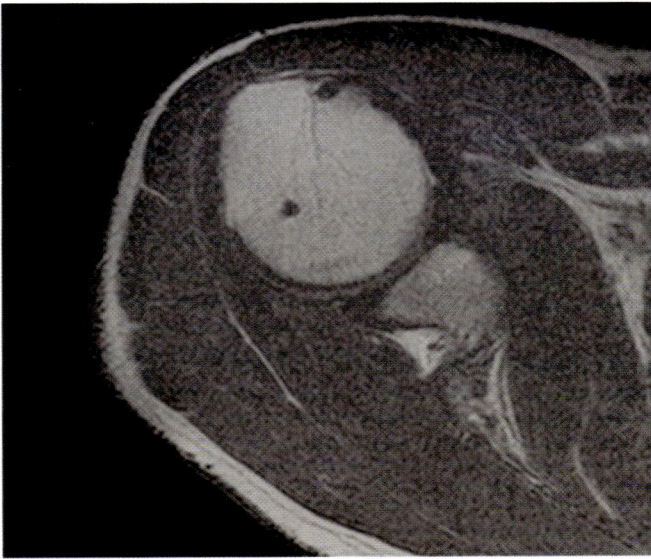
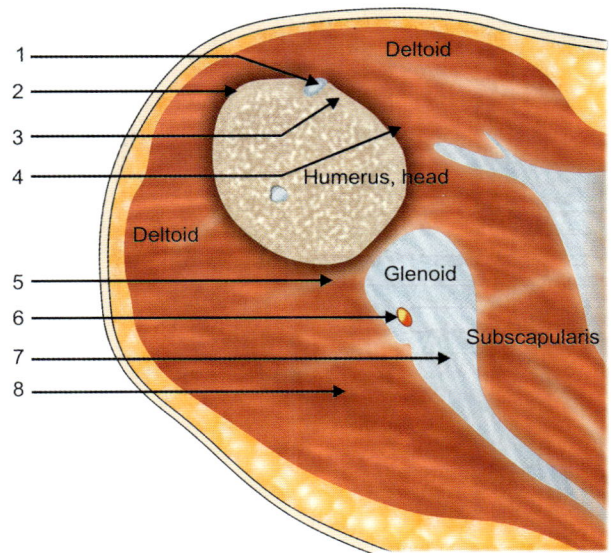

Figure 10.11

1. Biceps tendon, long head	5. Posterior labrum
2. Greater tuberosity	6. Suprascapular artery and nerve
3. Lesser tuberosity	7. Scapular body
4. Subscapularis, tendon	8. Infraspinatus

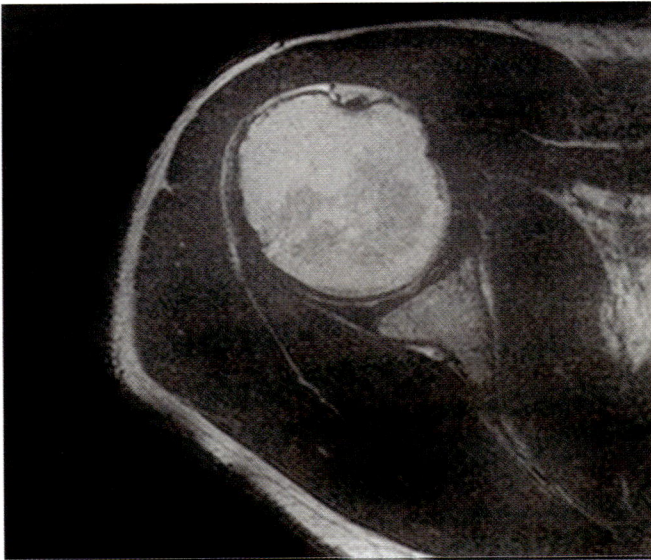
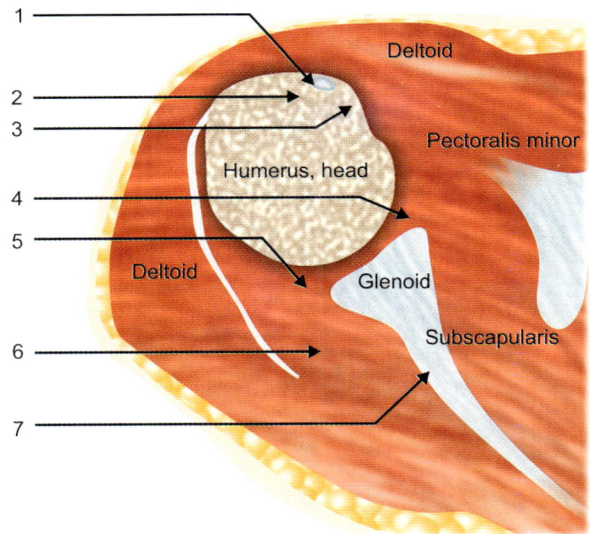

Figure 10.12

1. Biceps tendon, long head	5. Posterior labrum
2. Bicipital groove	6. Infraspinatus
3. Lesser tuberosity	7. Scapula
4. Anterior labrum	

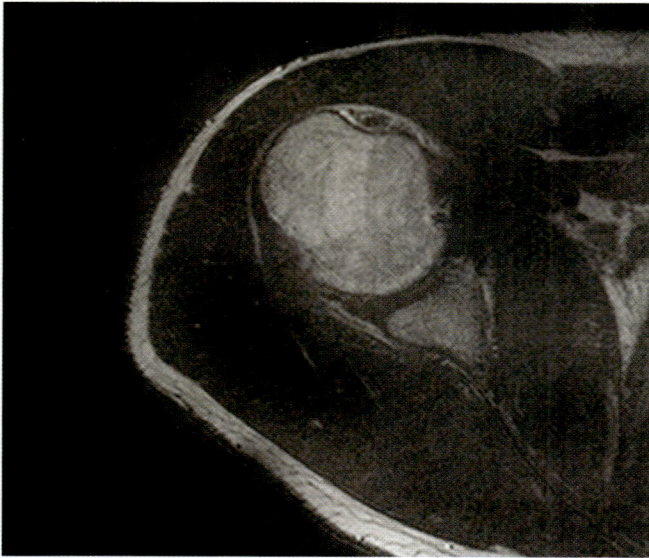

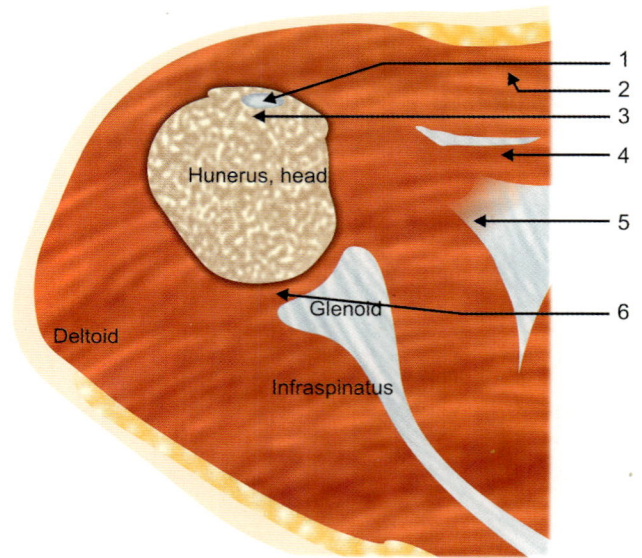

Figure 10.13

1. Biceps tendon, long head	4. Pectoralis minor
2. Pectoralis major	5. Neurovascular bundle
3. Bicipital groove	6. Inferior labrum

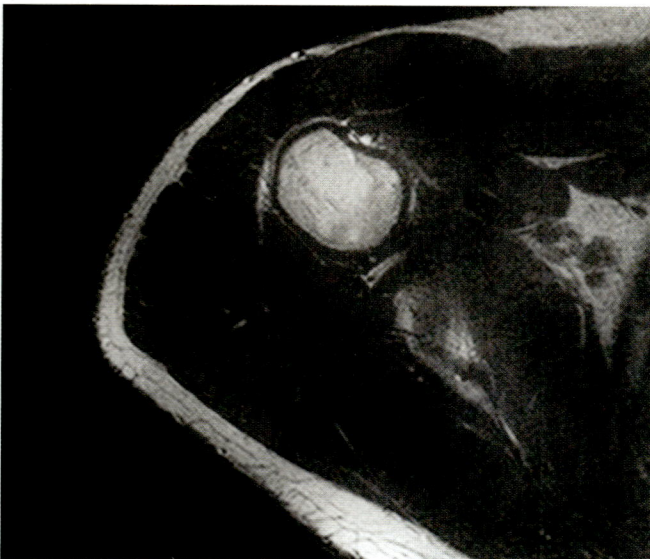

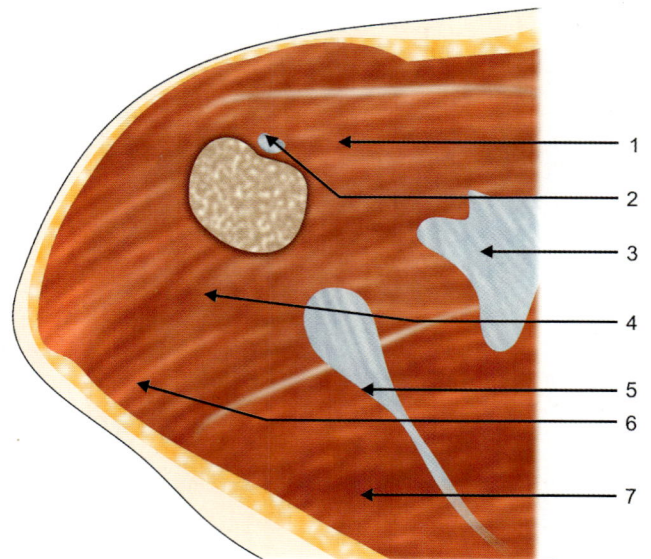

Figure 10.14

1. Coracobrachialis, short head biceps	5. Scapula
2. Biceps tendon, long head	6. Deltoid
3. Neurovascular bundle	7. Infraspinatus
4. Teres minor	

MR SHOULDER JOINT: CORONAL IMAGES—ANTERIOR TO POSTERIOR

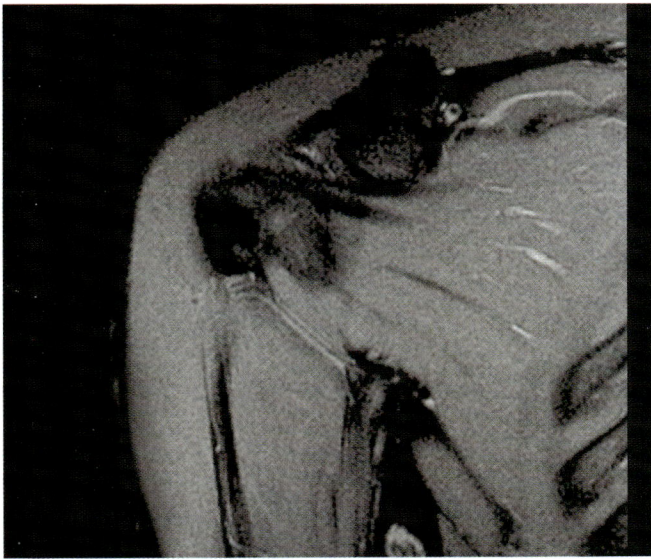

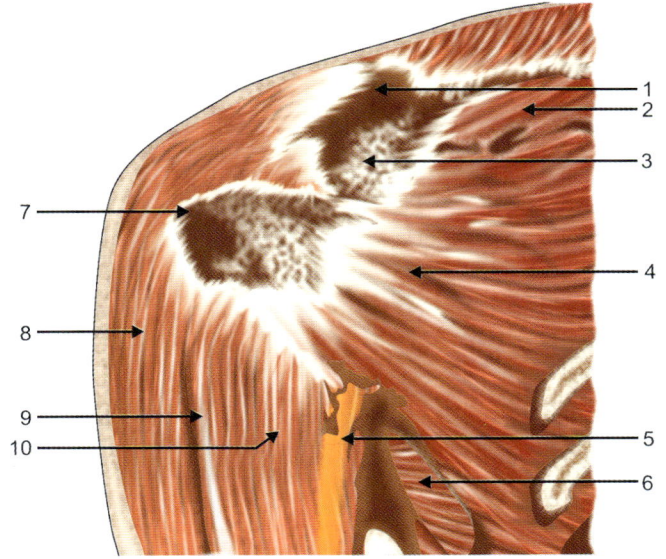

Figure 10.15

1. Clavicle	6. Latissimus dorsi
2. Supraspinatus	7. Lesser tuberosity
3. Coracoid process	8. Deltoid
4. Subscapularis muscle, tendon	9. Biceps tendon, long head
5. Neurovascular bundle	10. Biceps brachii

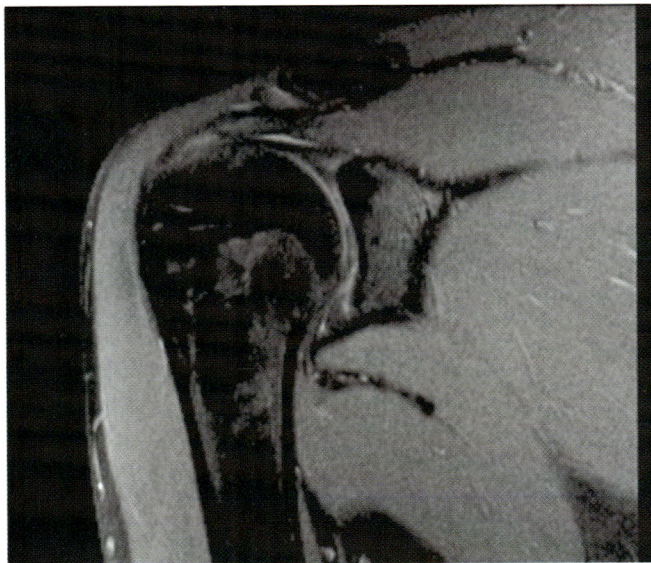

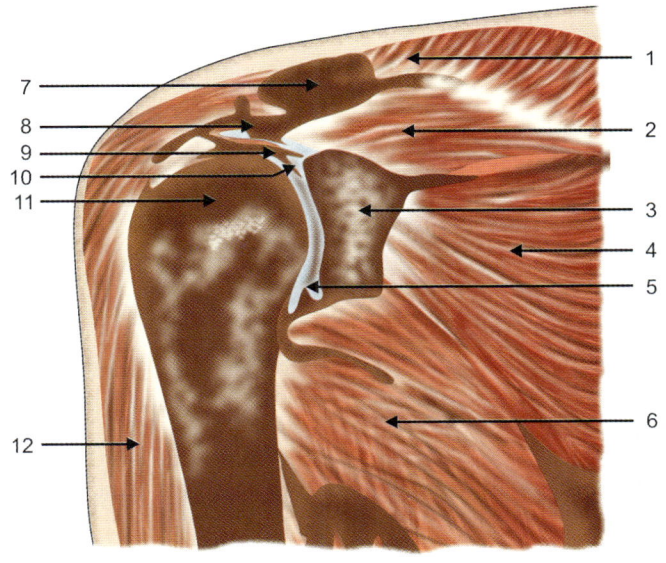

Figure 10.16

1. Trapezius	5. Inferior labrum	9. Biceps-labral complex
2. Supraspinatus muscle	6. Latissimus dorsi and teres major	10. Superior labrum
3. Glenoid	7. Clavicle	11. Humerus, head
4. Subscapularis	8. Supraspinatus tendon	12. Deltoid

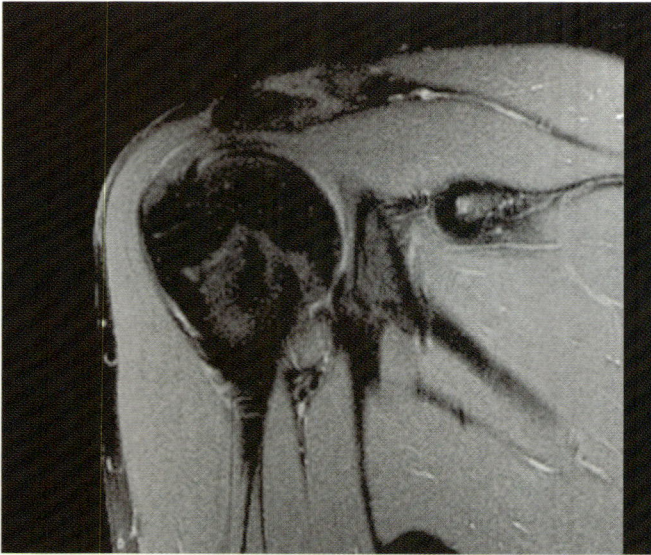

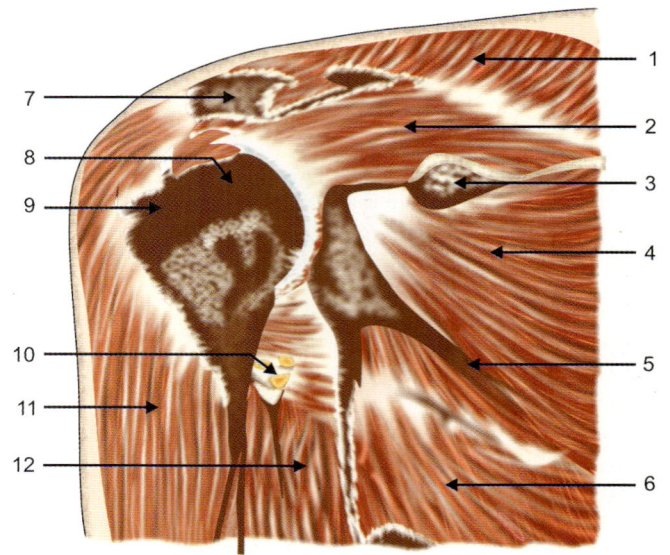

Figure 10.17

1. Trapezius	5. Scapula	9. Greater tuberosity
2. Supraspinatus	6. Teres minor	10. Profunda brachii vessels, radial nerve
3. Scapular spine	7. Acromion process	11. Deltoid
4. Infraspinatus	8. Humerus, head	12. Triceps, long head

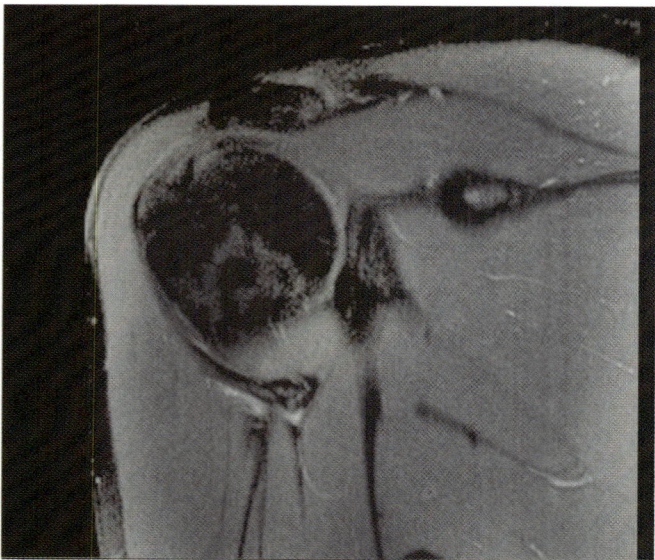

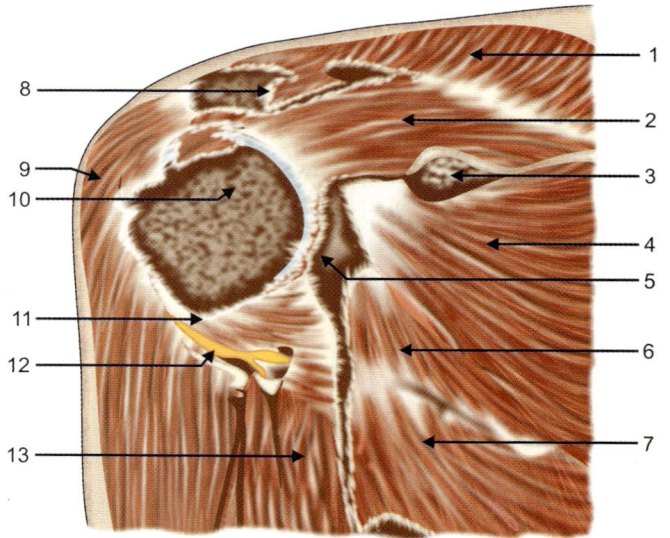

Figure 10.18

1. Trapezius	6. Teres minor	11. Surgical neck
2. Supraspinatus	7. Teres major	12. Posterior circumflex artery, axillary nerve
3. Scapular spine	8. Acromion process	13. Triceps, long head
4. Infraspinatus	9. Deltoid	
5. Labrum	10. Humerus, head	

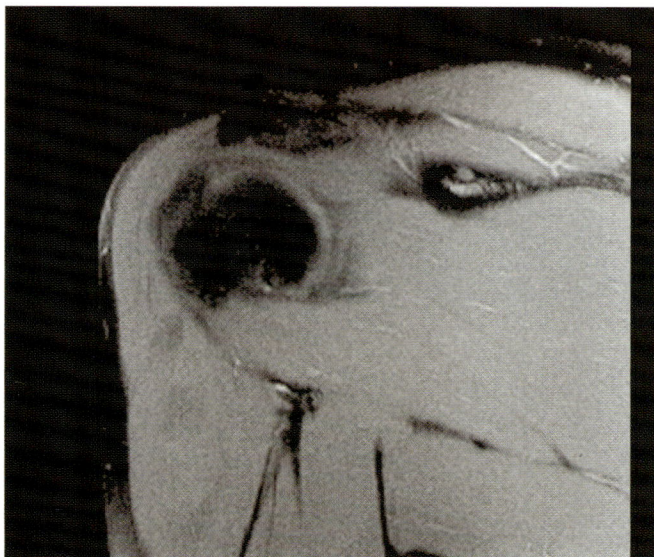

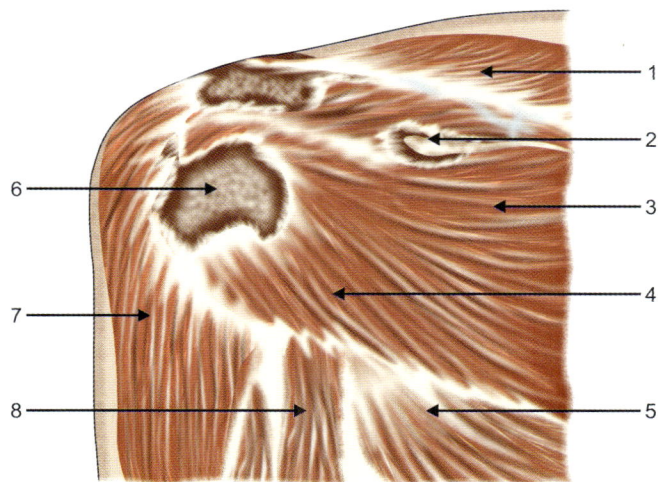

Figure 10.19

1. Trapezius	5. Teres major
2. Scapular spine	6. Humerus, head
3. Infraspinatus	7. Deltoid
4. Teres minor	8. Triceps

CHAPTER 11

Arm and Forearm

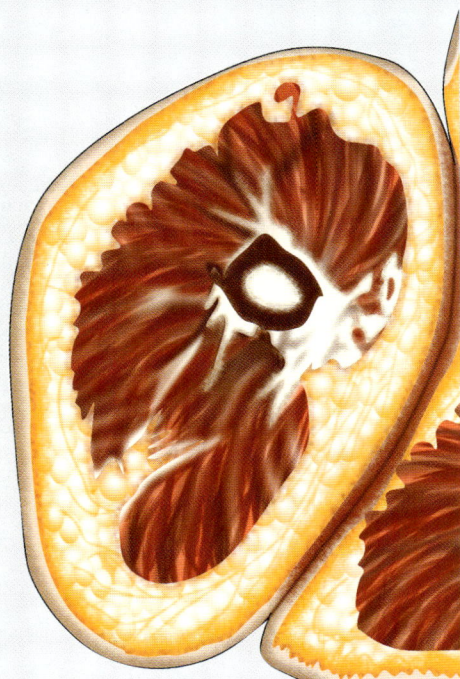

ARM

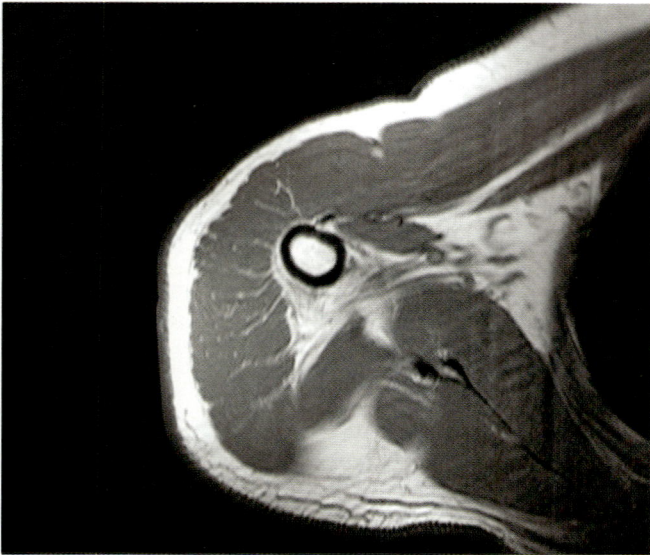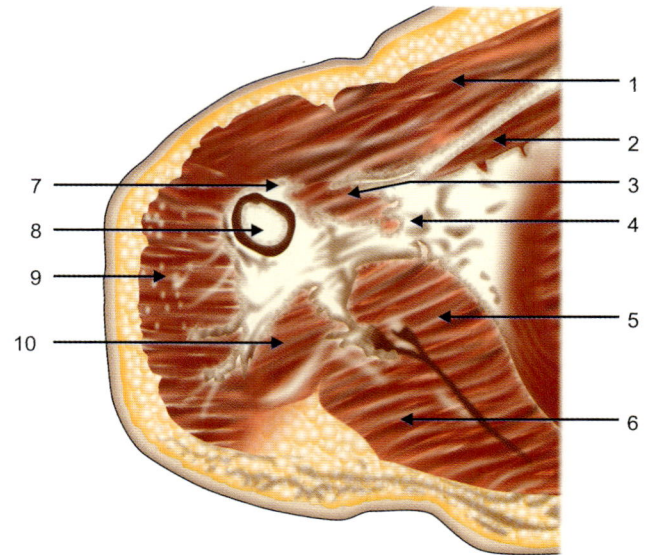

Figure 11.1

1. Pectoralis major	6. Infraspinatus
2. Pectoralis minor	7. Biceps, long head tendon
3. Biceps brachii, short head	8. Humerus
4. Neurovascular bundle	9. Deltoid
5. Subscapularis	10. Triceps

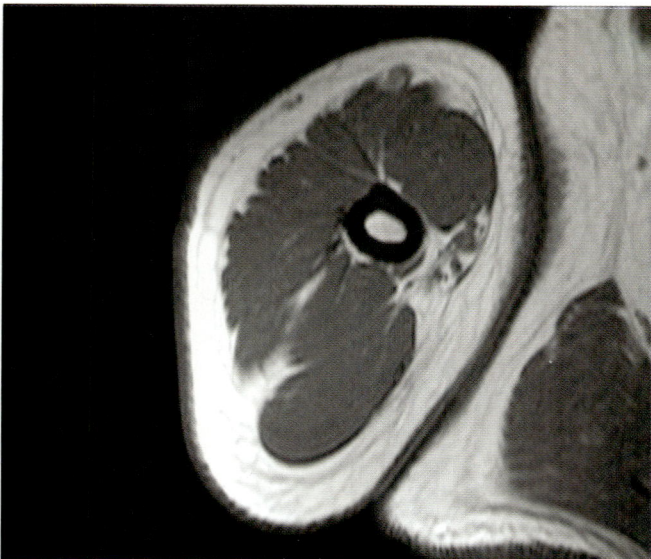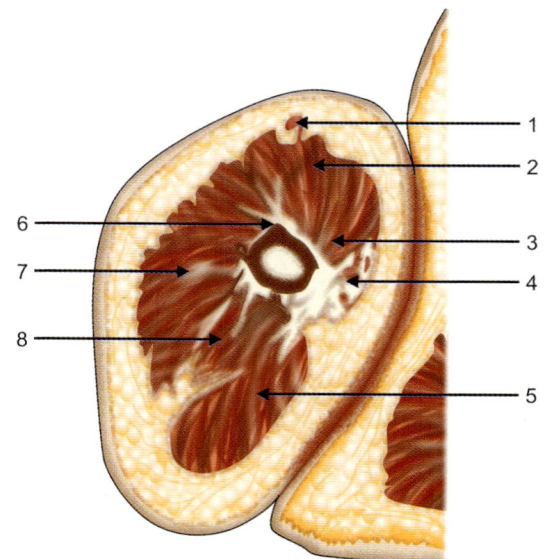

Figure 11.2

1. Cephalic vein	5. Triceps, long head
2. Biceps brachii	6. Deltoid tuberosity
3. Coracobrachialis	7. Deltoid
4. Neurovascular bundle	8. Triceps, lateral head
[Brachial artery, Brachial veins, Median and Ulnar nerves]	

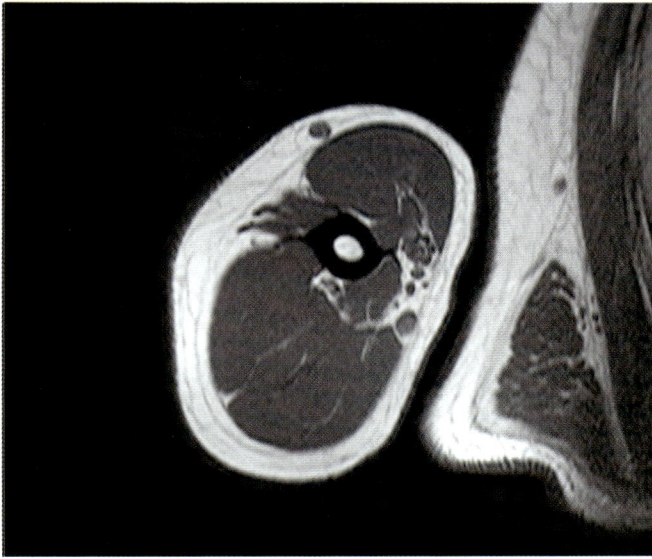
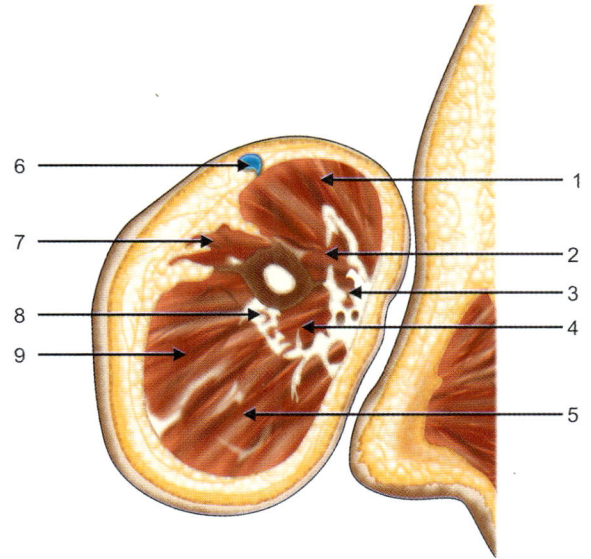

Figure 11.3

1. Biceps brachii	6. Cephalic vein
2. Brachialis	7. Deltoid insertion
3. Neurovascular bundle	8. Radial nerve, deep brachial artery
4. Triceps, medial head	9. Triceps, lateral head
5. Triceps, long head	

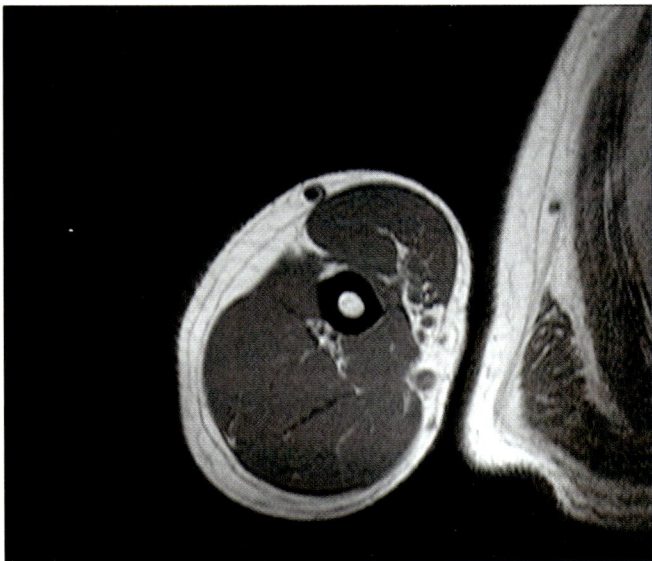
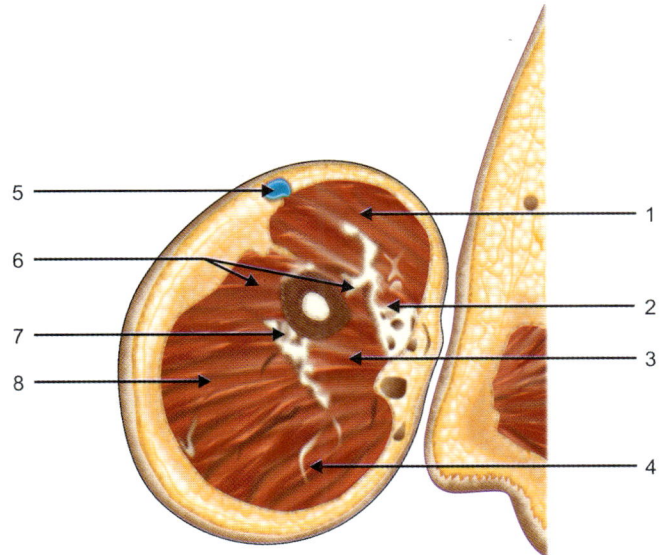

Figure 11.4

1. Biceps brachii	5. Cephalic vein
2. Neurovascular bundle	6. Brachialis
3. Triceps, medial head	7. Radial nerve, deep brachial artery
4. Triceps, long head	8. Triceps, lateral head

FOREARM

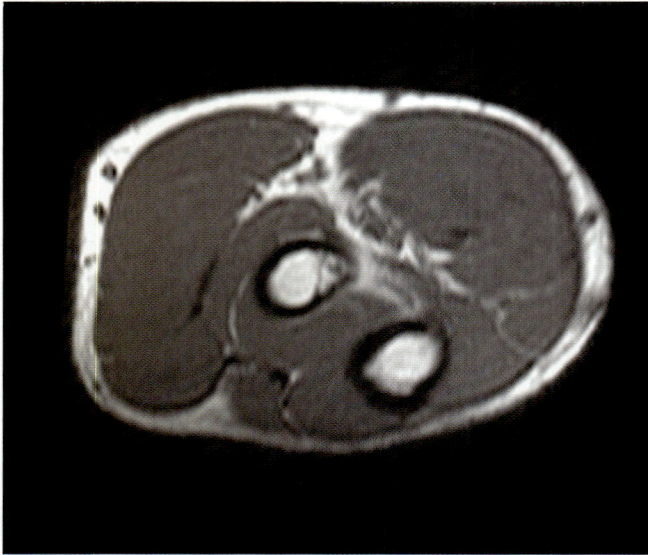
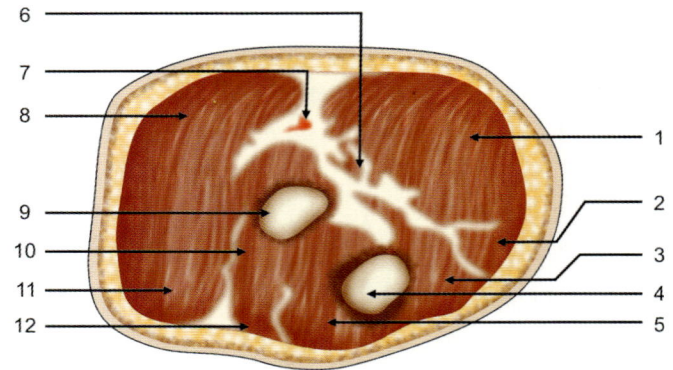

Figure 11.5

1. Flexor digitorum superficialis	5. Extensor carpi ulnaris	9. Radius
2. Flexor carpi ulnaris	6. Ulnar artery, nerve	10. Supinator
3. Flexor digitorum profundus	7. Radial artery	11. Extensor carpi radialis brevis
4. Ulna	8. Brachioradialis	12. Extensor digitorum

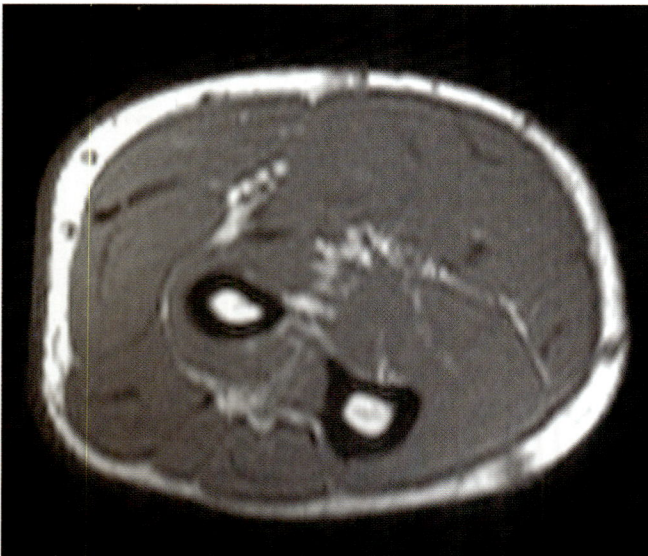
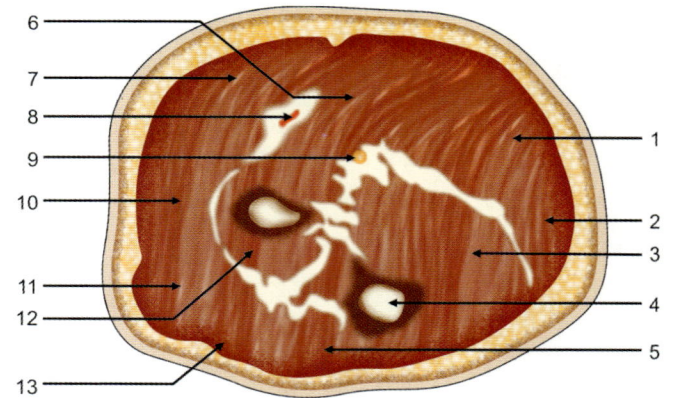

Figure 11.6

1. Flexor digitorum superficialis	8. Radial artery
2. Flexor carpi ulnaris	9. Median nerve
3. Flexor digitorum profundus	10. Extensor carpi longus
4. Ulna	11. Extensor carpi radialis brevis
5. Extensor carpi ulnaris	12. Supinator
6. Flexor carpi radialis	13. Extensor digitorum
7. Brachioradialis	

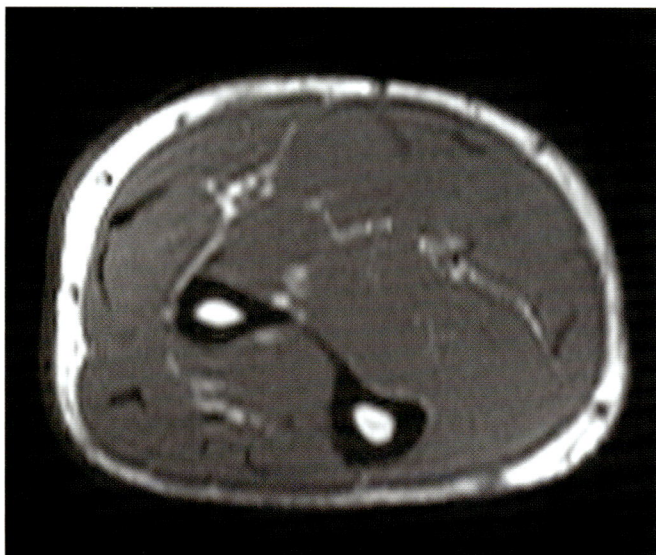

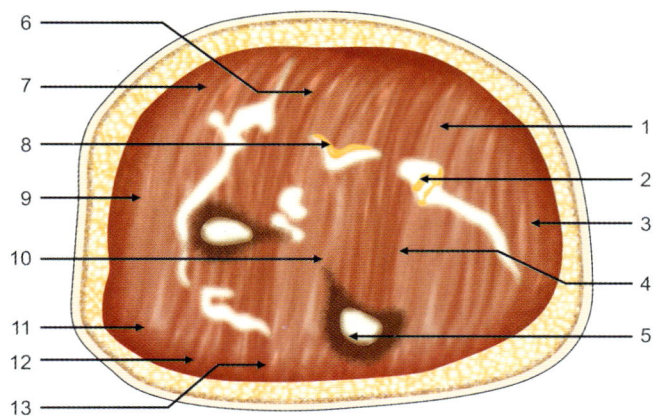

Figure 11.7

1. Flexor digitorum superficialis	6. Flexor carpi radialis	11. Extensor carpi radialis brevis
2. Ulnar nerve	7. Brachioradialis	12. Extensor digitorum
3. Flexor carpi ulnaris	8. Median nerve	13. Extensor carpi ulnaris
4. Flexor digitorum profundus	9. Extensor carpi radialis longus	
5. Ulna	10. Interosseous membrane	

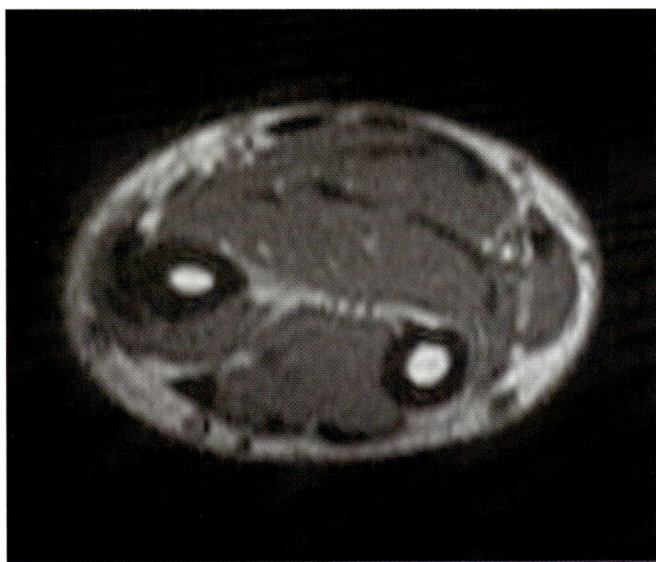

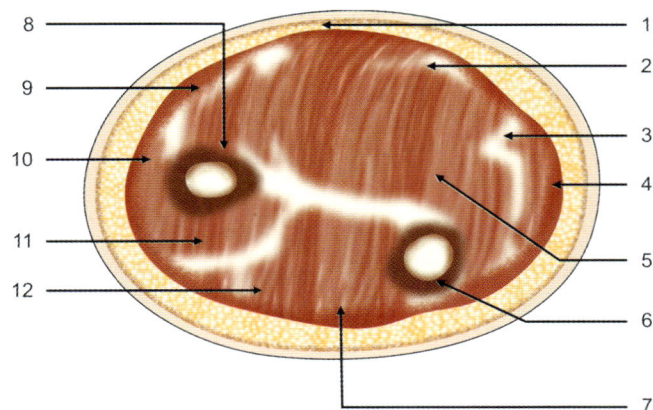

Figure 11.8

1. Palmaris longus	5. Flexor digitorum profundus	9. Radial artery
2. Flexor digitorum superficialis	6. Ulna	10. Extensor carpi radialis
3. Ulnar artery, nerve	7. Extensor carpi ulnaris	11. Abductor pollicis longus
4. Flexor carpi ulnaris	8. Radius	12. Extensor digitorum

CHAPTER 12

Elbow

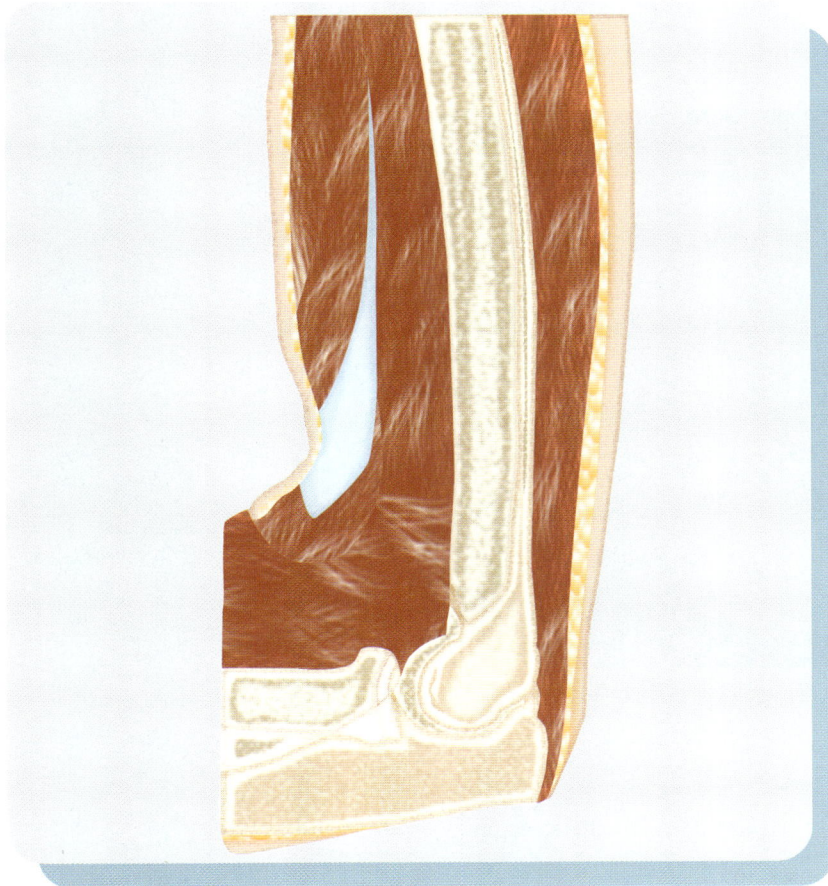

X-RAY IMAGES

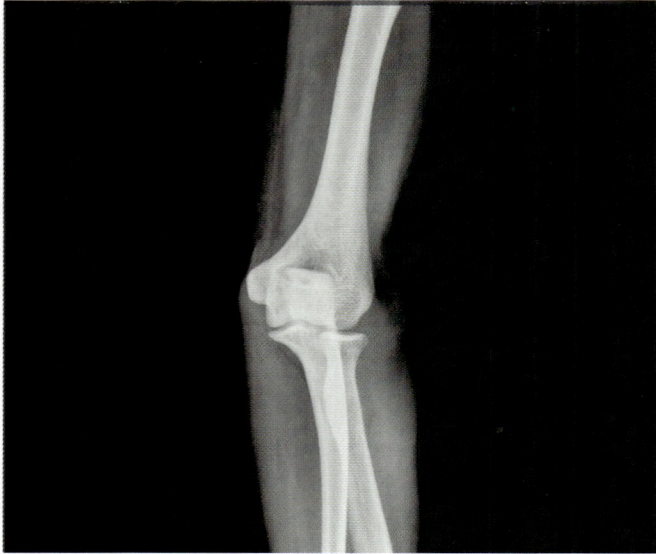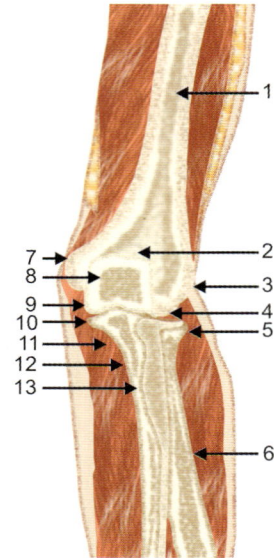

Figure 12.1

1. Humerus	6. Radius	11. Muscle
2. Olecranon fossa	7. Medial epicondyl	12. Ulna
3. Lateral epicondyle	8. Olecranon process	13. Radial tuberosity
4. Capitulum	9. Trochlea	
5. Radius, head	10. Coronoid process, ulna	

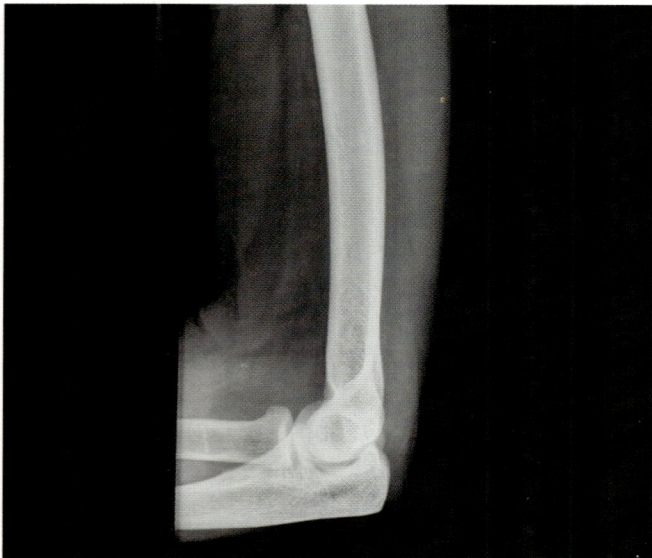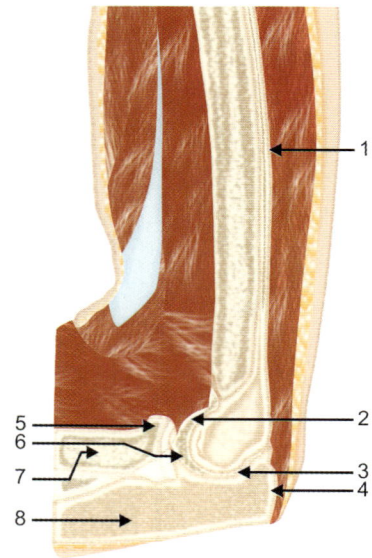

Figure 12.2

1. Humerus	5. Radius, head
2. Capitulum	6. Coronoid process
3. Trochlear notch	7. Radius
4. Olecranon process	8. Ulna

AXIAL VIEWS

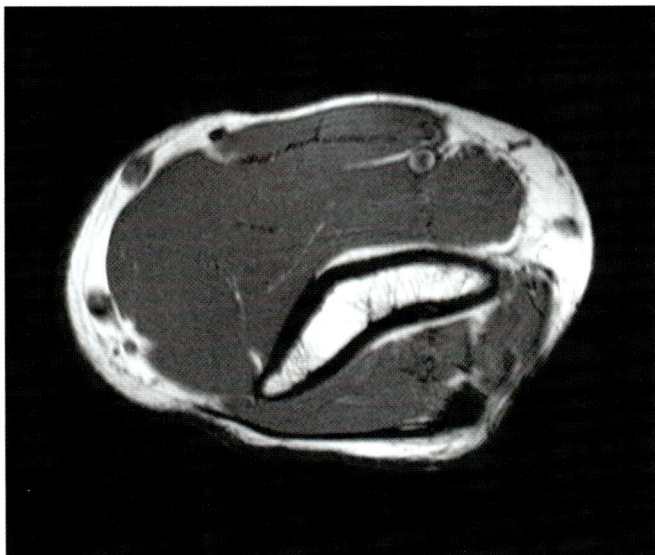

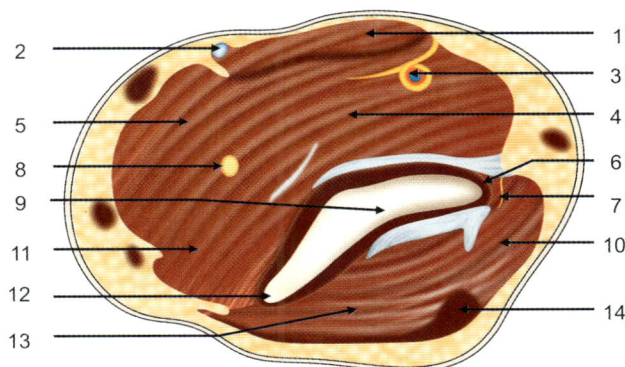

Figure 12.3

1. Biceps brachii	5. Brachioradialis	10. Triceps, long head
2. Cephalic vein	6. Medial supracondylar ridge	11. Extensor carpi radialis longus
3. Brachial artery, vein, median nerve	7. Ulnar nerve	12. Lateral supracondylar ridge
	8. Radial nerve	13. Tricep, medial and lateral heads
4. Brachialis	9. Humerus	14. Triceps tendon

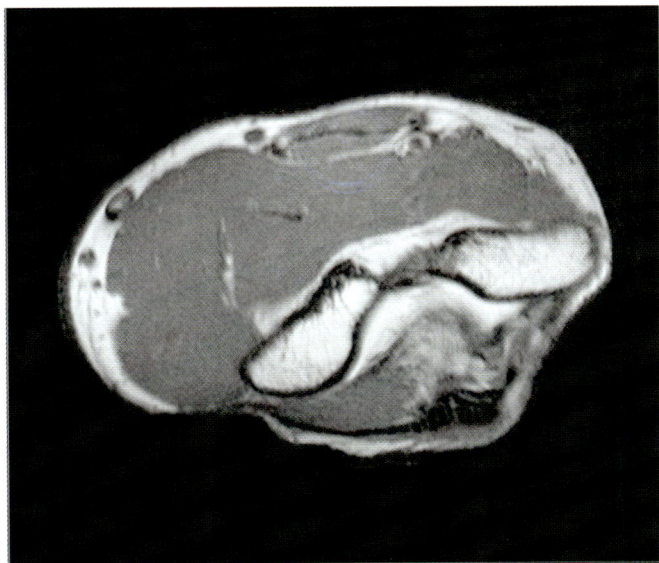

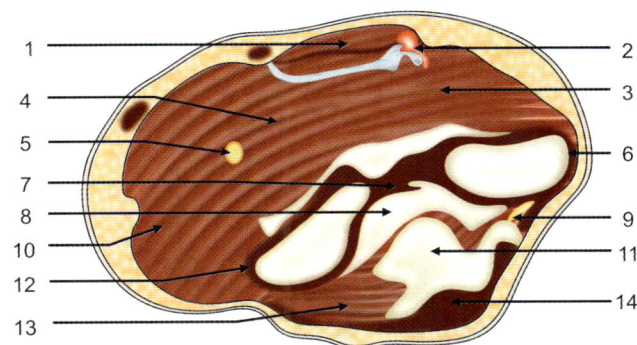

Figure 12.4

1. Biceps brachii	5. Radial nerve	10. Extensor carpi radialis longus
2. Neurovascular bundle (brachial artery, vein, medial nerve)	6. Medial supracondylar ridge	11. Olecranon process
	7. Olecranon fossa	12. Lateral supracondylar ridge
3. Brachialis	8. Post fat pad	13. Triceps muscle
4. Brachioradialis	9. Ulnar nerve	14. Triceps tendon

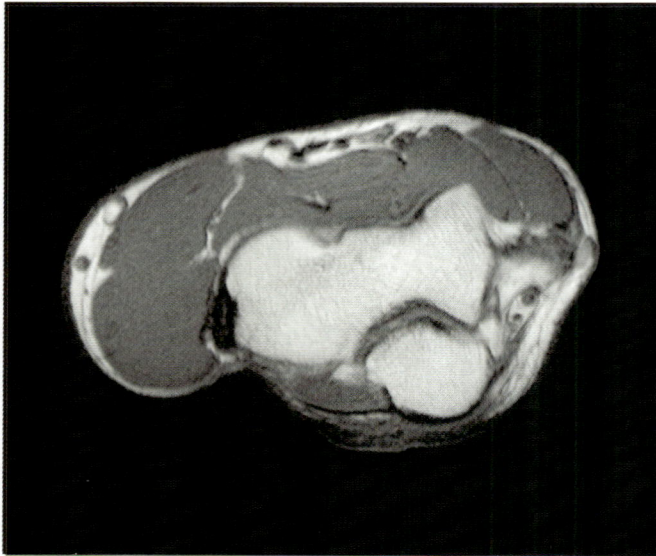

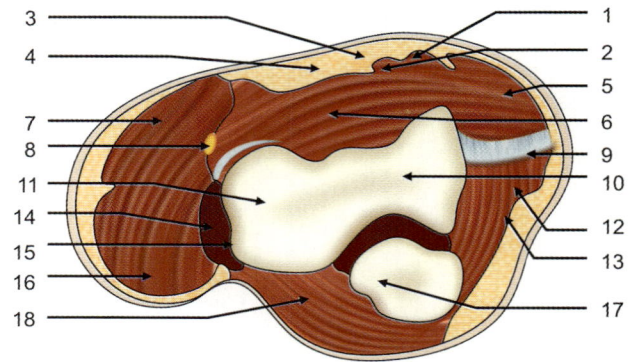

Figure 12.5

1. Median nerve	7. Brachioradialis	13. Ulnar nerve
2. Brachial artery	8. Radial nerve	14. Common extensor tendon
3. Bicipital aponeurosis	9. Common flexor tendon	15. Lateral epicondyle
4. Biceps brachii tendon	10. Trochlea	16. Extensor carpi radialis longus
5. Pronator teres	11. Capitulum	17. Olecranon process
6. Brachialis	12. Medial epicondyle	18. Anconeus

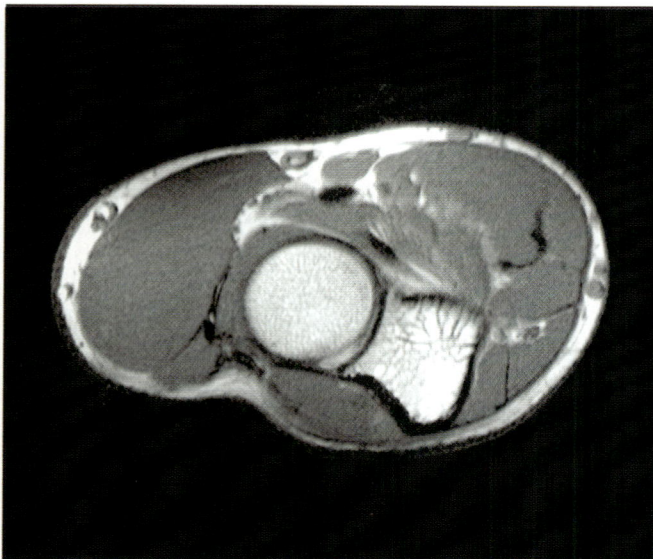

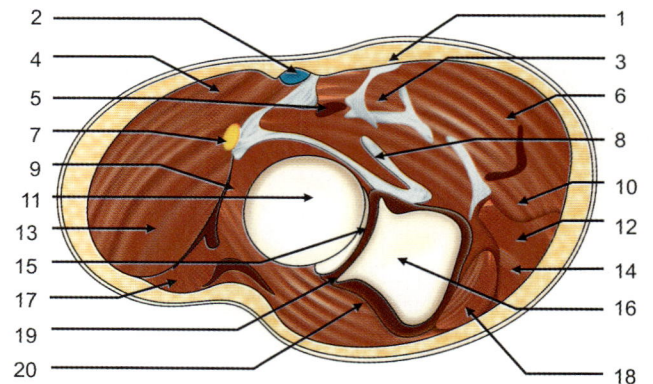

Figure 12.6

1. Bicipital aponeurosis	8. Brachialis muscle and tendon	15. Radial notch
2. Cephalic vein	9. Supinator	16. Ulna
3. Brachial artery	10. Palmaris longus	17. Extensor digitorum
4. Brachioradialis	11. Radius, head	18. Flexor carpi ulnaris
5. Biceps brachii tendon	12. Ulnar nerve	19. Supinator crest
6. Pronator teres	13. Extensor carpi radialis longus	20. Anconeus
7. Radial nerve	14. Flexor digitorum superficialis	

CORONAL VIEWS

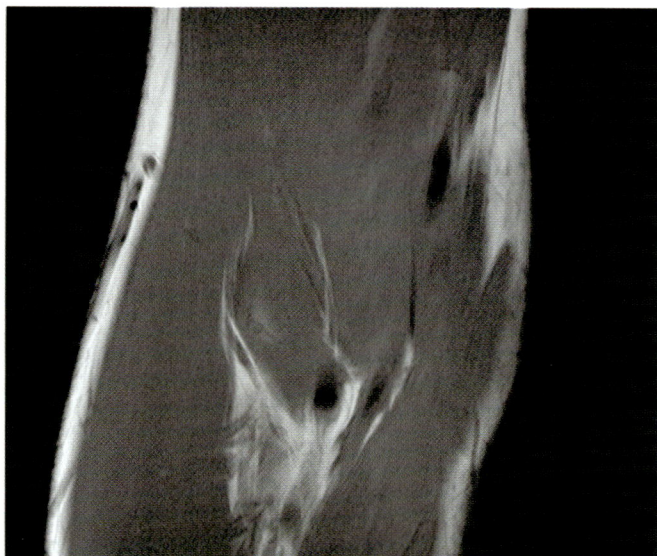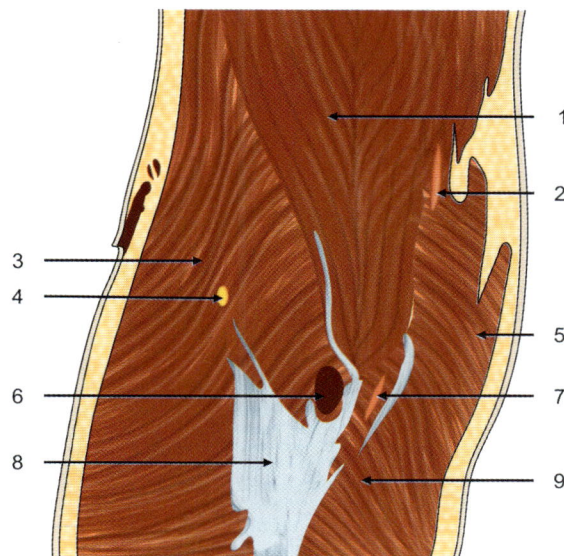

Figure 12.7

1. Brachialis	4. Radial nerve	7. Ulnar artery
2. Brachial artery	5. Pronator teres	8. Supinator
3. Brachioradialis	6. Biceps tendon	9. Flexor carpi radialis

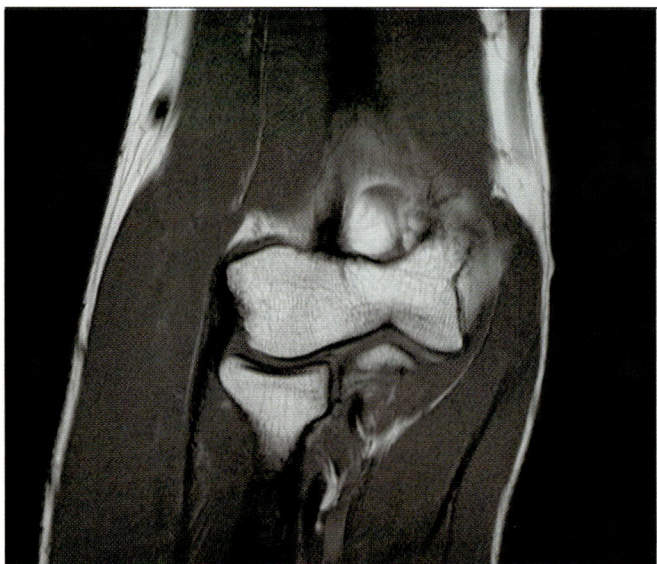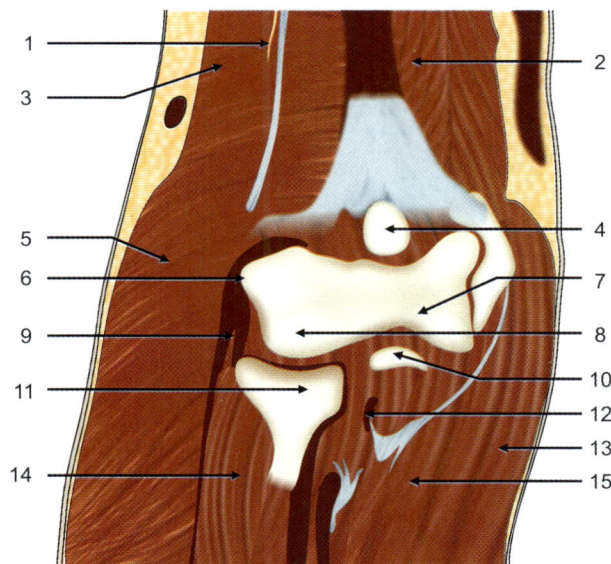

Figure 12.8

1. Radial nerve	6. Lateral epicondyle	11. Radius, head
2. Brachialis	7. Trochlea	12. Brachialis muscle, tendon
3. Brachioradialis	8. Capitulum	13. Flexor carpi ulnaris
4. Olecranon fossa	9. Common extensor tendon	14. Supinator muscle
5. Extensor carpi radialis longus	10. Coronoid process	15. Flexor digitorum superficialis

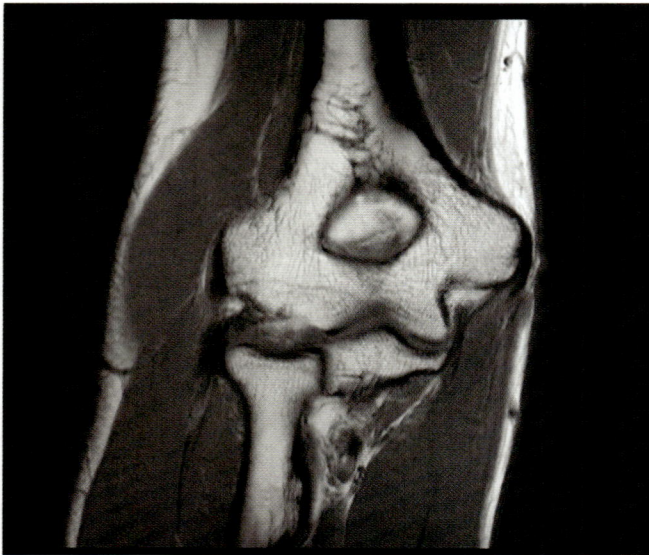

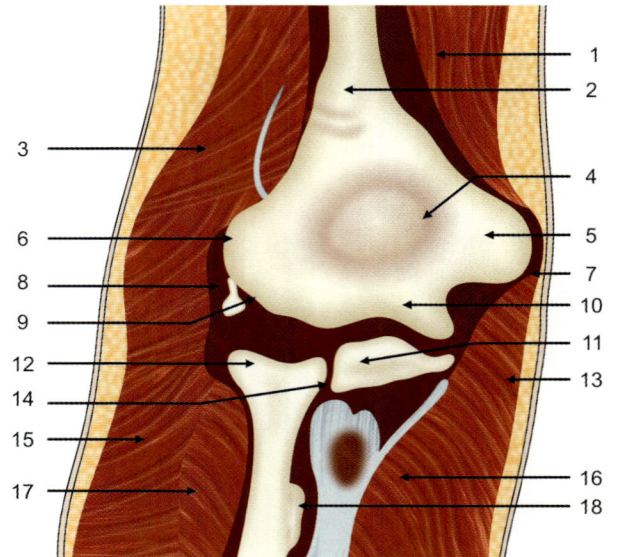

Figure 12.9

1. Triceps	7. Common flexor tendon	13. Flexor carpi ulnaris
2. Humerus	8. Common extensor tendon	14. Radioulnar joint
3. Extensor carpi radialis longus	9. Capitulum	15. Extensor carpi radialis brevis
4. Olecranon fossa	10. Trochlea	16. Flexor digitorum profundus
5. Medial epicondyle	11. Coronoid process	17. Supinator
6. Lateral epicondyle	12. Radius, head	18. Radial tuberosity

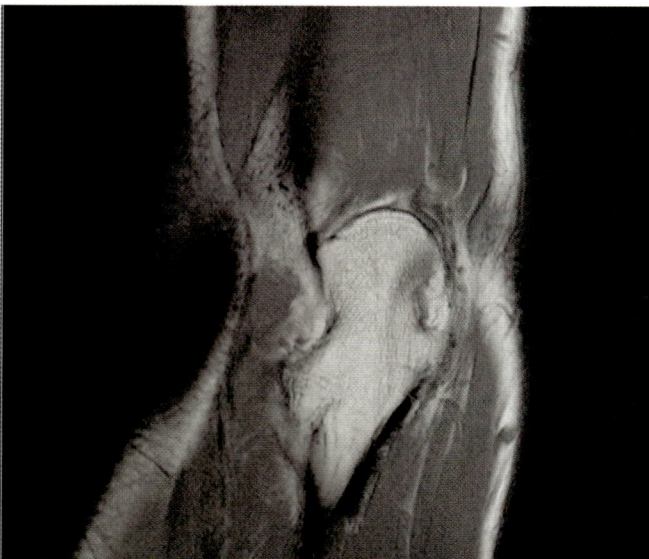

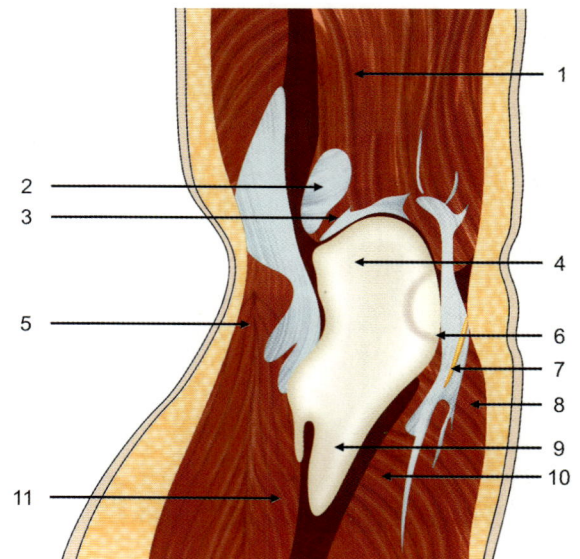

Figure 12.10

1. Triceps	5. Anconeus	9. Ulnar shaft
2. Humerus	6. Coronoid process	10. Flexor digitorum profundus
3. Olecranon fossa	7. Ulnar nerve	11. Extensor muscles
4. Olecranon process	8. Flexor carpi ulnaris	

SAGITTAL VIEWS

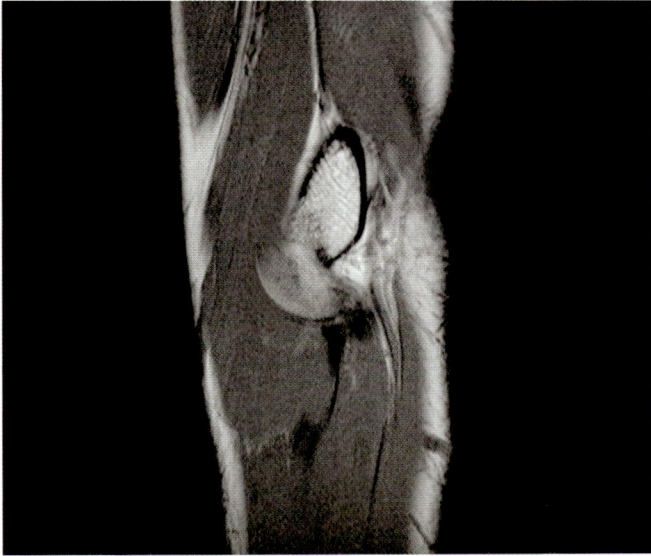

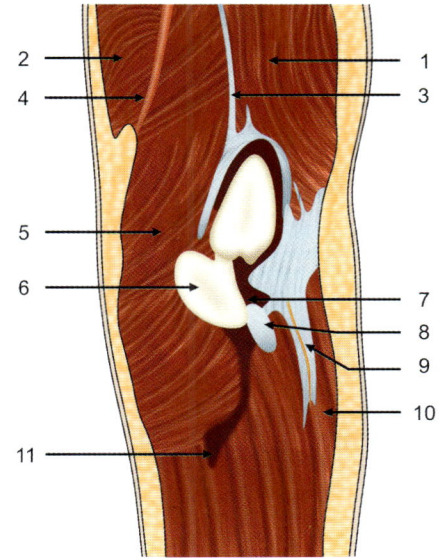

Figure 12.11

1. Triceps	5. Brachialis muscle	9. Ulnar nerve
2. Biceps brachii	6. Trochlea	10. Flexor carpi ulnaris
3. Medial intermuscular septum	7. Medial epicondyle	11. Superficial flexor muscles
4. Brachial artery	8. Common flexor tendon	

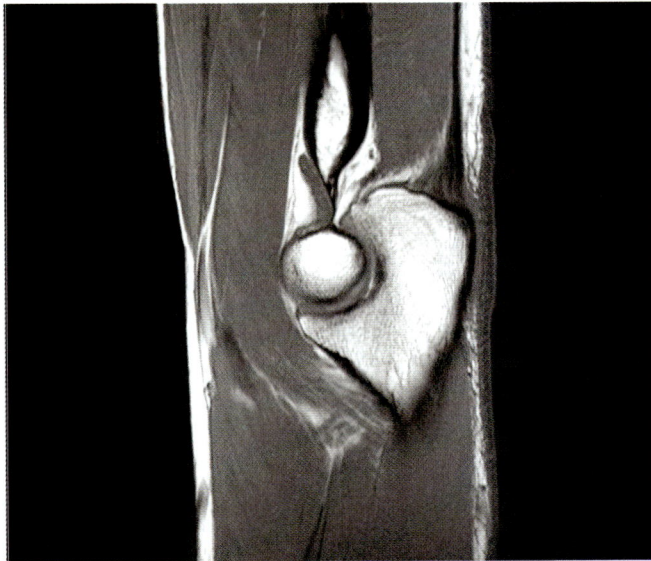

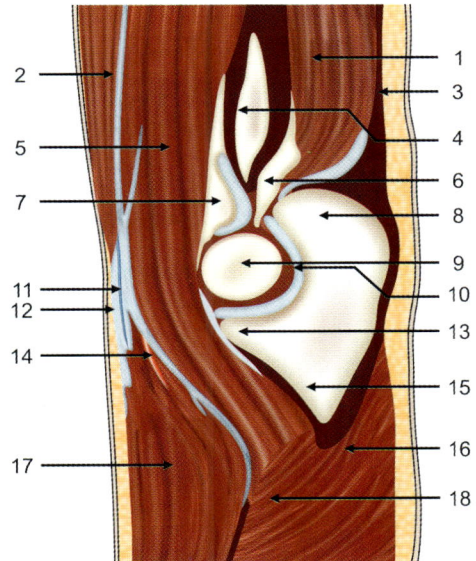

Figure 12.12

1. Triceps	7. Anterior fat pad	13. Coronoid process
2. Biceps brachii	8. Olecranon process	14. Brachial artery
3. Triceps tendon	9. Trochlea	15. Ulna
4. Humerus	10. Trochlear notch	16. Flexor carpi ulnaris
5. Brachialis	11. Cephalic vein	17. Superficial flexor muscles
6. Olecranon fossa and posterior fat pad	12. Bicipital aponeurosis	18. Flexor digitorum profundus

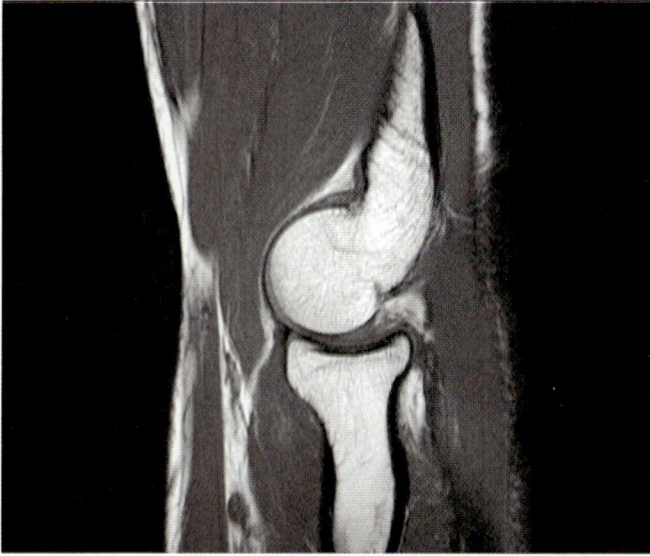

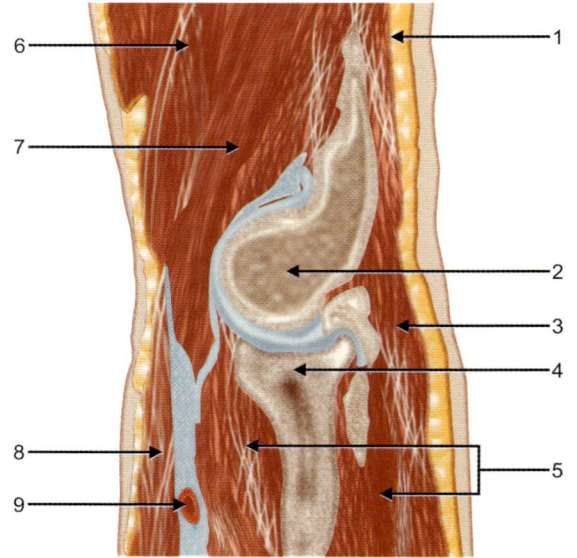

Figure 12.13

1. Triceps	6. Brachioradialis
2. Capitulum	7. Extensor carpi radialis longus
3. Anconeus	8. Brachioradialis
4. Radius, head	9. Radial artery
5. Supinator	

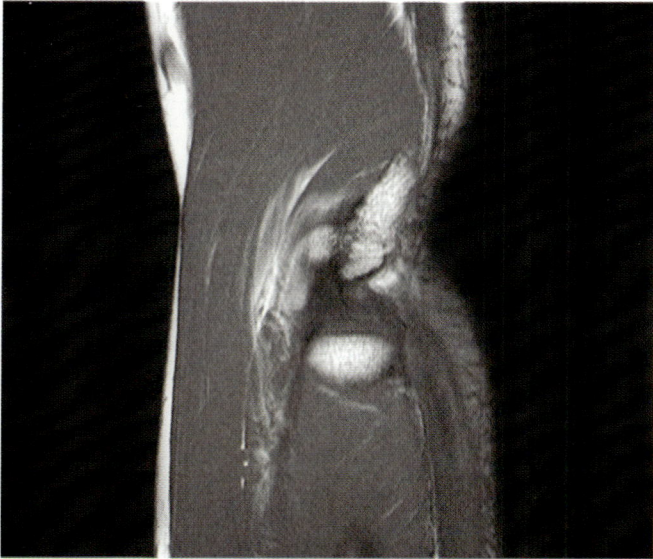

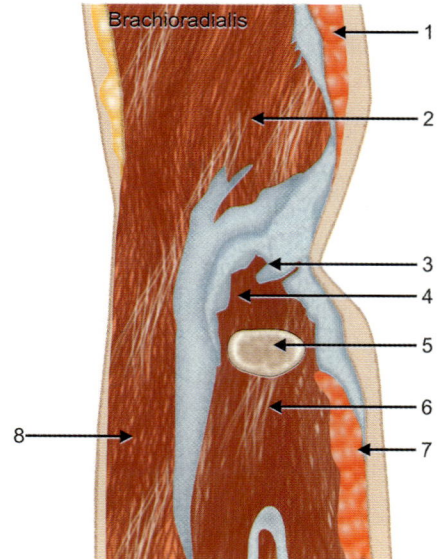

Figure 12.14

1. Triceps	5. Radius, head
2. Extensor carpi radialis longus	6. Supinator
3. Lateral epicondyle	7. Extensor digitorum
4. Common extensor tendon	8. Brachioradialis

CHAPTER 13

Wrist

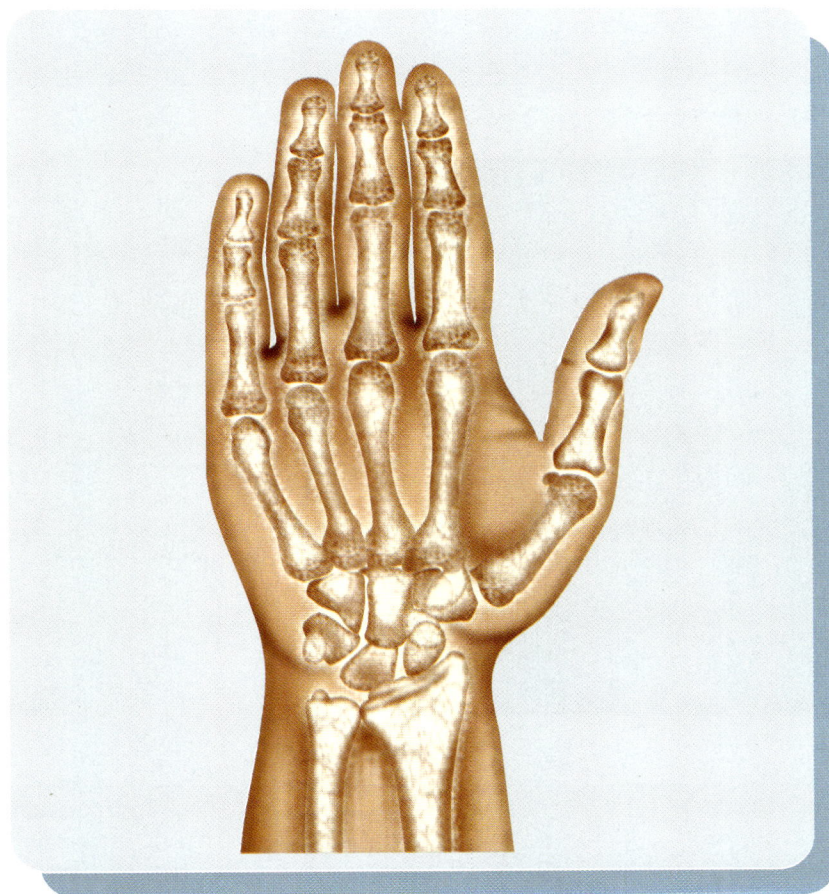

X-RAYS

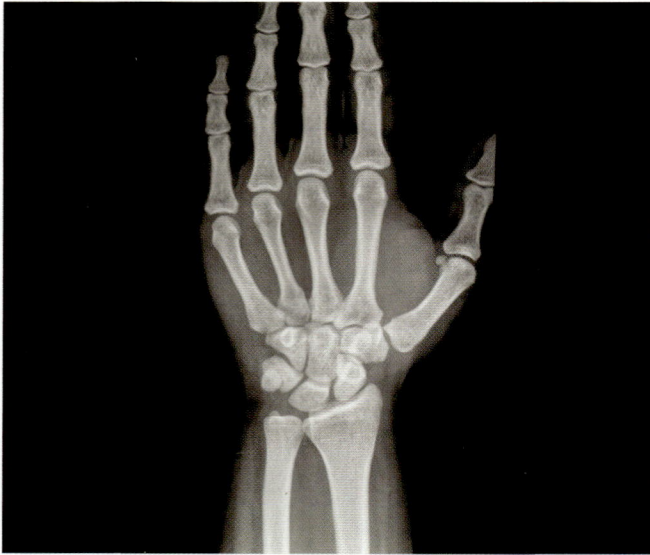
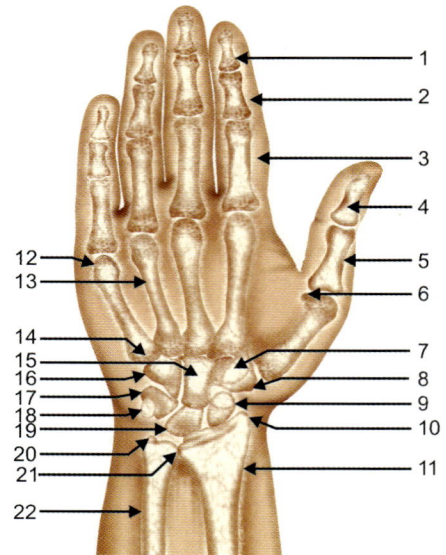

Figure 13.1

1. Distal phalanx	7. Trapezoid	13. Fourth metacarpal	19. Lunate
2. Middle phalanx	8. Trapezium	14. Base, fifth metacarpal	20. Styloid process of ulna
3. Proximal phalanx	9. Scaphoid	15. Capitate	21. Inferior radioulnar joint
4. Distal phalanx, thumb	10. Styloid process of radius	16. Hamate	22. Ulna
5. Proximal phalanx, thumb	11. Radius	17. Triquetral	
6. Sesamoid bone	12. Head, fifth metacarpal	18. Pisiform	

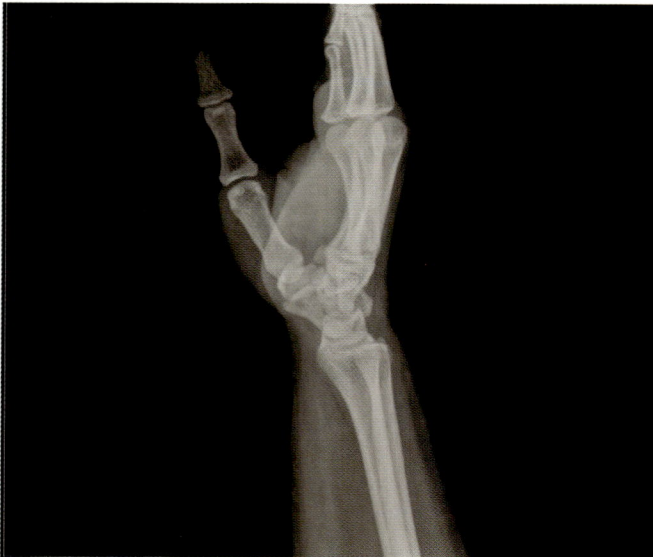
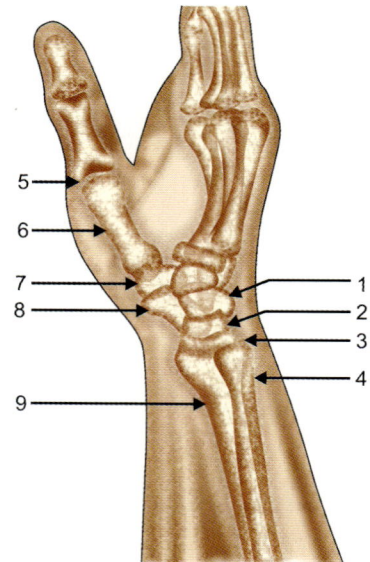

Figure 13.2

1. Capitate	4. Ulna	7. Trapezium
2. Lunate	5. Metacarpophalangeal joint	8. Scaphoid
3. Styloid process	6. First metacarpal	9. Radius

AXIAL IMAGES

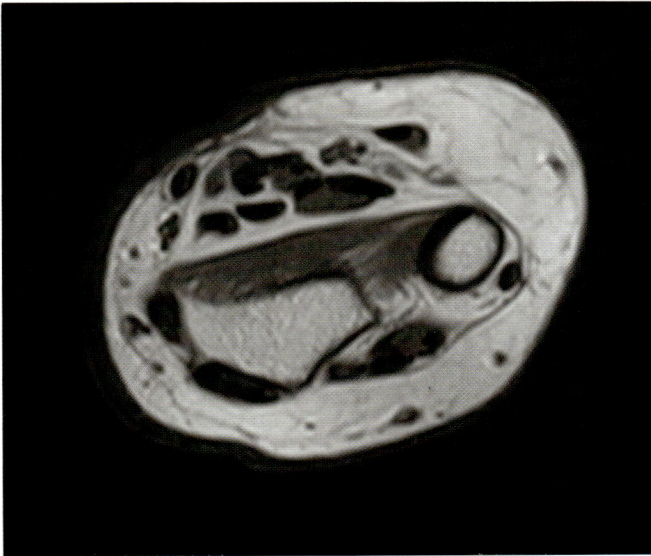
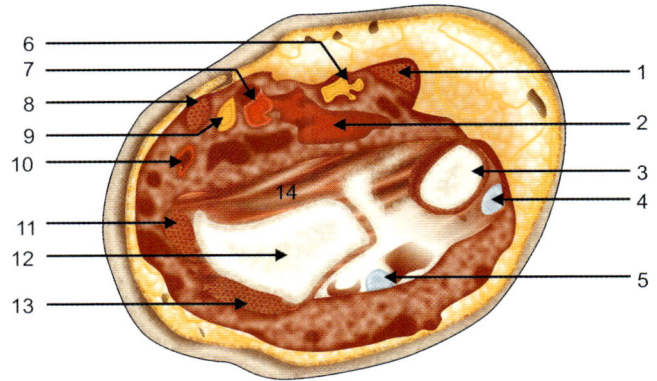

Figure 13.3

1. Flexor carpi ulnaris	6. Ulnar artery, nerve	11. Abductor pollicis longus
2. Flexor digitorum profundus	7. Flexor digitorum superficialis	12. Radius
3. Ulna	8. Flexor carpi radialis	13. Extensor carpi radialis longus, brevis
4. Extensor carpi ulnaris tendon	9. Median nerve	
5. Extensor digitorum tendons	10. Radial artery	14. Pronator quadratus

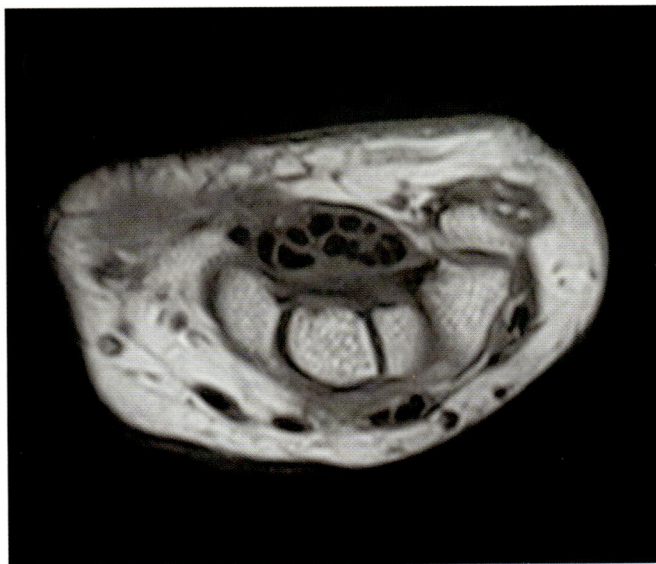
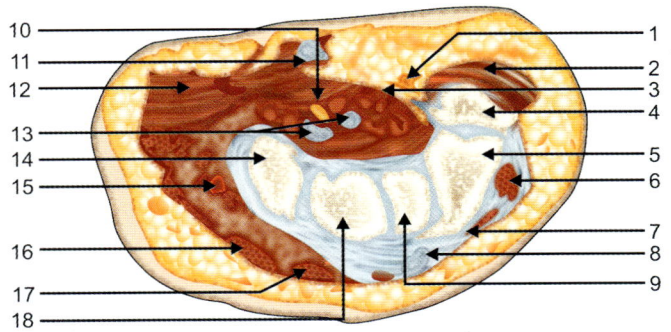

Figure 13.4

1. Ulnar artery, nerve	7. Extensor retinaculum	13. Flexor digitorum tendons
2. Abductor digiti minimi	8. Extensor digitorum tendons	14. Scaphoid
3. Flexor retinaculum	9. Hamate	15. Radial artery
4. Pisiform	10. Median nerve	16. Extensor carpi radialis longus, brevis
5. Triquetrum	11. Palmaris longus tendon	17. Extensor pollicis longus
6. Extensor carpi ulnaris	12. Abductor pollicis brevis	18. Capitate

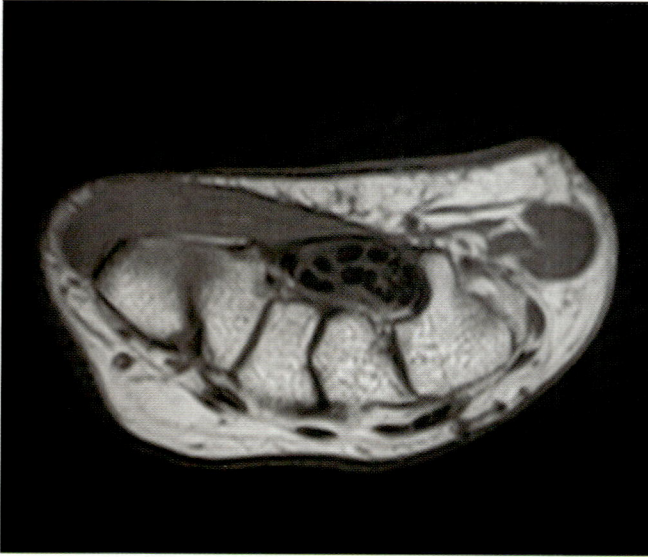

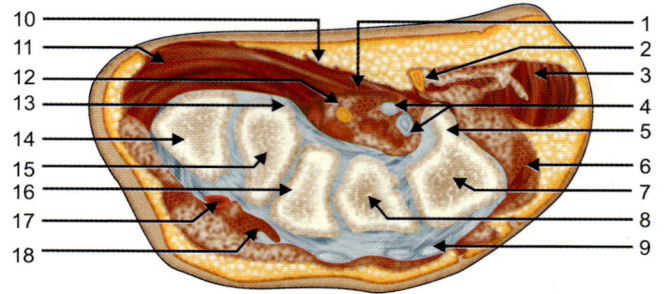

Figure 13.5

1. Flexor retinaculum	7. Hamate	13. Tubercle of trapezium
2. Ulnar nerve	8. Capitate	14. First metacarpal, base
3. Abductor digiti minimi	9. Extensor tendons	15. Trapezium
4. Flexor tendons	10. Palmar aponeurosis	16. Trapezoid
5. Hook of Hamate	11. Abductor pollicis brevis	17. Radial artery
6. Extensor carpi ulnaris	12. Median nerve	18. Extensor carpi radialis longus, brevis

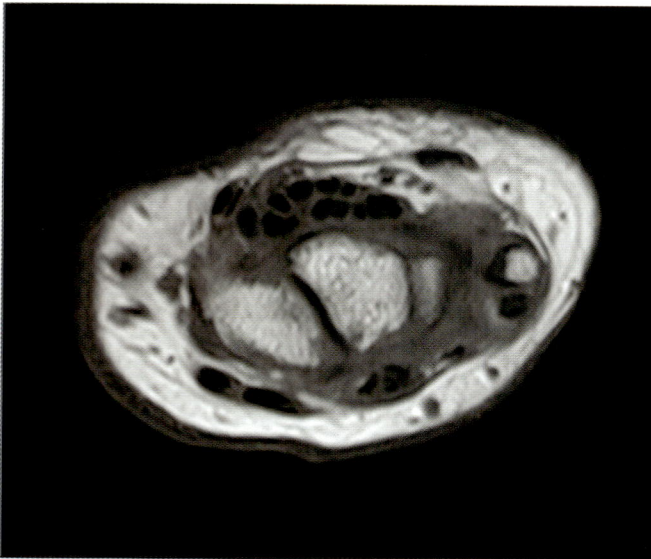

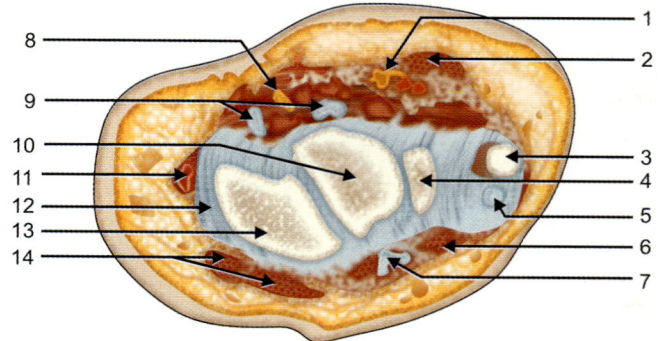

Figure 13.6

1. Ulnar nerve, artery	6. Extensor retinaculum	11. Radial artery
2. Flexor carpi ulnaris	7. Extensor tendons	12. Abductor pollicis longus
3. Ulnar styloid	8. Median nerve	13. Scaphoid
4. Triquetrum	9. Flexor digitorum tendons	14. Extensor carpi radialis longus, brevis
5. Extensor carpi ulnaris tendon	10. Lunate	

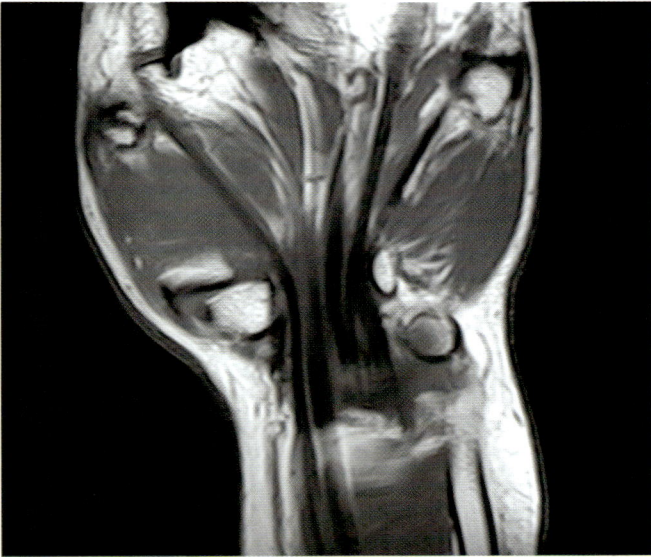
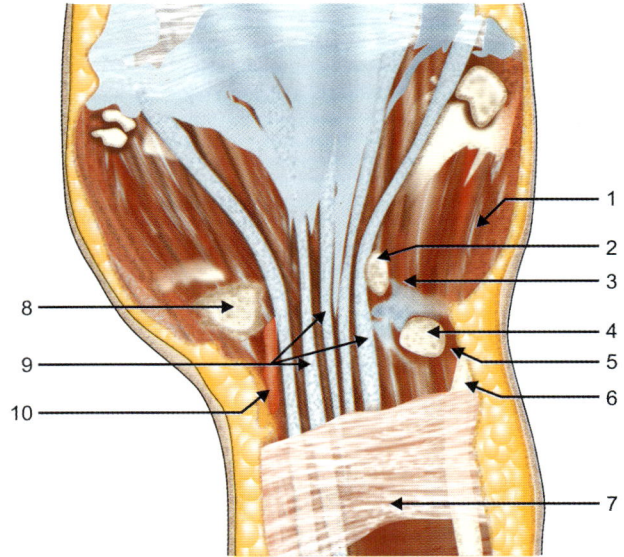

Figure 13.7

1. Abductor digiti minimi
2. Hook of hamate
3. Pisohamate ligament
4. Pisiform
5. Flexor carpi ulnaris (insertion)
6. Ulna
7. Pronator quadratus
8. Trapezium, tubercle
9. Flexor digitorum profundus and superficialis tendons
10. Radial artery

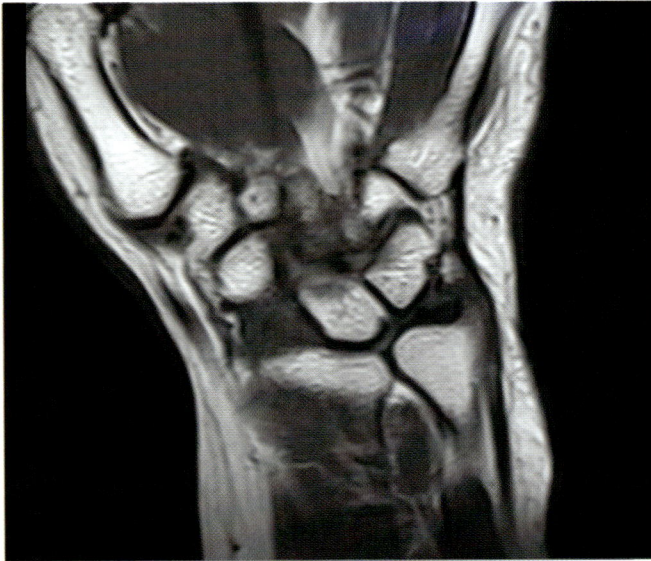
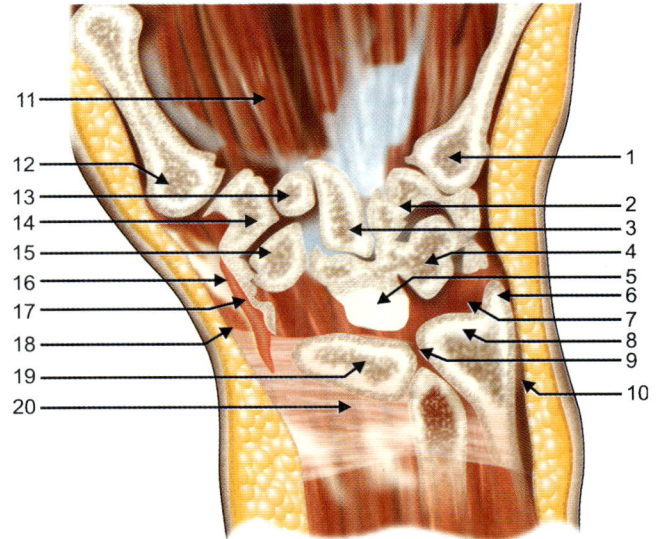

Figure 13.8

1. Fifth metacarpal base
2. Hamate
3. Capitate
4. Triquetrum
5. Lunate
6. Ulnar styloid
7. Triangular fibrocartilage
8. Ulna
9. Distal radioulnar joint
10. Extensor carpi ulnaris tendon
11. Abductor pollicis, oblique head
12. First metacarpal base
13. Trapezoid
14. Trapezium
15. Scaphoid, distal pole
16. Snuff box
17. Radial artery
18. Extensor pollicis brevis and abductor pollicis longus tendons
19. Radius
20. Pronator quadratus

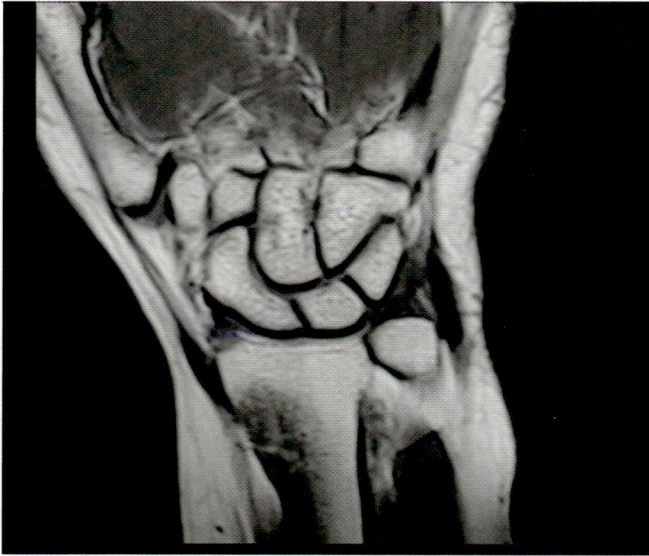
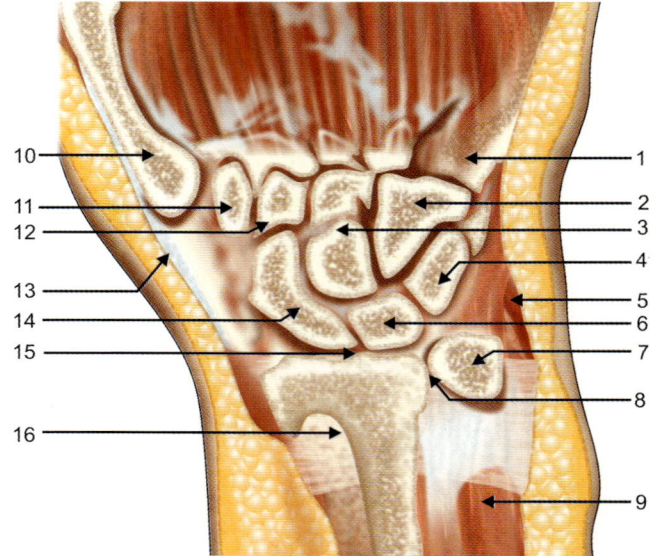

Figure 13.9

1. Fifth metacarpal base
2. Hamate
3. Capitate
4. Triquetrum
5. Extensor carpi ulnaris tendon
6. Lunate
7. Ulna
8. Distal radioulnar joint
9. Pronator quadratus
10. First metacarpal
11. Trapezium
12. Trapezoid
13. Extensor pollicis brevis and abductor pollicis longus tendons
14. Scaphoid
15. Scapholunate ligament
16. Radius

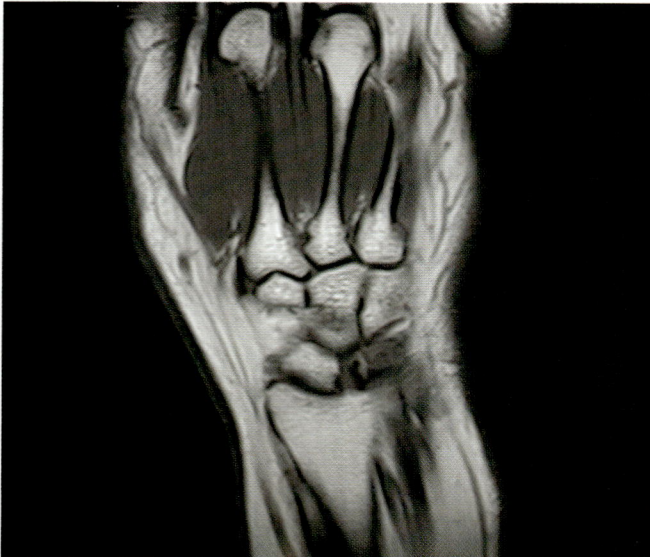
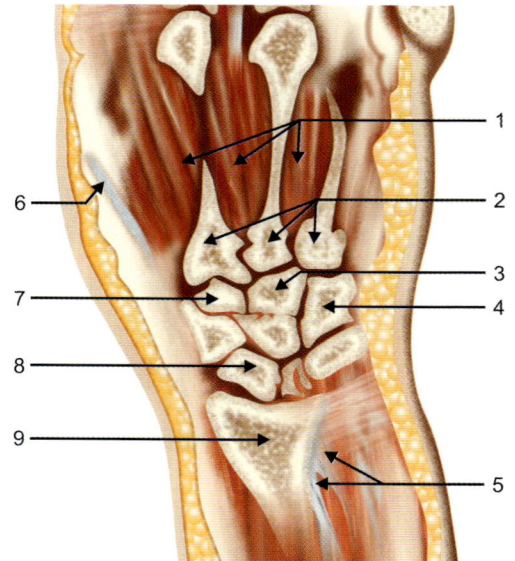

Figure 13.10

1. Interosseous muscles
2. Second, third, fourth metacarpals
3. Capitate
4. Hamate
5. Extensor tendons
6. Extensor pollicis longus
7. Trapezoid
8. Scaphoid, proximal pole
9. Radius

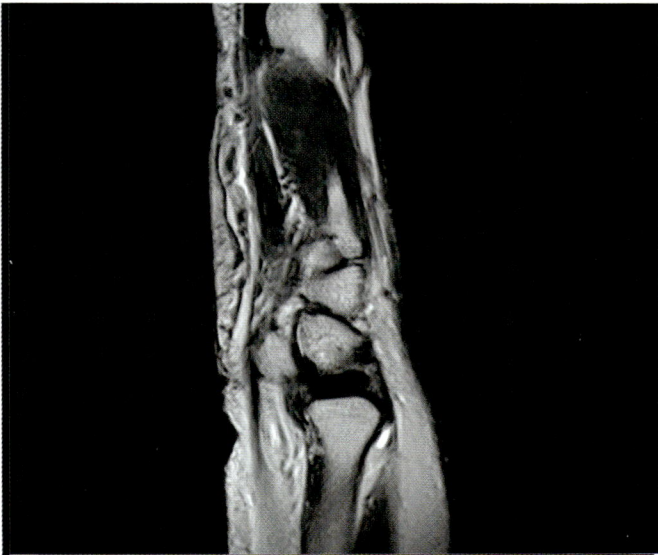
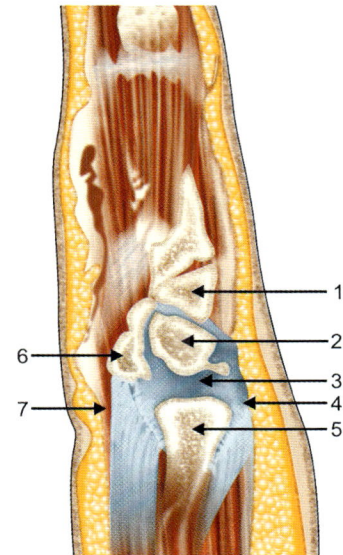

Figure 13.11

1. Hamate	5. Ulna
2. Triquetrum	6. Pisiform
3. Triangular fibrocartilage	7. Flexor carpi ulnaris
4. Extensor carpi ulnaris	

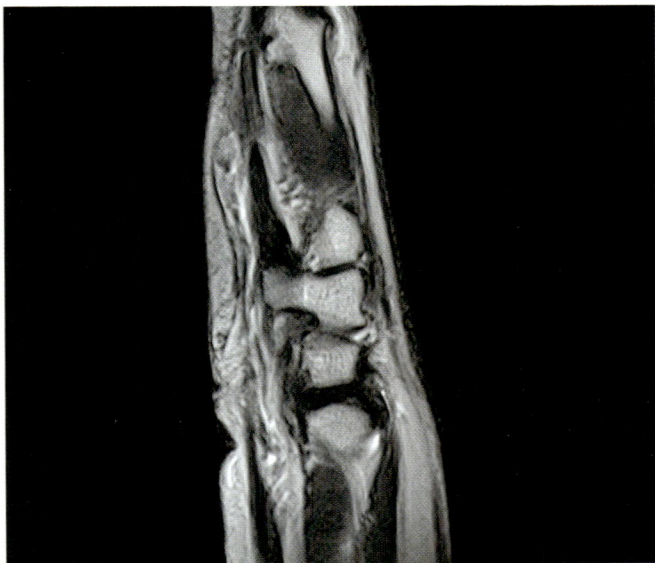
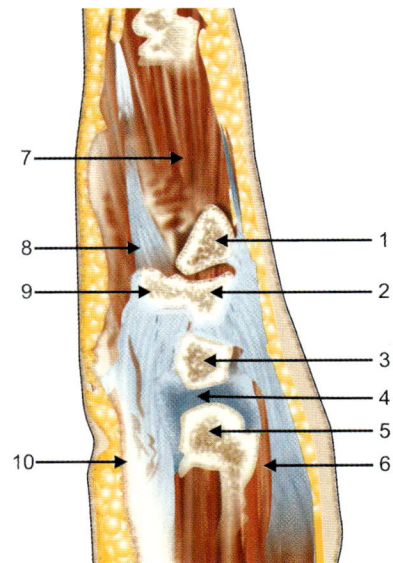

Figure 13.12

1. Fourth metacarpal base	5. Ulna, head	9. Hook of hamate
2. Hamate	6. Extensor carpi ulnaris	10. Flexor carpi ulnaris
3. Triquetrum	7. Interosseous muscle	
4. Triangular fibrocartilage	8. Flexor tendons	

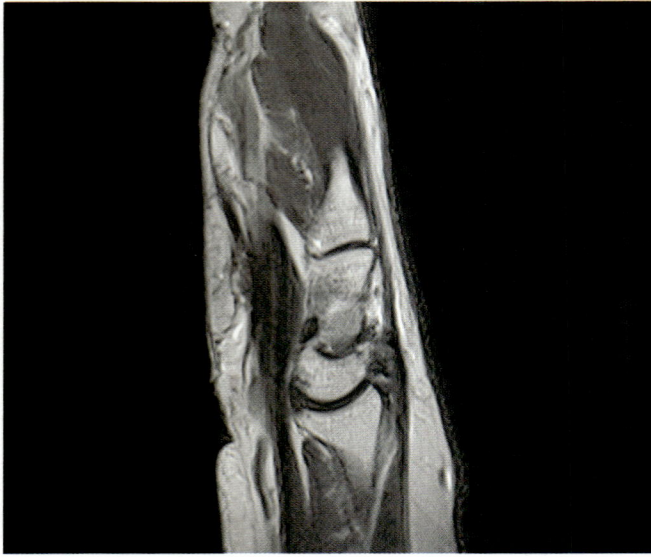

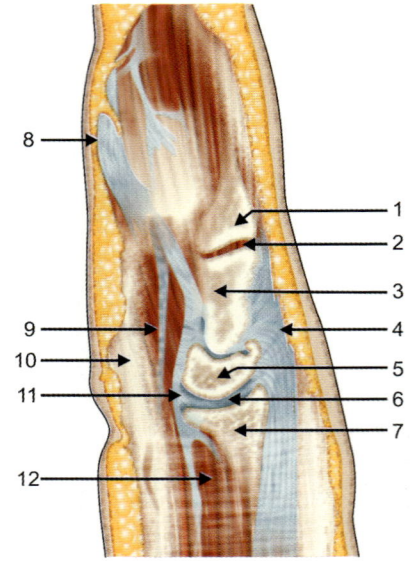

Figure 13.13

1. Third metacarpal base	5. Lunate	9. Flexor tendon
2. Carpometacarpal joint	6. Radiocarpal joint	10. Flexor retinaculum
3. Capitate	7. Radius	11. Palmar radiocarpal ligament
4. Extensor digitorum tendon	8. Palmar aponeurosis	12. Pronator quadratus

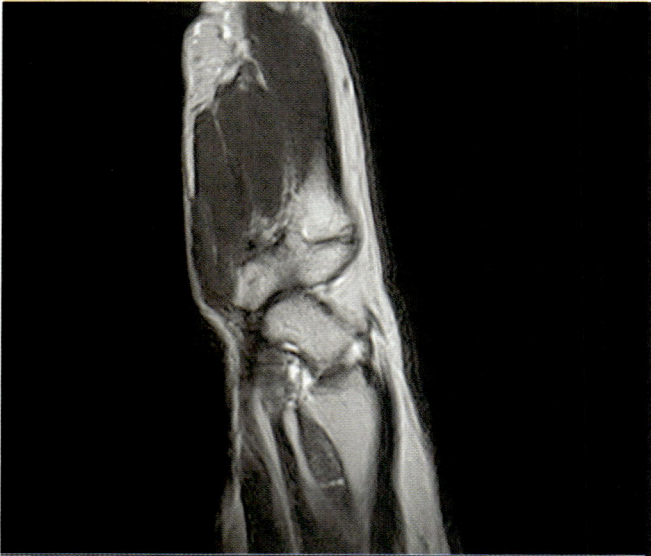

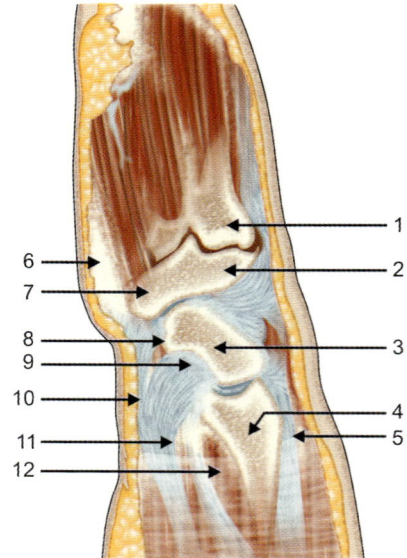

Figure 13.14

1. Second metacarpal, base	5. Extensor pollicis longus tendon	9. Palmar radiocarpal ligaments
2. Trapezoid	6. Thenar muscle	10. Flexor carpi radialis tendon
3. Scaphoid	7. Trapezium	11. Flexor pollicis longus tendon
4. Radius	8. Scaphoid tuberosity	12. Pronator quadratus

CHAPTER 14

Upper Extremity Vessels

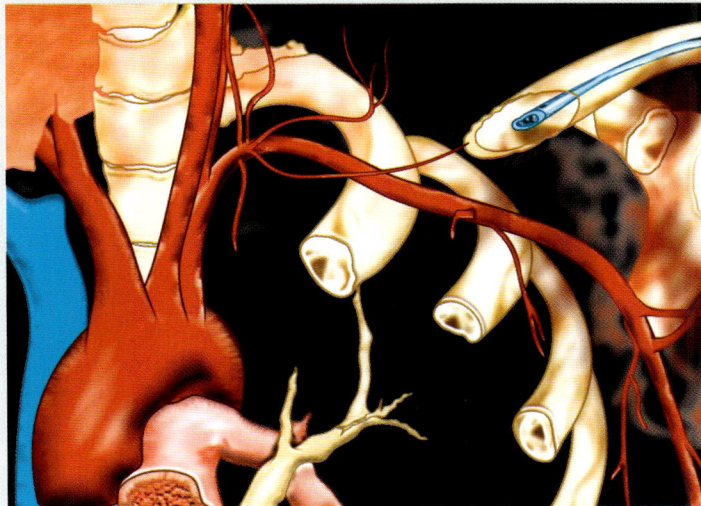

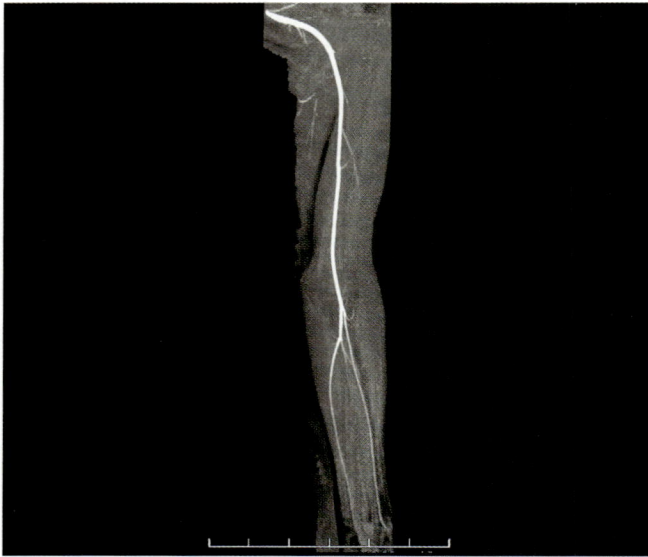

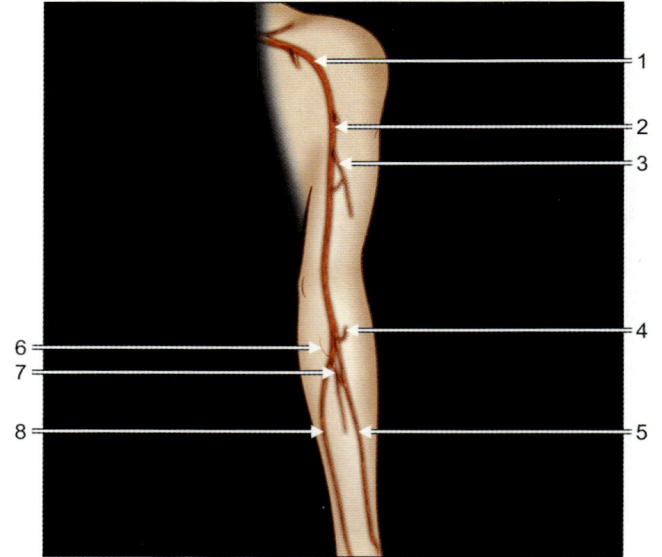

Figure 14.1

1. Axillary artery	5. Radial artery
2. Brachial artery	6. Ulnar recurrent artery
3. Profunda brachii artery	7. Common interosseous artery
4. Radial recurrent artery	8. Ulnar artery

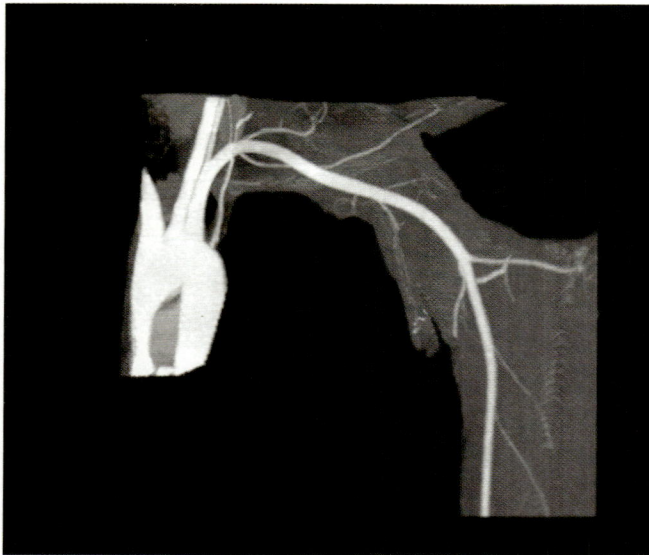

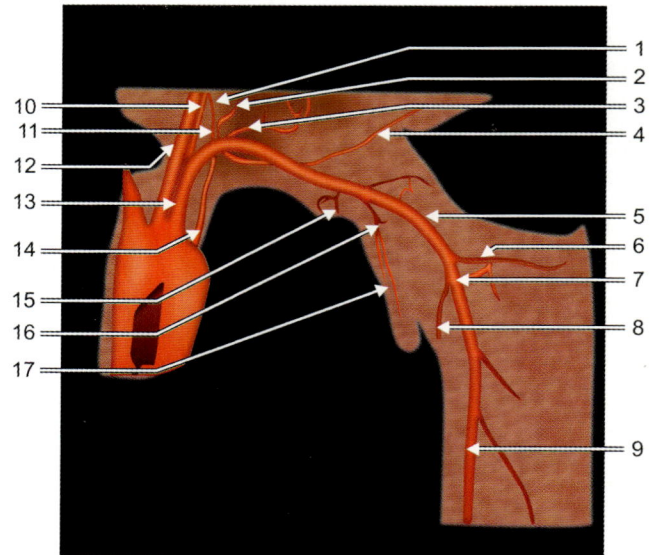

Figure 14.2

1. Inferior thyroid artery	7. Post circumflex humeral artery	13. Left subclavian artery
2. Transverse cervical artery	8. Subscapular artery	14. Internal mammary artery
3. Costocervical trunk	9. Brachial artery	15. Superior thoracic artery
4. Supracapsular artery	10. Vertebral artery	16. Thoracoacromial artery
5. Axillary artery	11. Thyrocervical trunk	17. Lateral thoracic artery
6. Ant circumflex humeral artery	12. Left carotid artery	

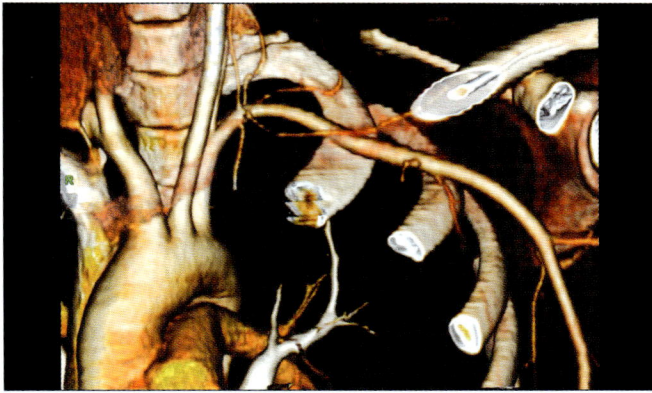

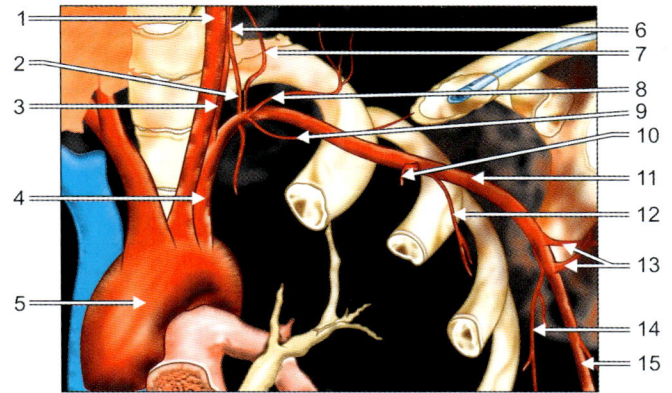

Figure 14.3

1. Left carotid artery	6. Inferior thyroid artery	11. Axillary artery
2. Thyrocervical trunk	7. Transverse cervical artery	12. Lateral thoracic artery
3. Left vertebral artery	8. Costocervical trunk	13. Circumflex humeral arteries
4. Left subclavian artery	9. Suprascapular artery	14. Subscapular artery
5. Arch of aorta	10. Superior thoracic artery	15. Brachial artery

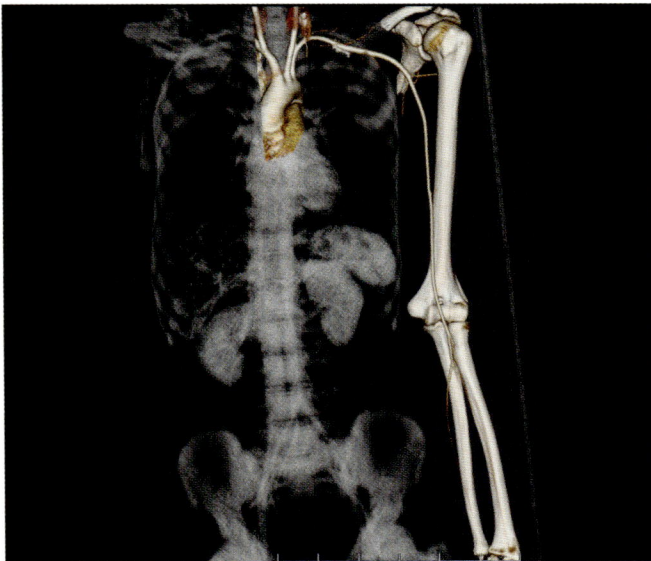

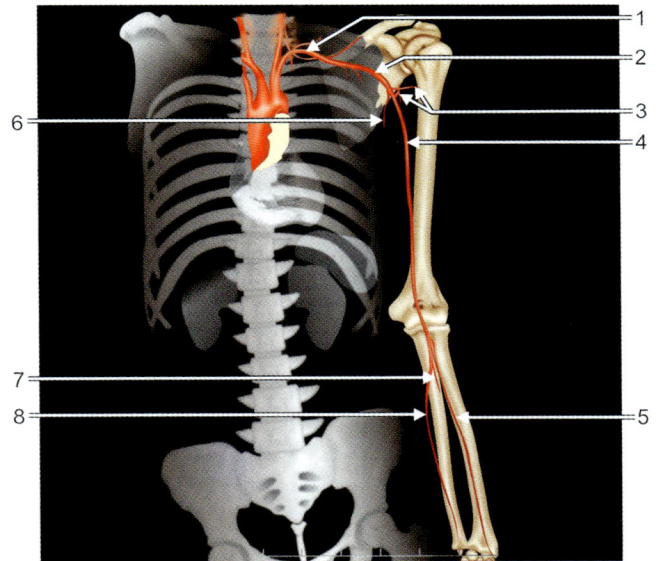

Figure 14.4

1. Subclavian artery	5. Radial artery
2. Axillary artery	6. Subscapular artery
3. Circumflex humeral artery	7. Interosseous artery
4. Brachial artery	8. Ulnar artery

Section 5

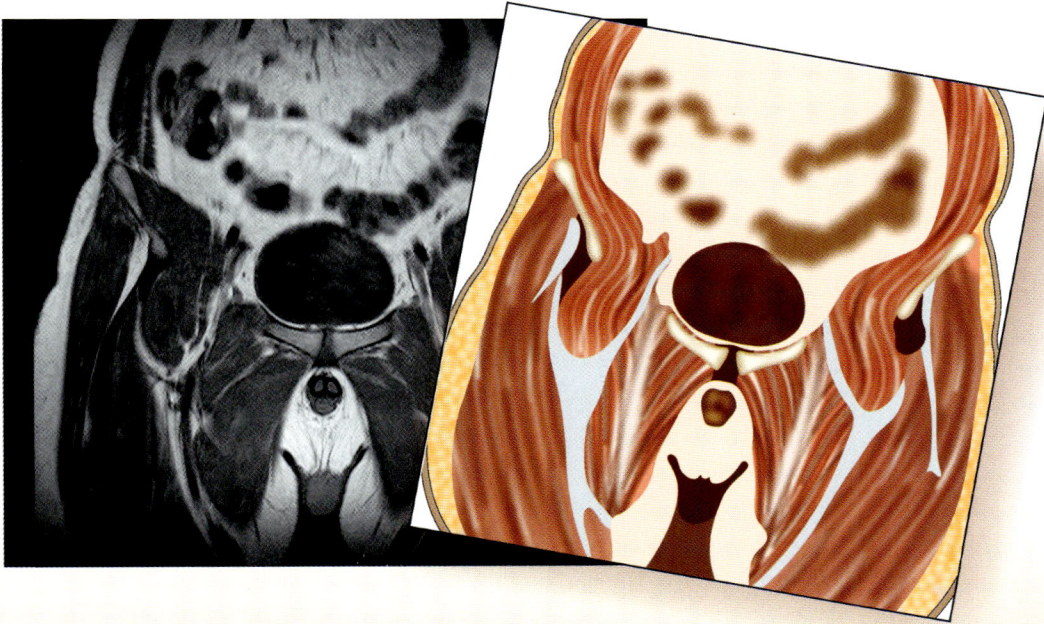

Lower Extremity

- Hips
- Thigh and Calf
- Knee
- Ankle and Foot
- Lower Extremity Vessels

Hips

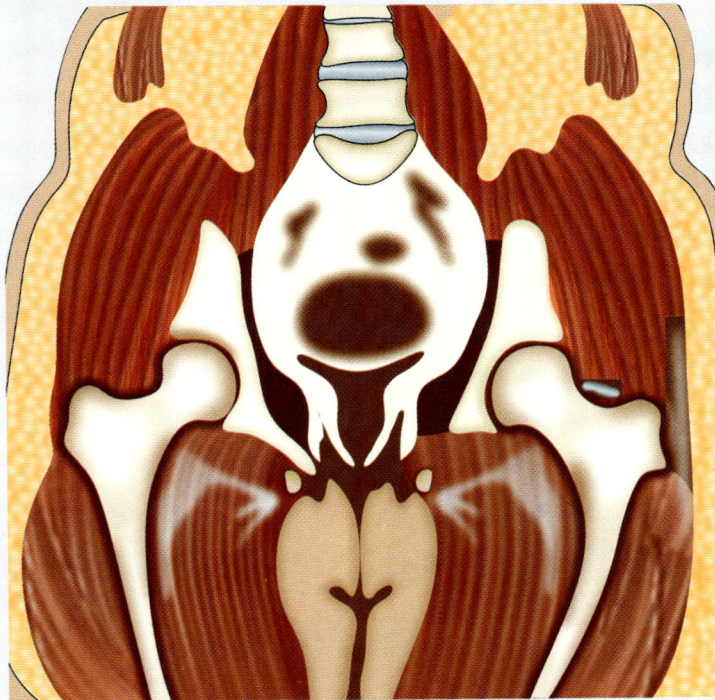

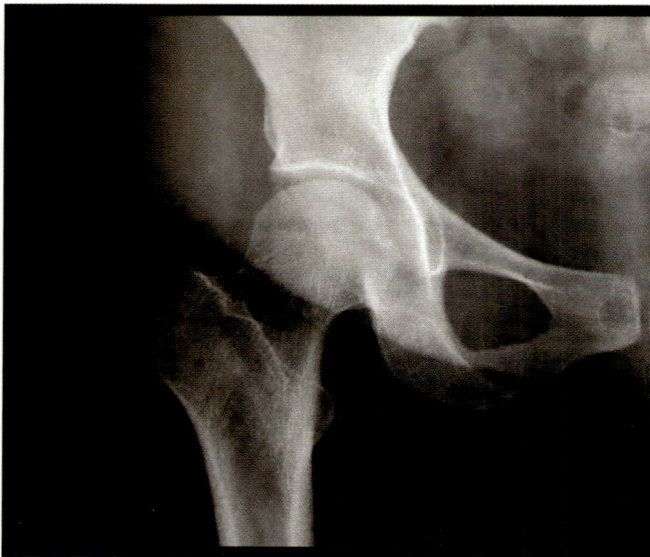

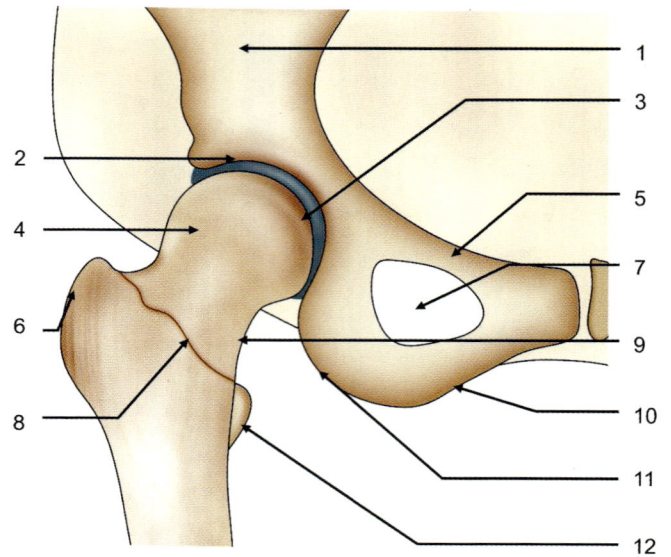

Figure 15.1

1. Ilium	7. Obturator foramen
2. Acetabulum	8. Intertrochanteric line
3. Fovea capitis	9. Femoral neck
4. Femoral head	10. Inferior pubic ramus
5. Superior pubic ramus	11. Ischial tuberosity
6. Greater trochanter	12. Lesser trochanter

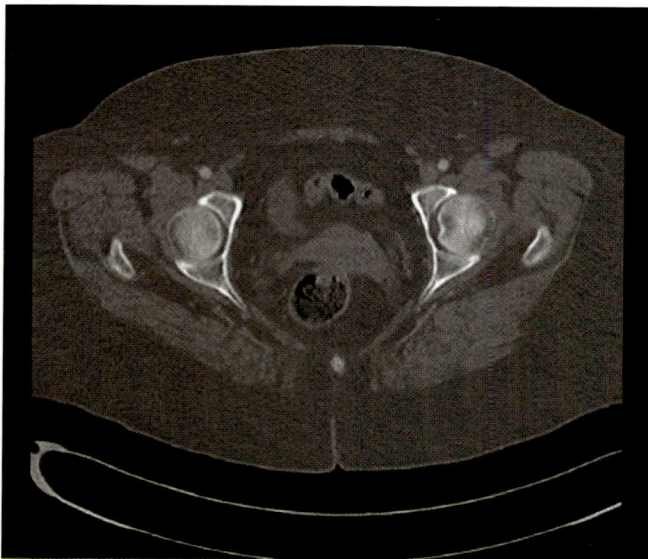

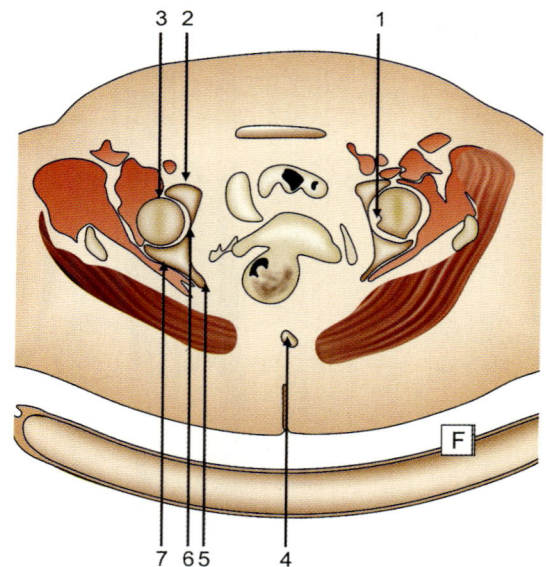

Figure 15.2

1. Fovea capitis	4. Coccyx
2. Anterior pillar acetabulum	5. Ischial spine
3. Femoral head	6. Quadrilateral plate
	7. Posterior pillar acetabulum

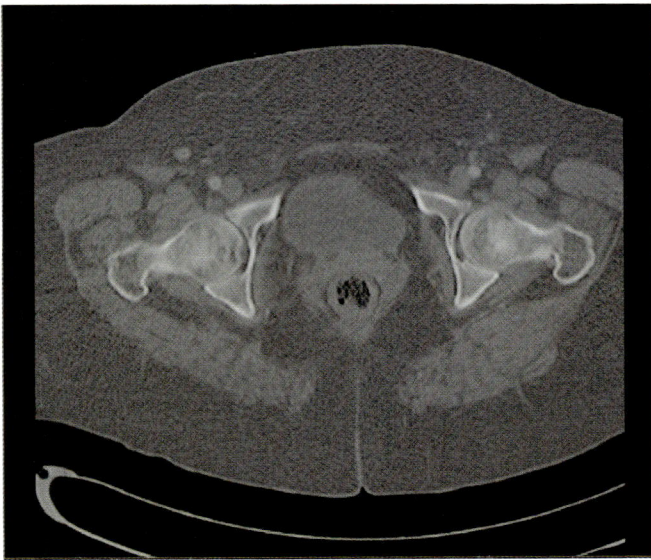

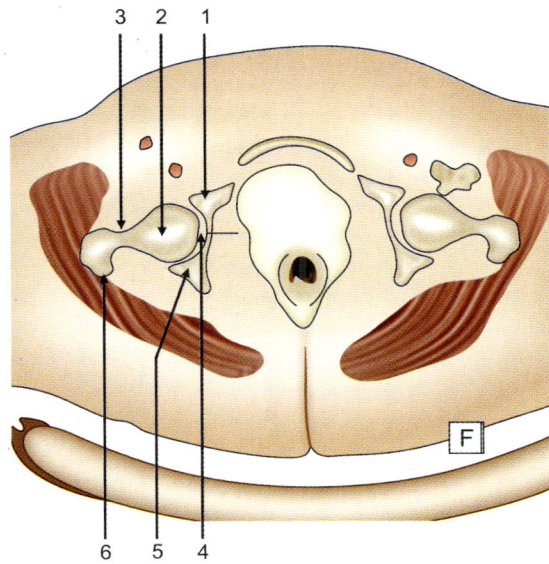

Figure 15.3

1.	Acetabulum	4.	Joint space
2.	Femoral head	5.	Ischium
3.	Neck	6.	Greater trochanter

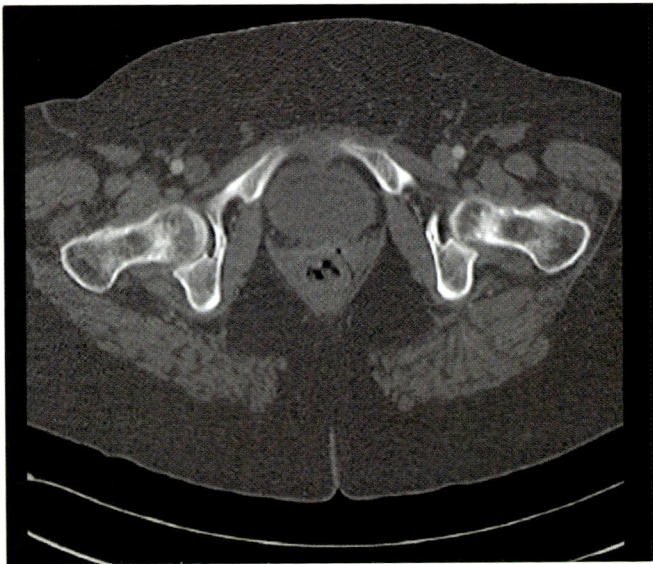

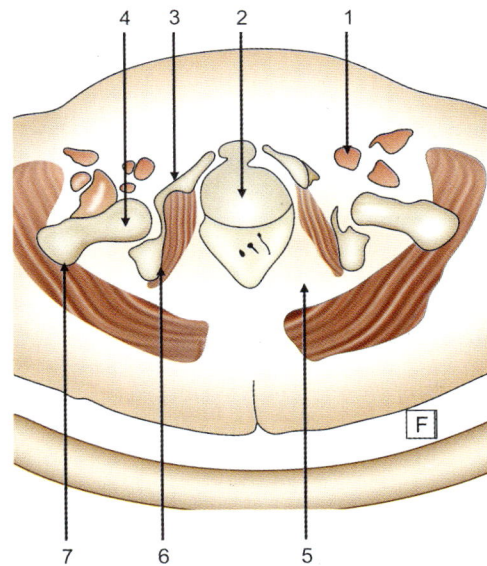

Figure 15.4

1.	Femoral vessels	5.	Ischio-anal fossa
2.	Bladder	6.	Ischium
3.	Superior ramus of pubis	7.	Greater trochanter
4.	Head of femur		

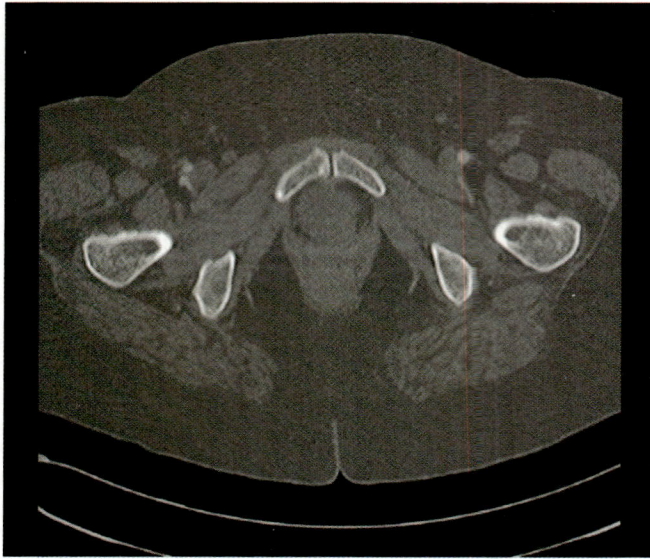

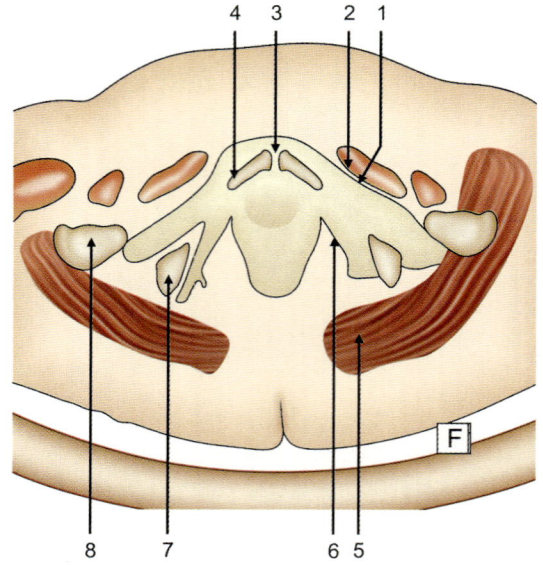

Figure 15.5

1. Obturator externus	5. Gluteus maximus
2. Pectineus	6. Obturator internus
3. Pubic symphysis	7. Ischium
4. Body of pubis	8. Femur

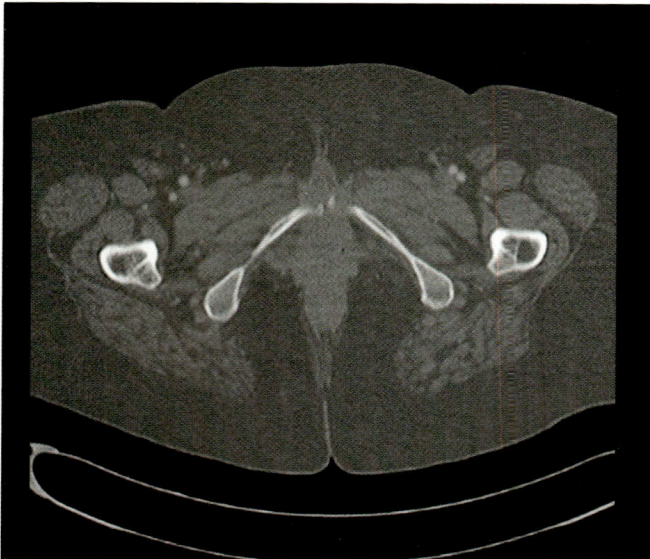

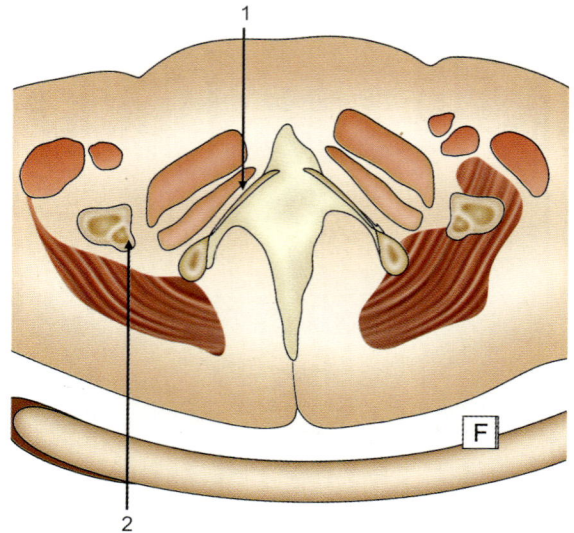

Figure 15.6

1. Inferior ramus of pubi	2. Lesser trochanter

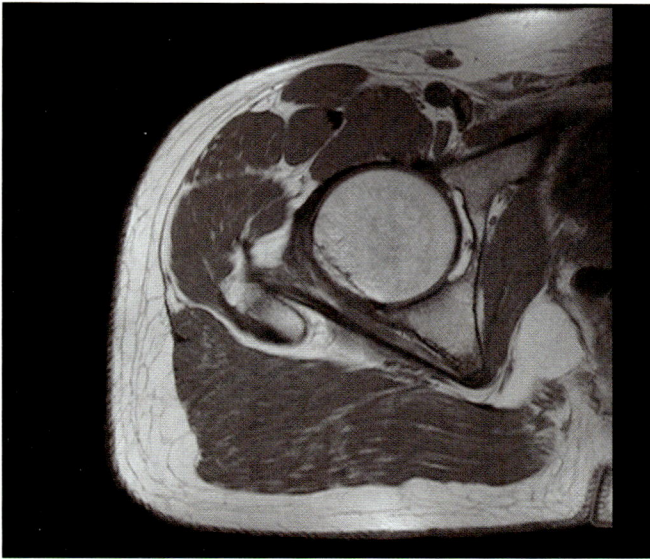

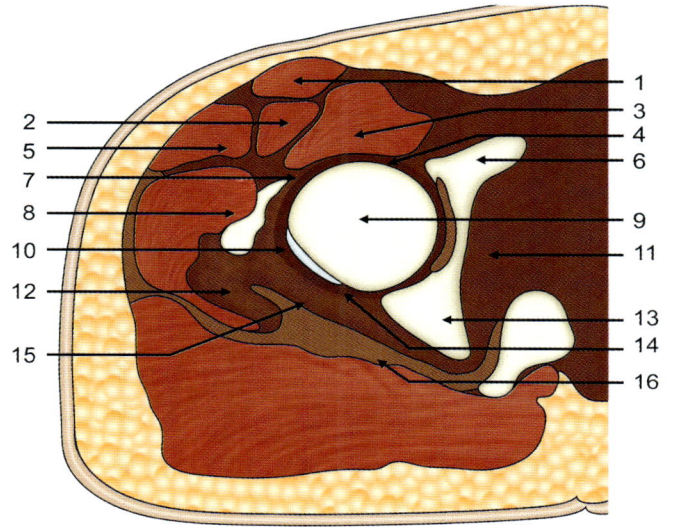

Figure 15.7

1. Sartorius	7. Iliofemoral ligament	13. Ischium
2. Rectus femoris	8. Gluteus medius	14. Posterior labrum
3. Iliopsoas	9. Femoral head	15. Obturator internus tendon
4. Anterior labrum	10. Iliofemoral ligament	16. Sciatic nerve
5. Tensor fascia lata	11. Obturator internus	
6. Pubis	12. Greater trochanter	

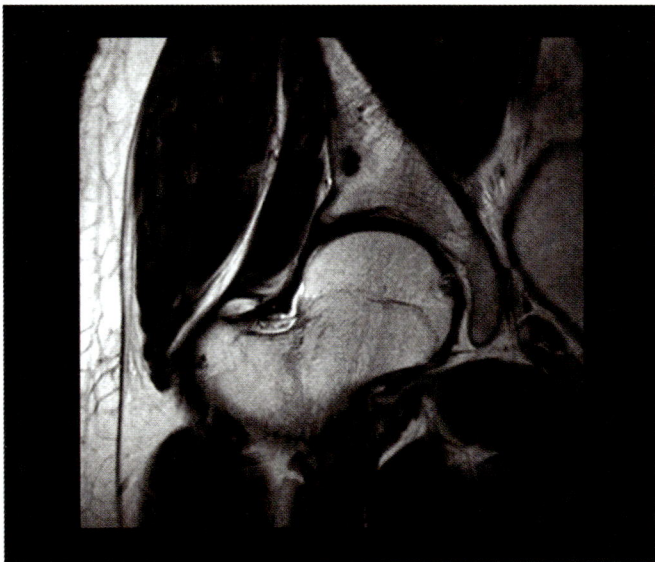

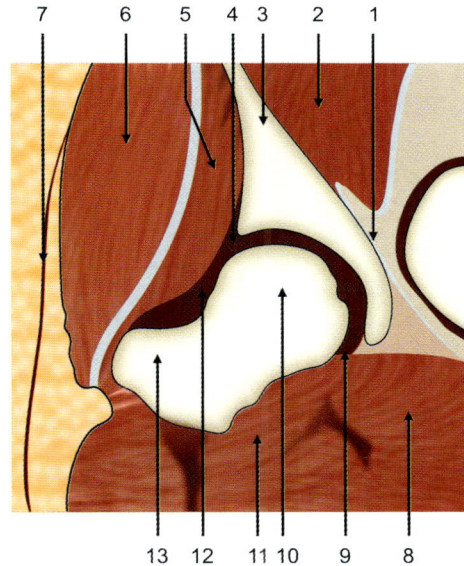

Figure 15.8

1. Acetabulum	6. Gluteus medius	11. Iliopsoas
2. Iliopsoas	7. Iliotibial tract	12. Iliofemoral ligament
3. Ilium	8. Obturator externus	13. Greater trochanter
4. Superior labrum	9. Joint space	
5. Gluteus minimus	10. Femoral head	

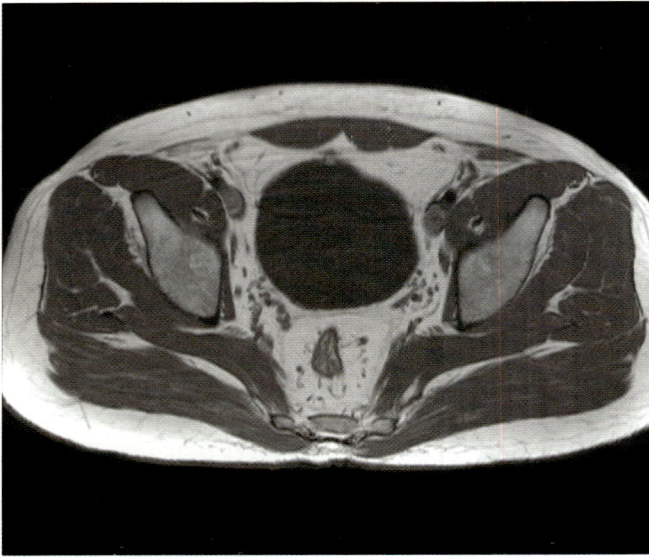

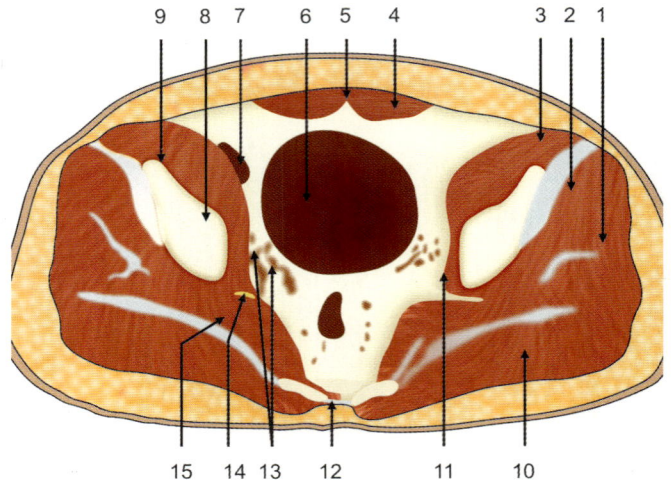

Figure 15.9

1. Gluteus medius	6. Urinary bladder	11. Obturator internus
2. Gluteus minimus	7. External iliac vessels	12. Sacrum
3. Iliopsoas	8. Acetabulum	13. Obturator and inferior gluteal vessels
4. Rectus abdominis	9. Anterior inferior iliac spine	14. Sciatic nerve
5. Linea alba	10. Gluteus maximus	15. Piriformis

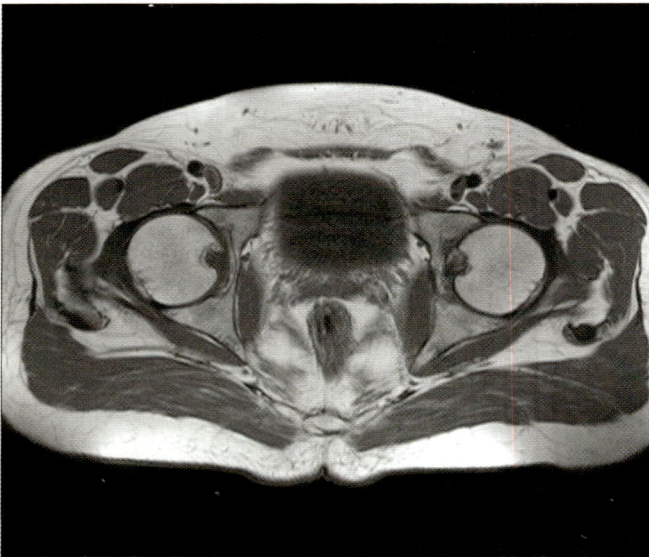

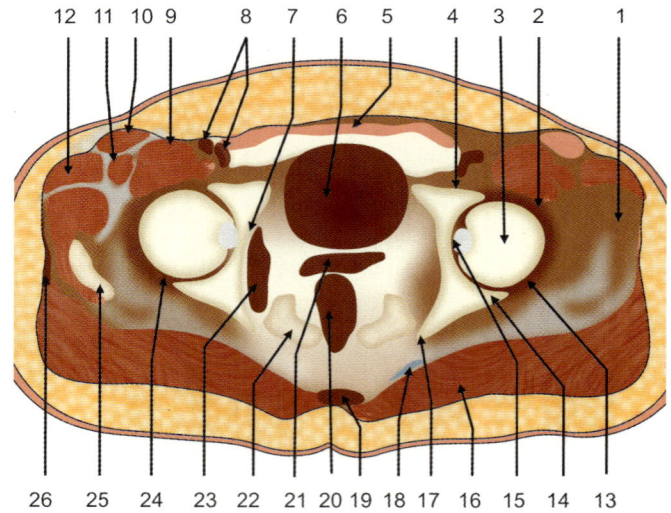

Figure 15.10

1. Gluteus medius	8. Femoral vessels	15. Ligamentum teres	22. Ischiorectal fossa
2. Iliofemoral ligament	9. Iliopsoas	16. Gluteus maximus	23. Obturator internus
3. Femoral head	10. Sartorius	17. Ischial spine	24. Posterior labrum
4. Anterior pillar, acetabulum	11. Rectus femoris	18. Sacrotuberous ligament	25. Greater trochanter
5. Rectus abdominis	12. Tensor fascia lata	19. Coccyx	26. Iliotibial tract
6. Urinary bladder	13. Ischiofemoral ligament	20. Rectum	
7. Quadrilateral plate	14. Posterior pillar, acetabulum	21. Seminal vesicles	

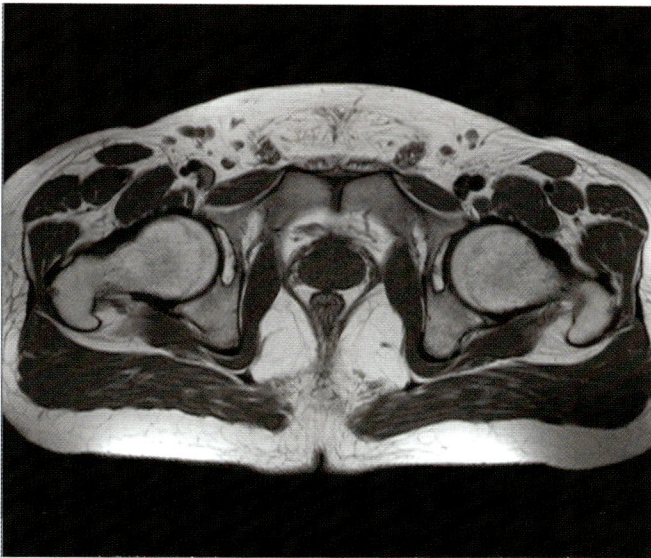

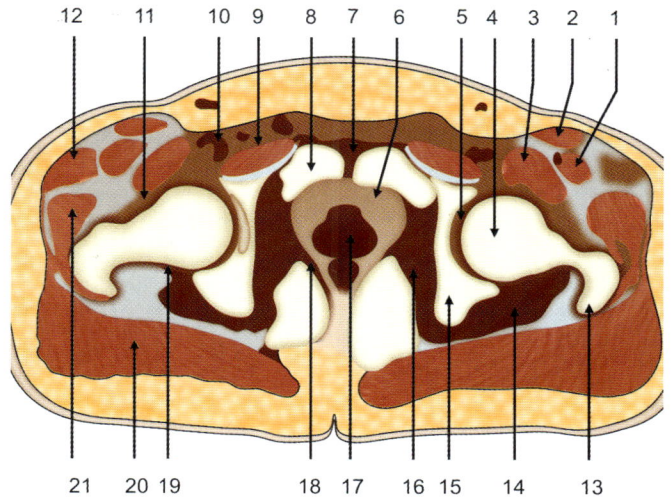

Figure 15.11

1. Rectus femoris	8. Pubis	15. Ischium
2. Sartorius	9. Pectineus	16. Obturator internus
3. Iliopsoas	10. Femoral vessels	17. Prostate
4. Femoral head	11. Iliofemoral ligament	18. Levator ani
5. Labrum	12. Tensor fascia lata	19. Ischiofemoral ligament
6. Retropubic space of Retzius	13. Greater trochanter	20. Gluteus maximus
7. Symphysis pubis	14. Inferior gemellus	21. Gluteus medius minimus

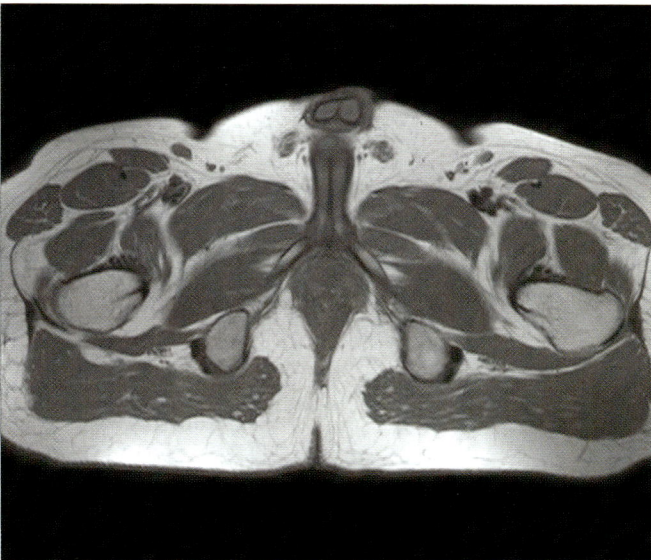

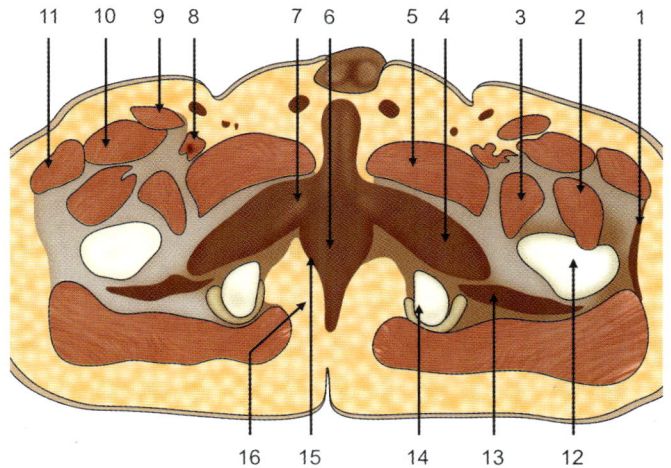

Figure 15.12

1. Ilio-tibial tract	7. Inferior pubic ramus	13. Quadratus femoris
2. Vastus lateralis	8. Femoral vessels	14. Ischial tuberosity
3. Iliopsoas	9. Sartorius	15. Levator ani
4. Obturator externus	10. Rectus femoris	16. Ischioanal fossa
5. Pectineus	11. Tensor fascia lata	
6. Anal canal	12. Femur	

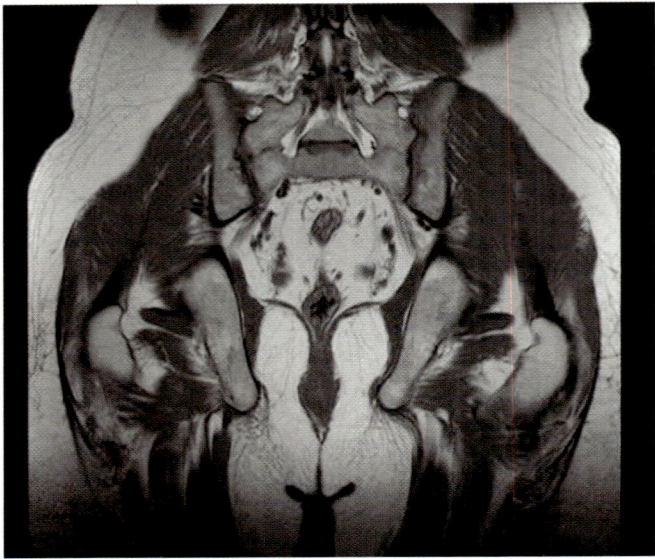

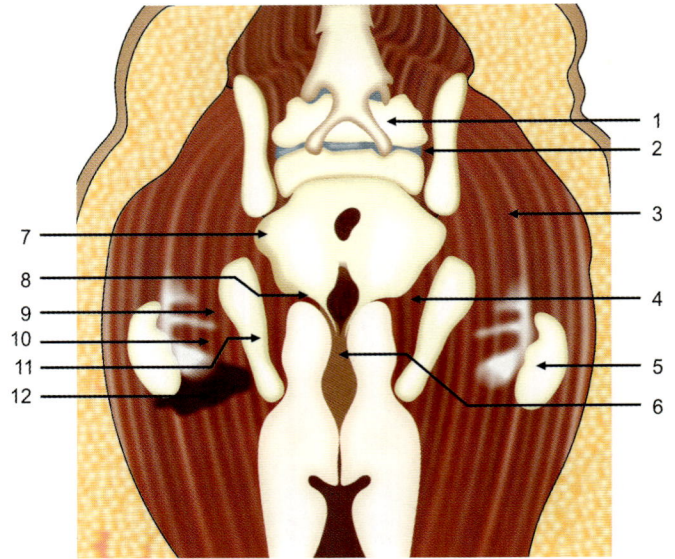

Figure 15.13

1. Sacrum	7. Sciatic nerve
2. Sacroiliac joint	8. Levator ani
3. Gluteus maximus	9. Gemelli
4. Obturator internus	10. Obturator externus
5. Greater trochanter	11. Ischium
6. Anal canal	12. Quadratus femoris

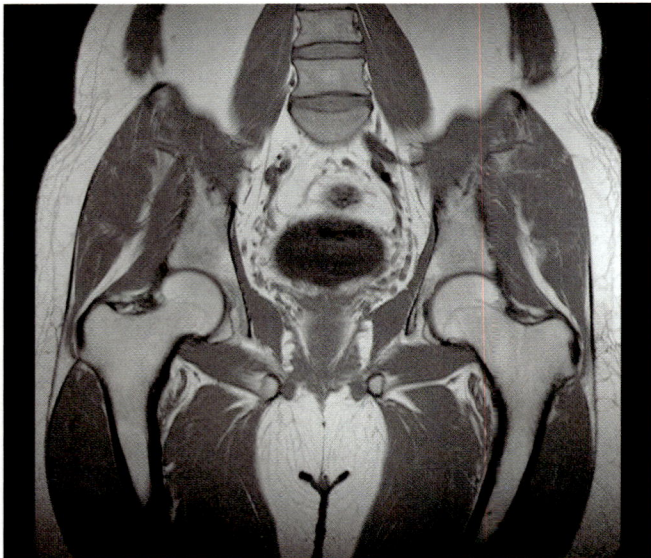

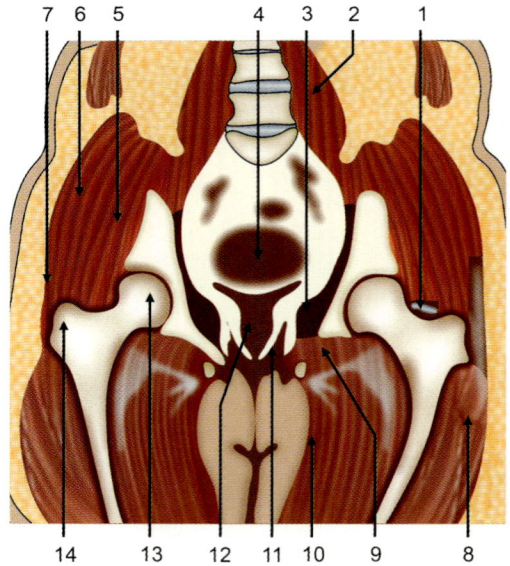

Figure 15.14

1. Iliofemoral ligament	6. Gluteus medius	11. Levator ani
2. Psoas	7. Iliofemoral tract	12. Prostate
3. Obturator internus	8. Vastus lateralis	13. Femoral head
4. Bladder	9. Obturator externus	14. Greater trochanter
5. Gluteus minimus	10. Adductor magnus	

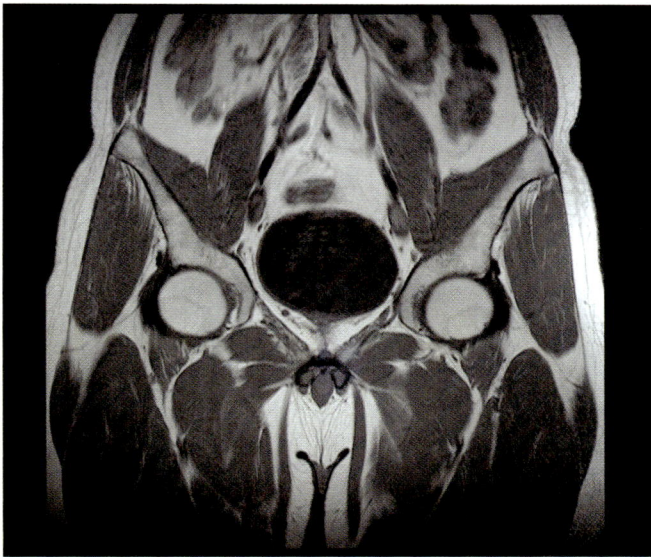

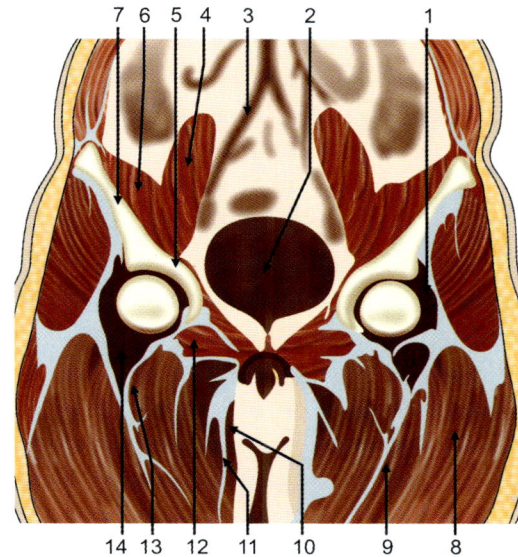

Figure 15.15

1. Iliofemoral ligament	6. Iliacus	11. Adductor brevis
2. Urinary bladder	7. Iliac bone	12. Obturator externus
3. Common iliac vessels	8. Vastus lateralis	13. Pectineus
4. Psoas	9. Vastus intermedius	14. Iliopsoas
5. Acetabulum	10. Gracilis	

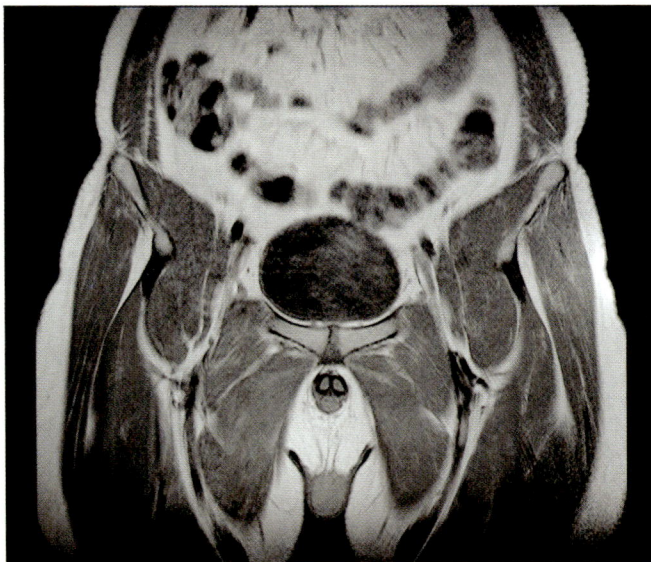

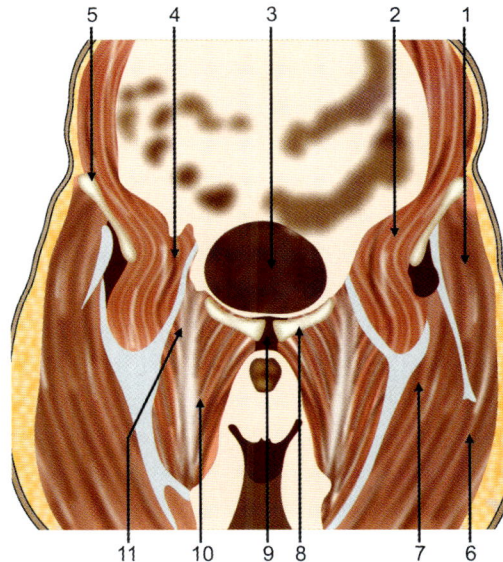

Figure 15.16

1. Gluteus medius	5. Ilium	9. Pubic symphysis
2. Iliopsoas	6. Vastus lateralis	10. Adductor longus
3. Urinary bladder	7. Rectus femoris	11. Pectineus
4. External iliac vessels	8. Superior ramus pubis	

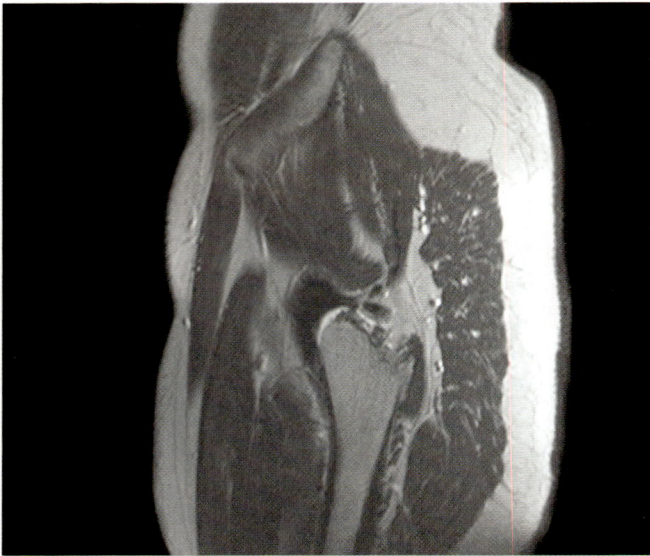

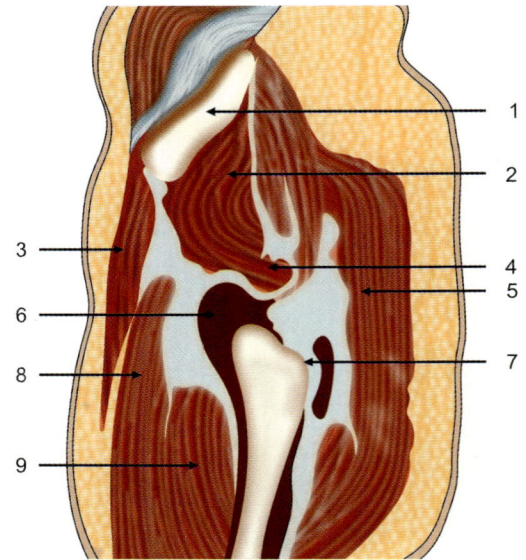

Figure 15.17

1. Ilium	6. Obturator internus
2. Gluteus medius	7. Greater trochanter
3. Sartorius	8. Rectus femoris
4. Piriformis	9. Vastus intermedius
5. Gluteus maximus	

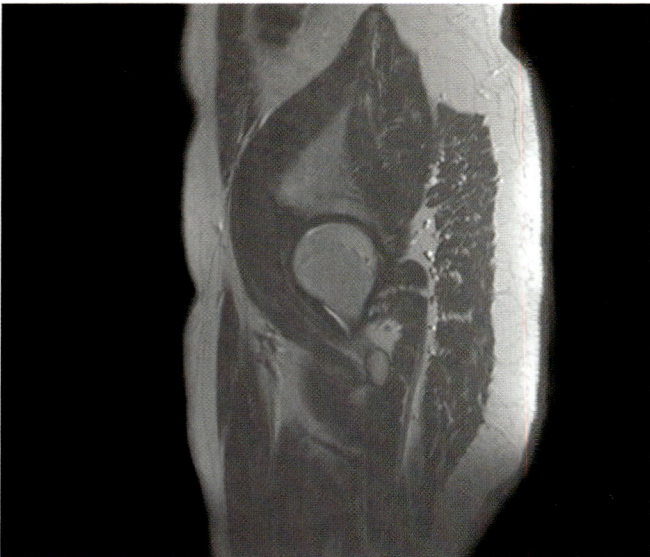

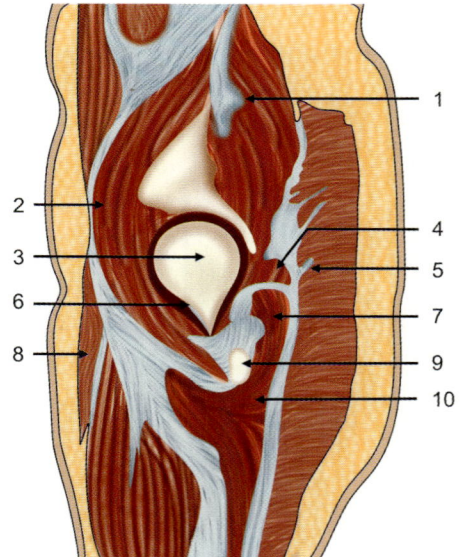

Figure 15.18

1. Gluteus minimus	6. Iliofemoral ligament
2. Iliopsoas	7. Quadratus femoris
3. Head, femur	8. Sartorius
4. Gemelli	9. Lesser trochanter
5. Gluteus maximus	10. Sciatic nerve

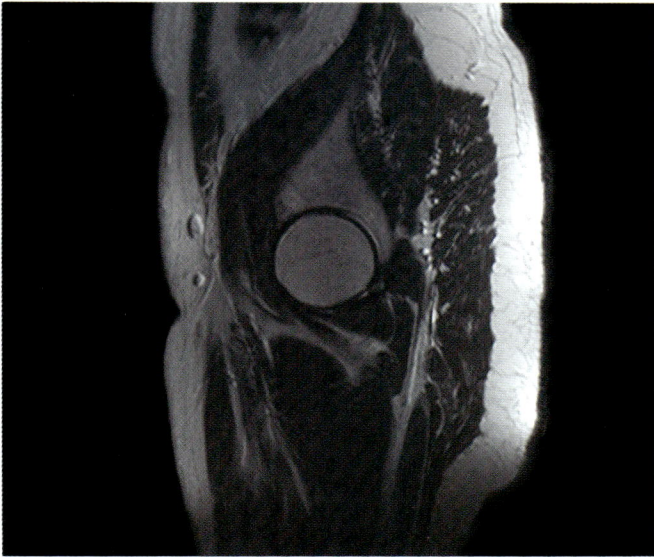

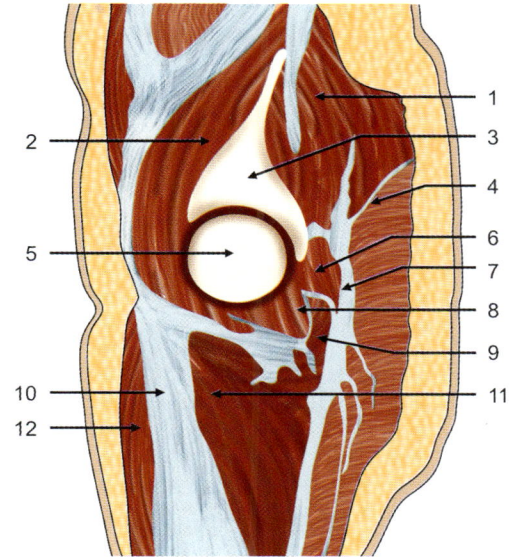

Figure 15.19

1. Gluteus minimus	7. Sciatic nerve
2. Iliopsoas	8. Obturator externus
3. Acetabular roof	9. Quadratus femoris
4. Gluteus maximus	10. Femoral vessels
5. Head, femur	11. Pectineus
6. Gemelli	12. Sartorius

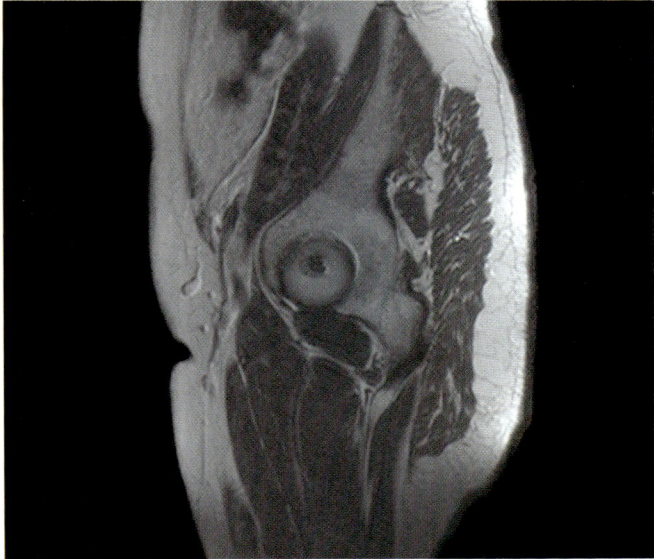

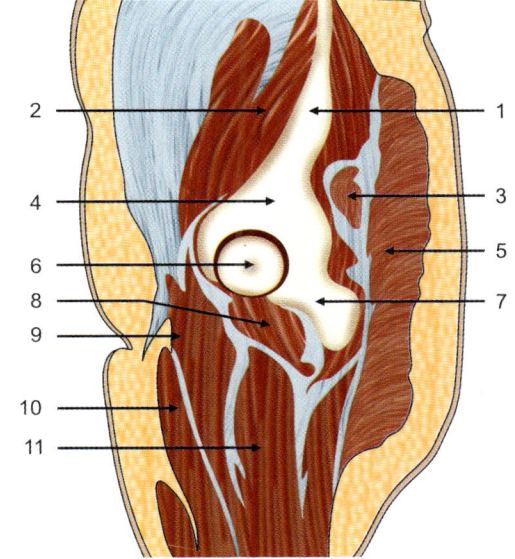

Figure 15.20

1. Ilium	7. Ischium
2. Iliopsoas	8. Obturator externus
3. Piriformis	9. Pectineus
4. Acetabulum	10. Adductor longus
5. Gluteus maximus	11. Adductor magnus
6. Head, femur	

CHAPTER 16

Thigh and Calf

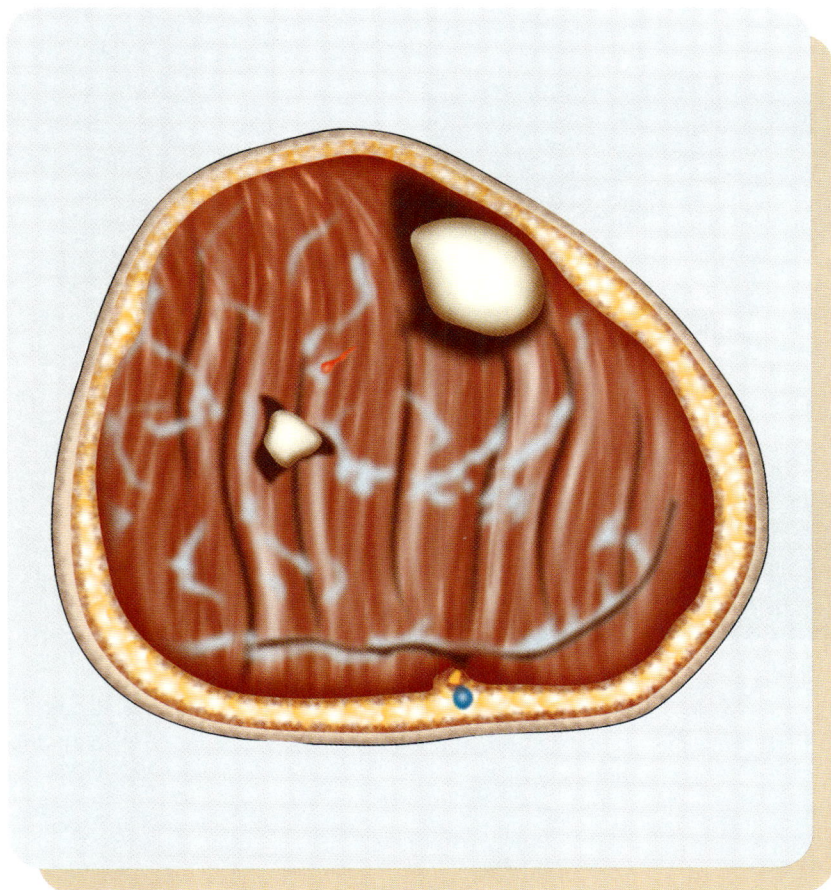

THIGH FIGURES

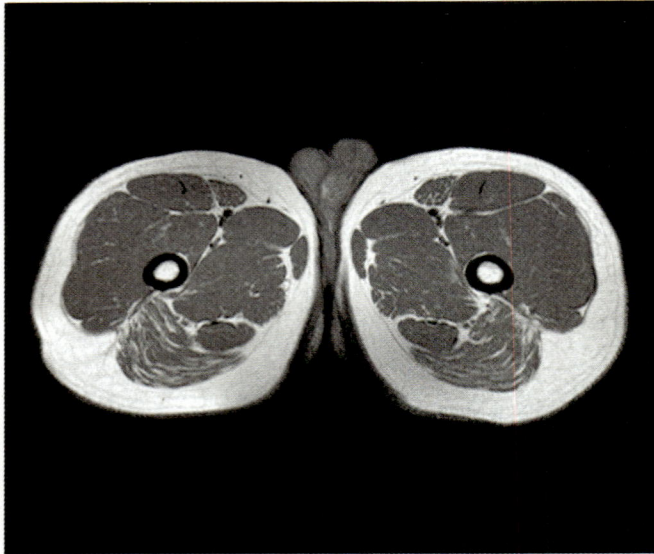

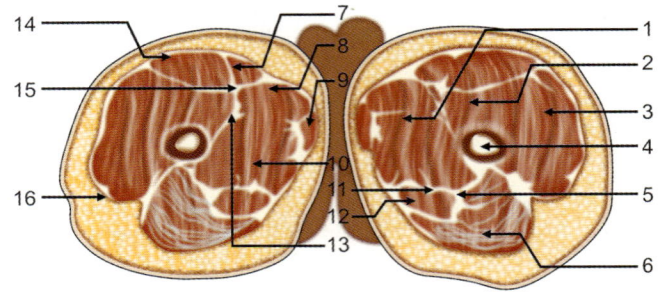

Figure 16.1

1. Adductor brevis	7. Sartorius	13. Deep femoral vessels
2. Vastus intermedius	8. Adductor longus	14. Rectus femoris
3. Vastus lateralis	9. Gracilis	15. Femoral vessels
4. Femur	10. Adductor magnus	16. Ilio-tibial tract
5. Sciatic nerve	11. Semimembranosis	
6. Gluteus maximus	12. Semitendinosis	

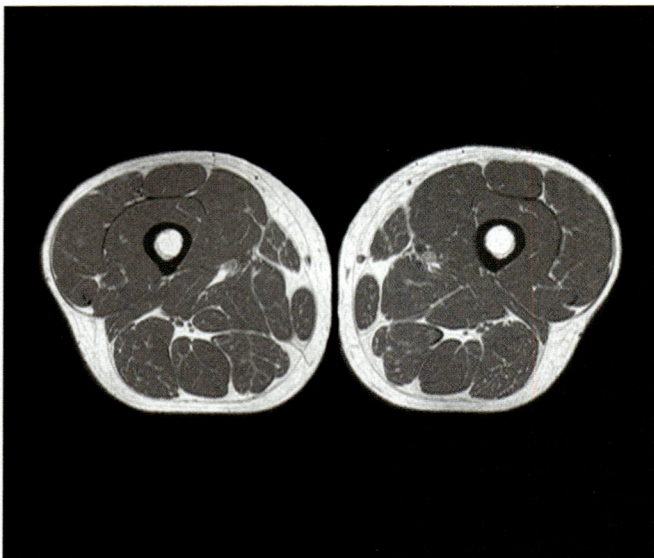

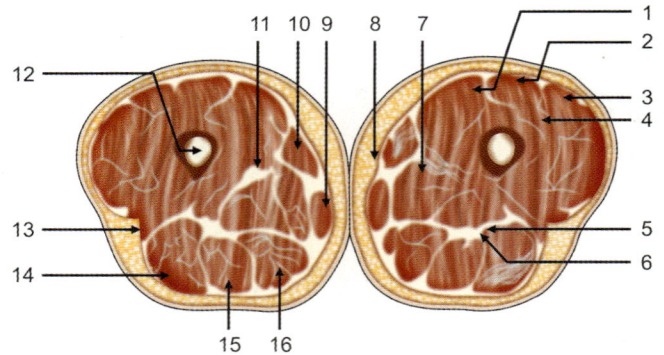

Figure 16.2

1. Vastus medialis	7. Adductor magnus	13. Biceps femoris (Short head)
2. Rectus femoris	8. Great saphenous vein	14. Biceps femoris (Long head)
3. Vastus lateralis	9. Gracilis	15. Semitendinosis
4. Vastus intermedius	10. Sartorius	16. Semimembranosis
5. Common peroneal nerve	11. Femoral vessels	
6. Tibial nerve	12. Femur	

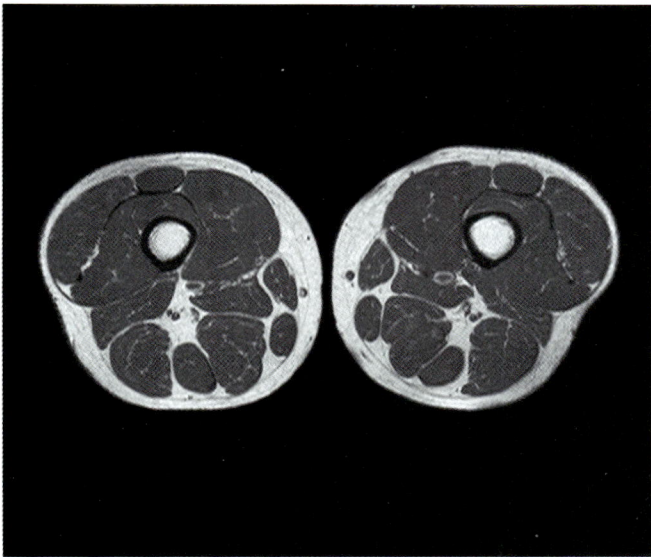

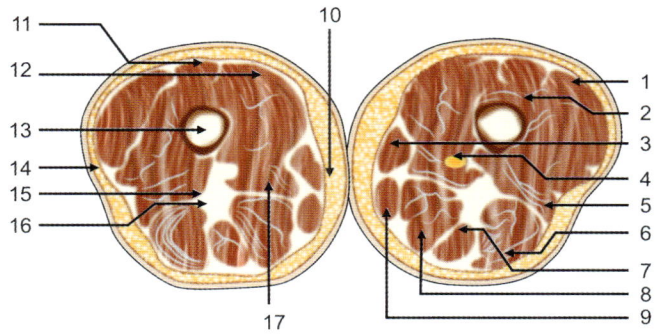

Figure 16.3

1. Vastus lateralis	7. Semitendinosis	13. Femur
2. Vastus intermedius	8. Semimembranosis	14. Ilio-tibial tract
3. Sartorius	9. Gracilis	15. Common peroneal nerve
4. Femoral vessels	10. Great saphenous vein	16. Tibial nerve
5. Biceps femoris (short head)	11. Rectus femoris	17. Adductor magnus
6. Biceps femoris	12. Vastus medialis	

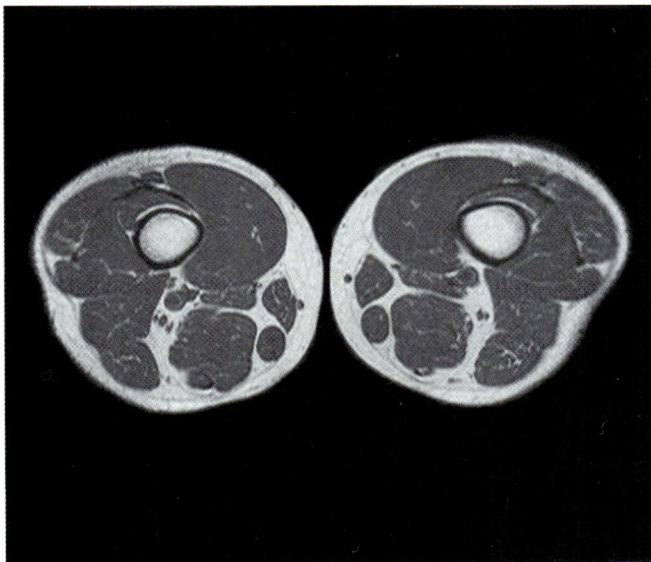

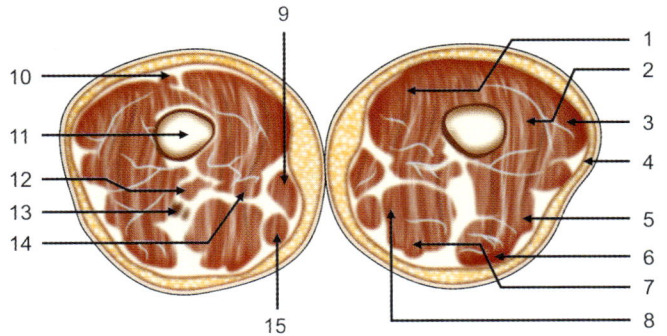

Figure 16.4

1. Vastus medialis	6. Biceps femoris (long head)	11. Femur
2. Vastus intermedius	7. Semitendinosis	12. Popliteal vessels
3. Vastus lateralis	8. Semimembranosis	13. Common peroneal nerve
4. Ilio-tibial tract	9. Sartorius	14. Adductor magnus
5. Biceps femoris (short head)	10. Quadriceps femoris	15. Gracilis

CORONAL IMAGES

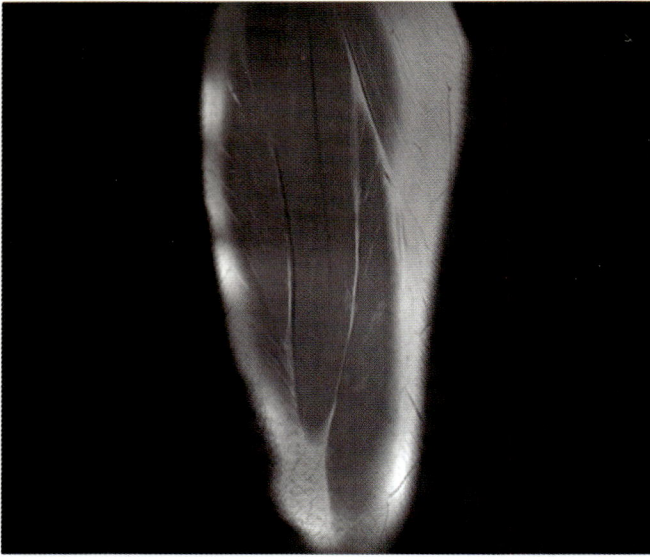

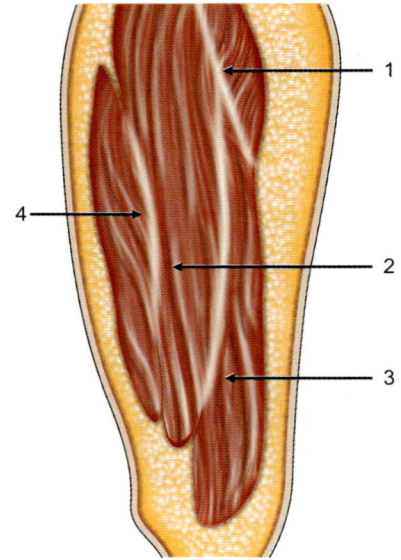

Figure 16.5

1. Sartorius	3. Vastus medialis
2. Rectus femoris	4. Vastus lateralis

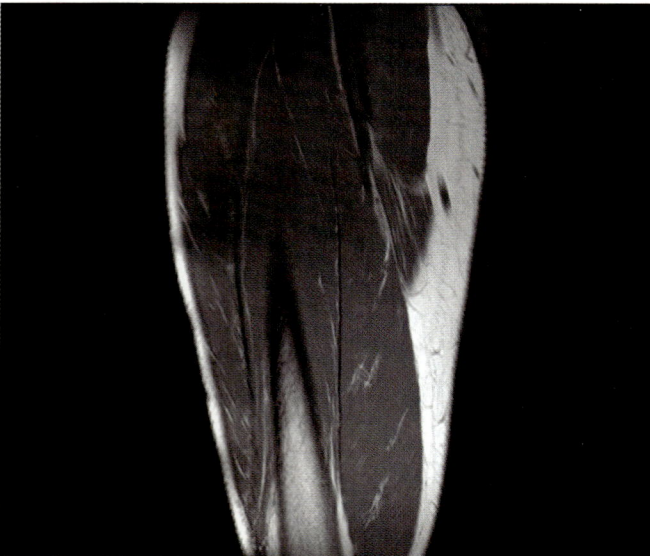

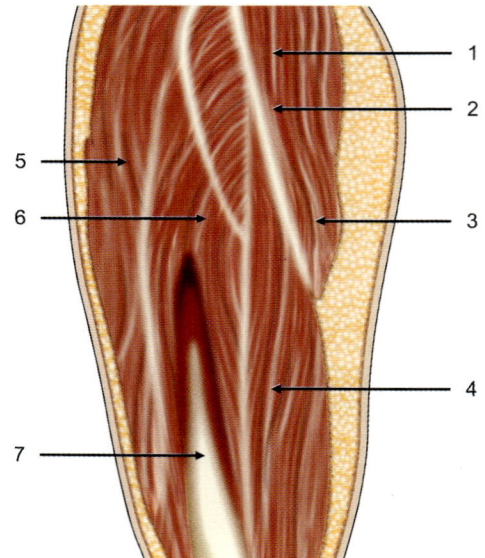

Figure 16.6

1. Adductor longus	5. Vastus lateralis
2. Femoral vessels	6. Vastus intermedius
3. Sartorius	7. Femur
4. Vastus medialis	

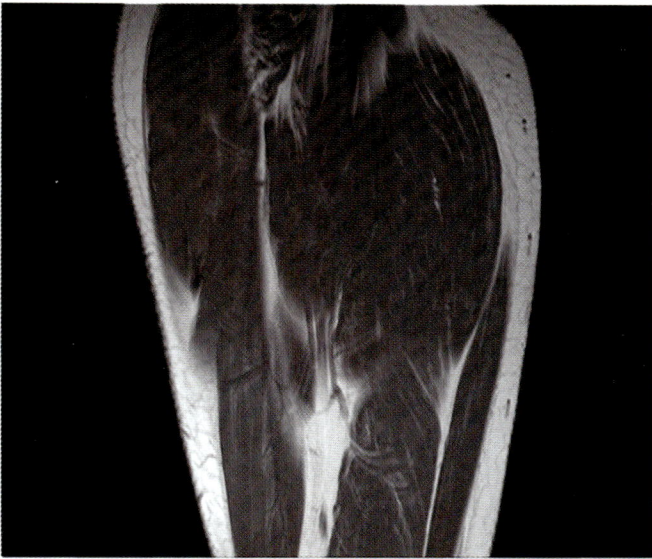

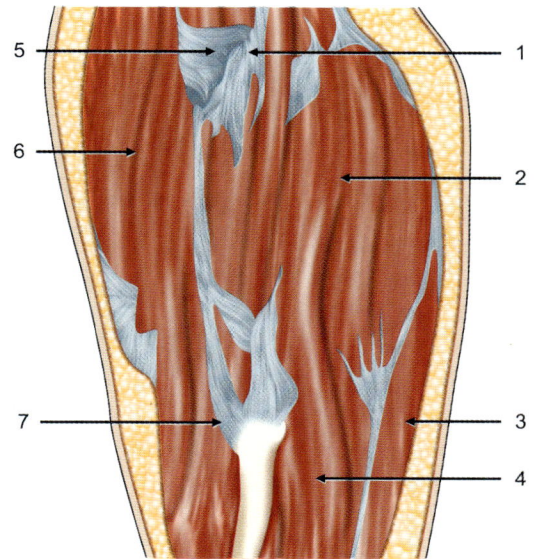

Figure 16.7

1.	Femoral vessels	5.	Gluteus maximus
2.	Adductor magnus	6.	Vastus lateralis
3.	Gracilis	7.	Biceps femoris
4.	Semimembranosus		

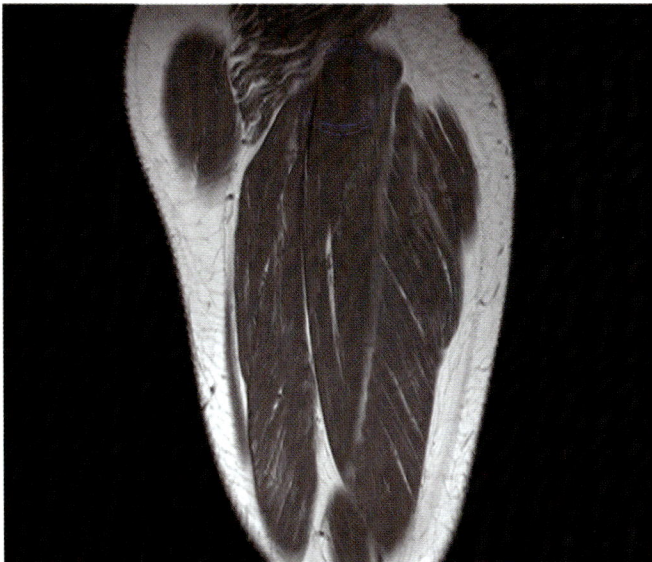

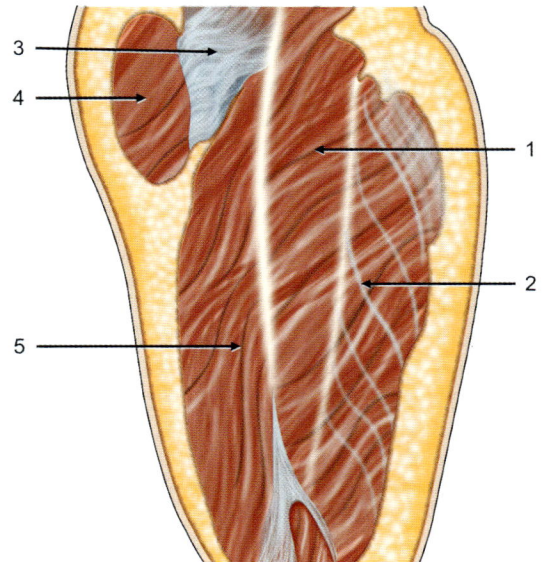

Figure 16.8

1.	Semitendinosus	4.	Vastus lateralis
2.	Semimembranosus	5.	Biceps femoris
3.	Gluteus maximus		

SAGITTAL IMAGES

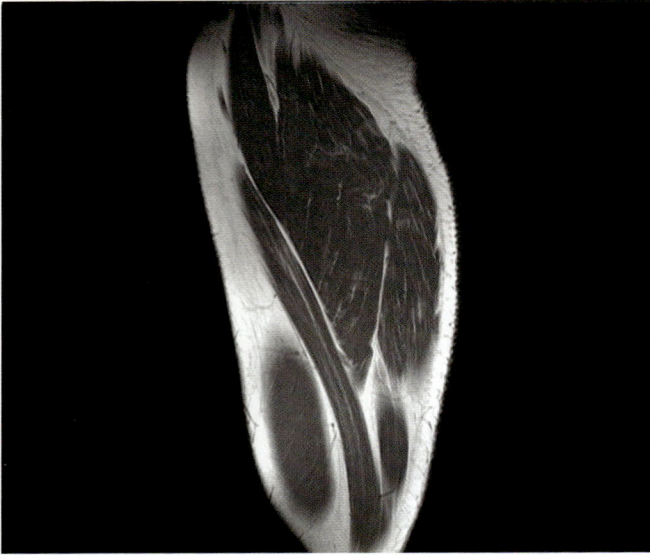

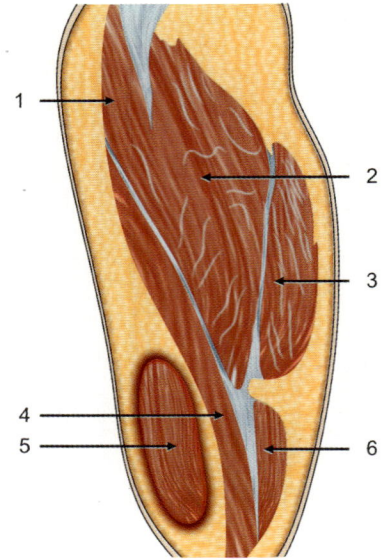

Figure 16.9

1. Adductor longus	4. Sartorius
2. Adductor magnus	5. Vastus medialis
3. Semimembranosus	6. Gracilis

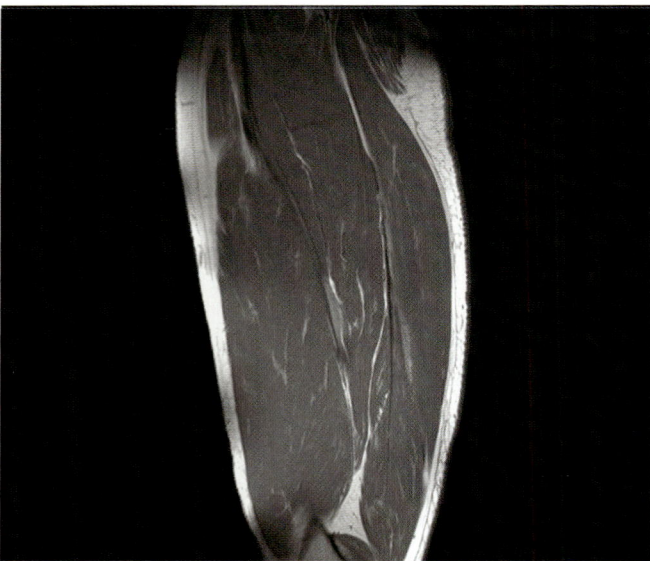

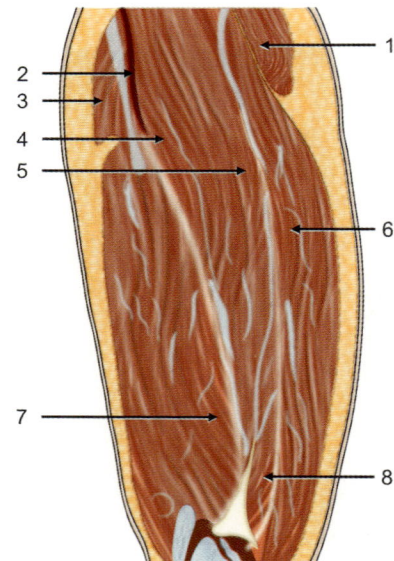

Figure 16.10

1. Gluteus maximus	5. Adductor magnus
2. Femoral vessels	6. Semitendinosus
3. Sartorius	7. Vastus medialis
4. Adductor longus	8. Semimembranosus

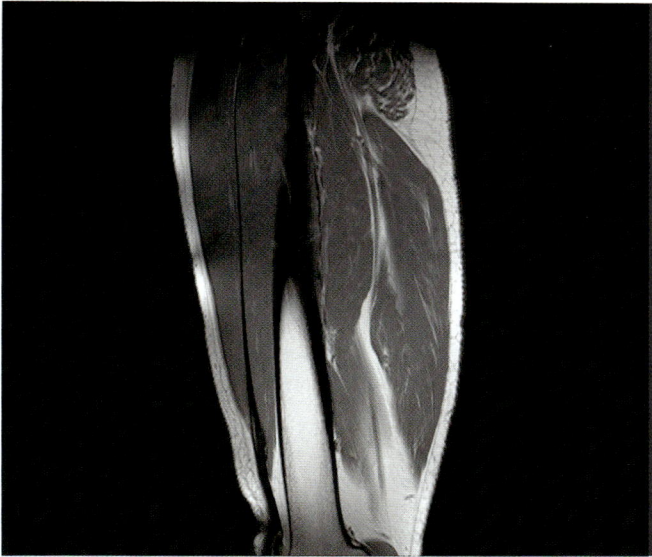

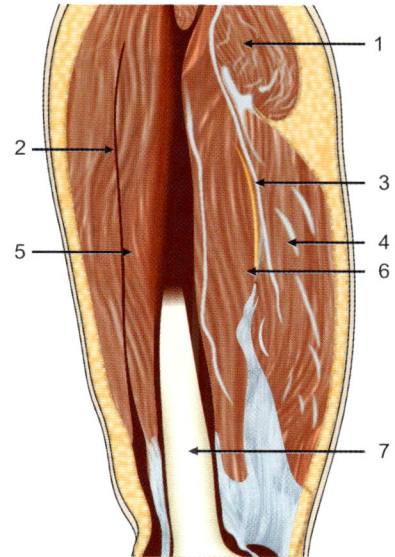

Figure 16.11

1. Gluteus maximus   5. Vastus intermedius
2. Rectus femoris   6. Adductor magnus
3. Sciatic nerve   7. Femur
4. Biceps femoris

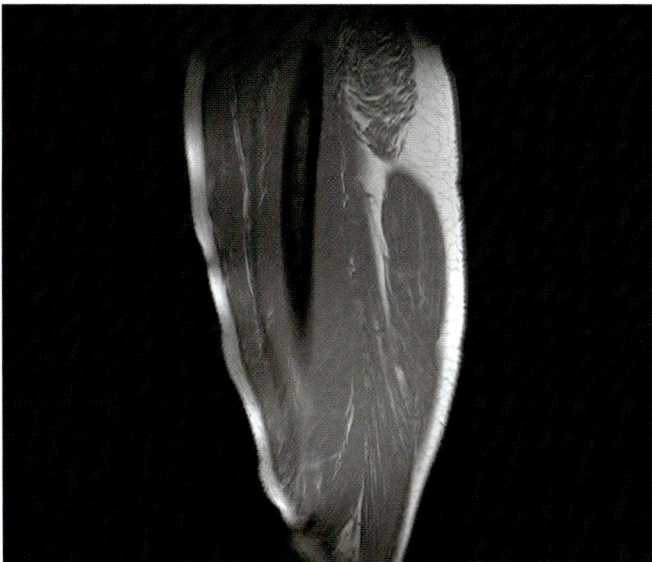

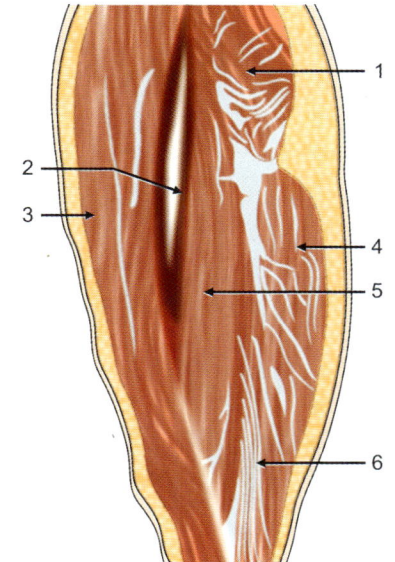

Figure 16.12

1. Gluteus maximus   4. Biceps femoris
2. Femur   5. Vastus intermedius
3. Vastus lateralis   6. Biceps femoris (short head)

CALF FIGURES

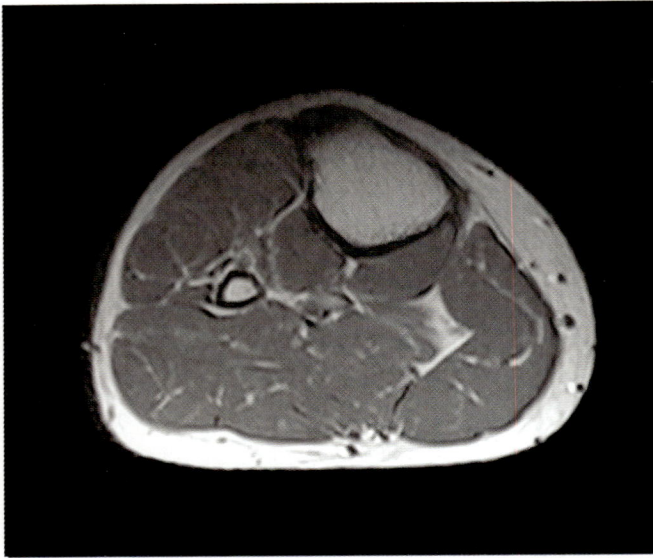
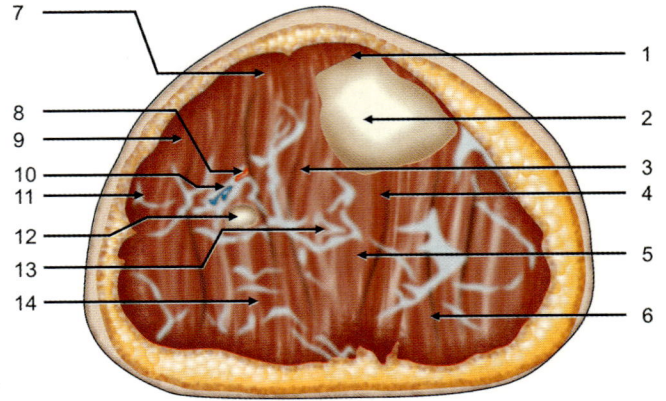

Figure 16.13

1. Tibial tuberosity	6. Gastrocnemius, medial head	11. Peroneus longus
2. Tibia	7. Tibialis anterior	12. Fibula
3. Tibialis posterior	8. Anterior tibial artery	13. Posterior tibial, peroneal artery
4. Popliteus	9. Extensor digitorum longus	14. Gastrocnemius, lateral head
5. Soleus	10. Common peroneal nerve	

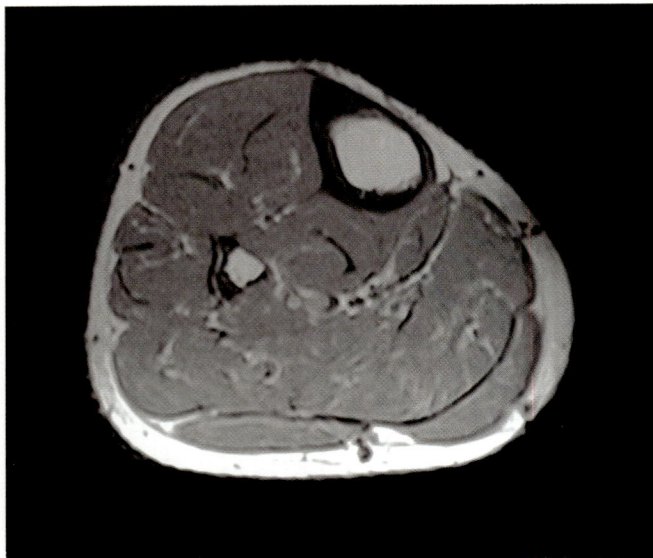
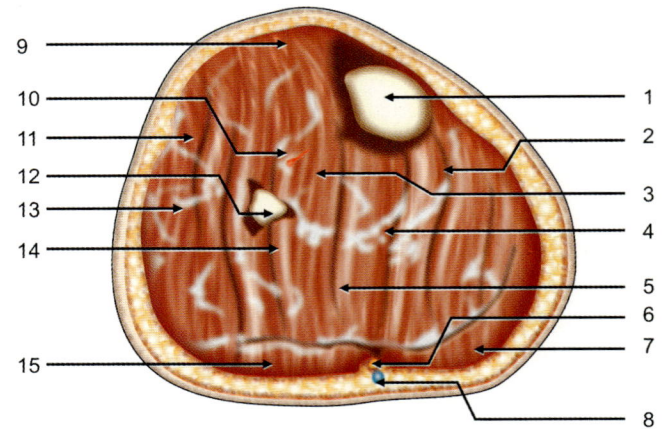

Figure 16.14

1. Tibia	7. Gastrocnemius, medial head	11. Extensor hallucis and digitorum longus
2. Flexor digitorum longus	8. Lesser saphenous vein	12. Fibula
3. Tibialis posterior	9. Tibialis anterior	13. Peroneus longus, brevis
4. Posterior tibial artery, tibial nerve	10. Anterior tibial artery, Deep peroneal nerve	14. Flexor hallucis longus
5. Soleus		15. Gastrocnemius, lateral head
6. Sural nerve		

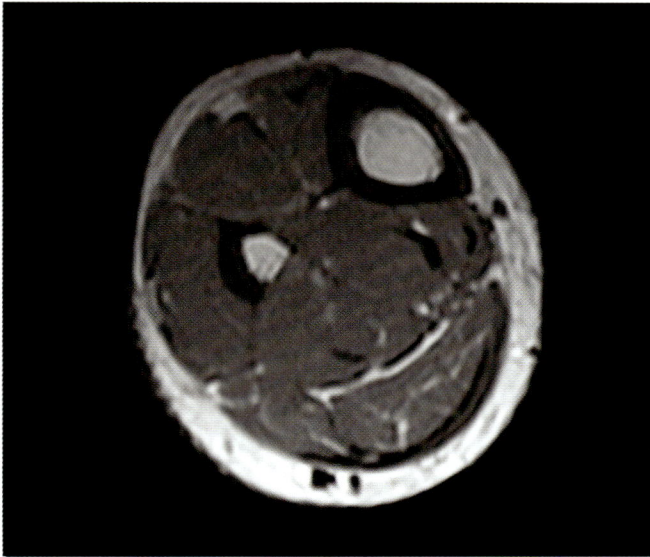

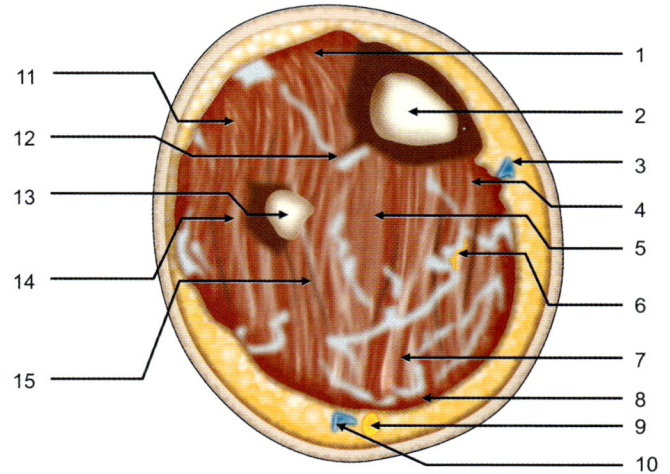

Figure 16.15

1. Tibialis anterior	6. Posterior tibial artery, tibial nerve	11. Extensor hallucis and digitorum longus
2. Tibia	7. Soleus	12. Interosseous membrane
3. Greater saphenous vein	8. Gastrocnemius tendon	13. Fibula
4. Flexor digitorum longus	9. Sural nerve	14. Peroneus longus and brevis
5. Tibialis posterior	10. Lesser saphenous vein	15. Flexor hallucis longus

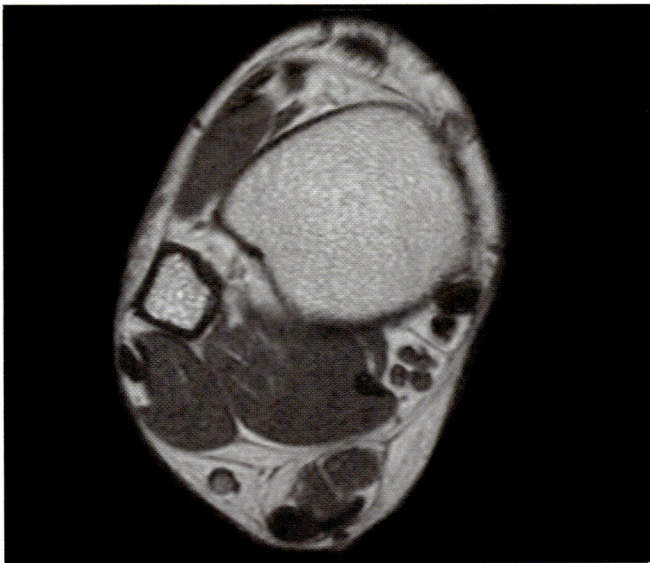

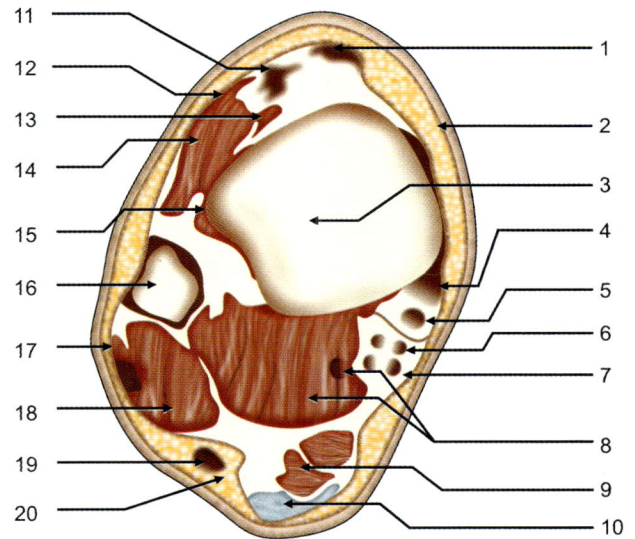

Figure 16.16

1. Tibialis anterior tendon	8. Flexor hallucis longus muscle and tendon	15. Anterior tubercle, tibia
2. Great saphenous vein	9. Soleus	16. Fibula
3. Tibia	10. Achilles tendon	17. Peroneus longus tendon
4. Tibialis posterior tendon	11. Extensor hallucis longus tendon	18. Peroneus brevis
5. Flexor digitorum longus tendon	12. Extensor digitorum longus tendon	19. Lesser saphenous vein
6. Posterior tibial artery	13. Anterior tibial artery	20. Sural nerve
7. Tibial nerve	14. Peroneus tertius	

CORONAL IMAGES

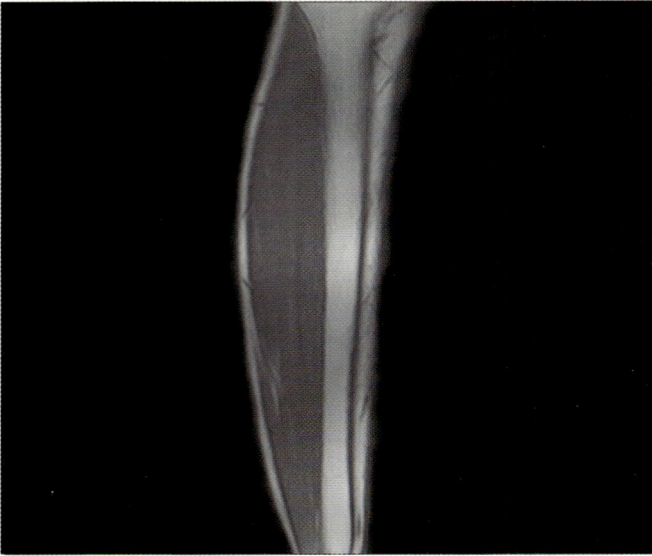

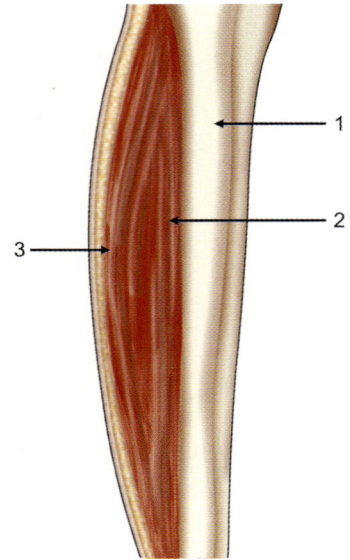

Figure 16.17

1. Tibia
2. Tibialis anterior
3. Extensor digitorum and extensor hallucis longus

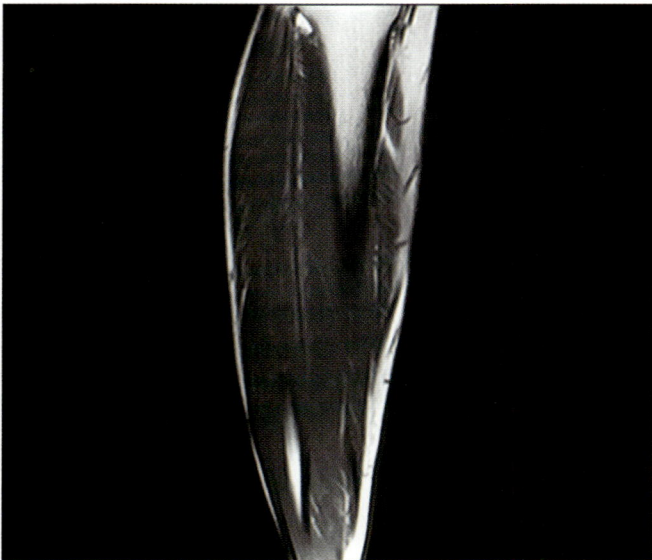

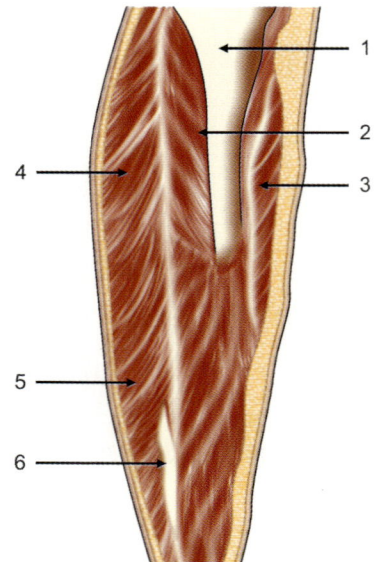

Figure 16.18

1. Tibia
2. Tibialis posterior
3. Soleus
4. Peroneus longus
5. Peroneus brevis
6. Fibula

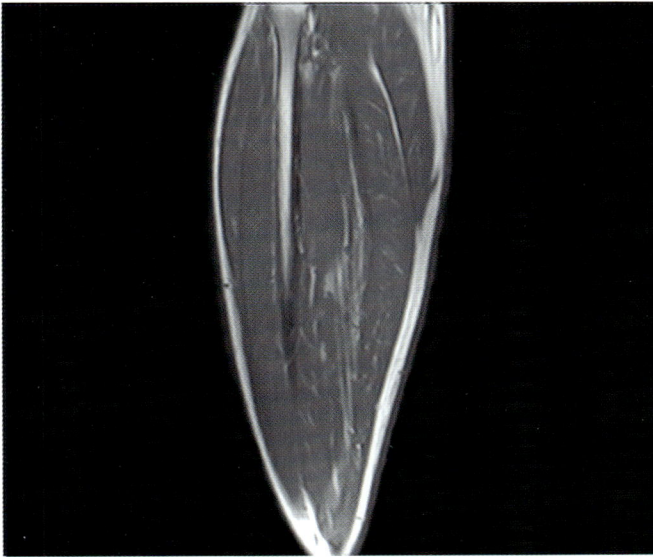
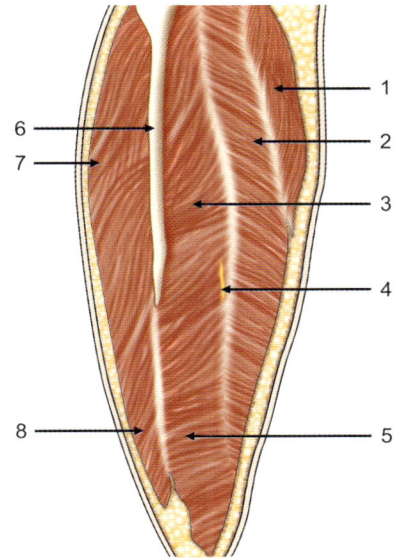

Figure 16.19

1. Gastrocnemius, medial head
2. Soleus
3. Tibialis posterior
4. Posterior tibial artery, tibial nerve
5. Flexor hallucis longus
6. Fibula
7. Peroneus longus
8. Peroneus brevis

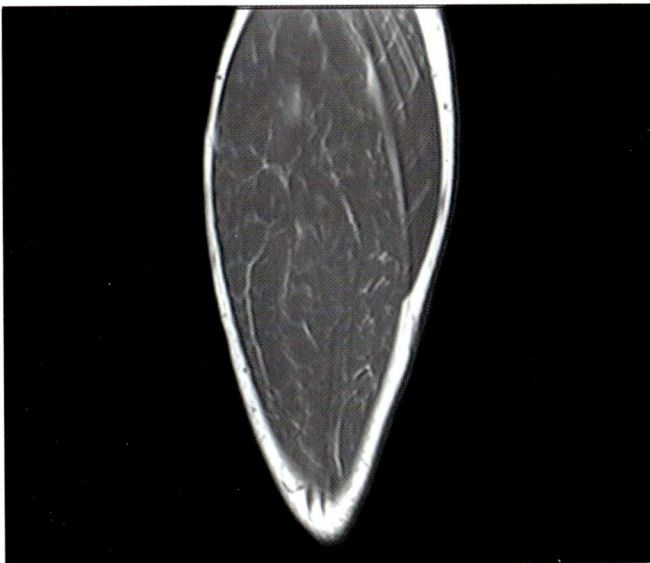
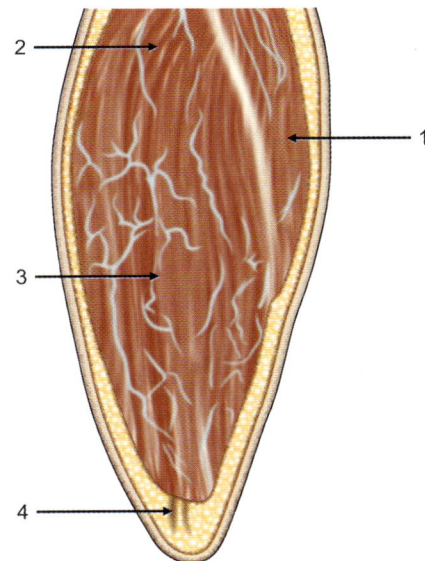

Figure 16.20

1. Gastrocnemius, medial head
2. Gastrocnemius, lateral head
3. Soleus
4. Lesser saphenous vein

SAGITTAL IMAGES

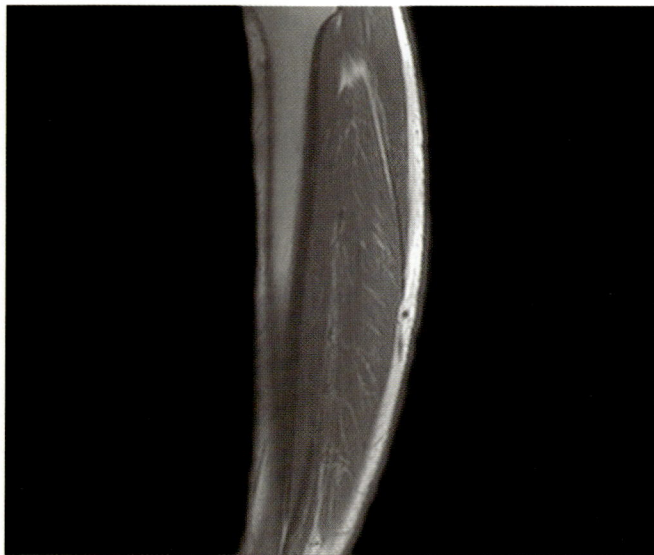

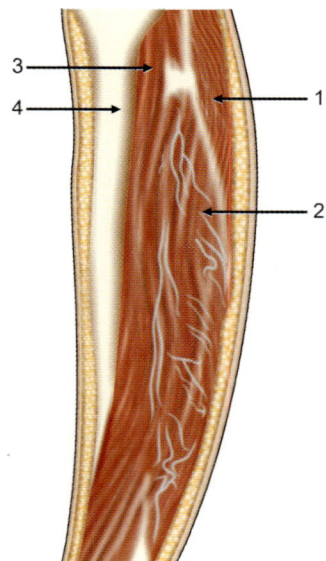

Figure 16.21

1. Gastrocnemius, medial head	3. Popliteus muscle
2. Soleus	4. Tibia

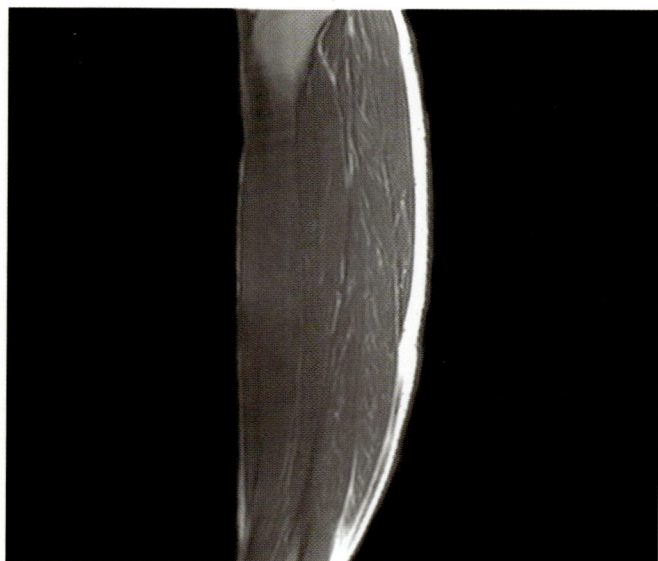

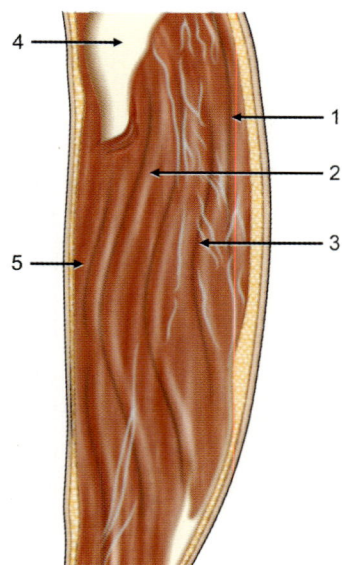

Figure 16.22

1. Gastrocnemius, medial head	4. Tibia
2. Tibialis posterior	5. Tibialis anterior
3. Soleus	

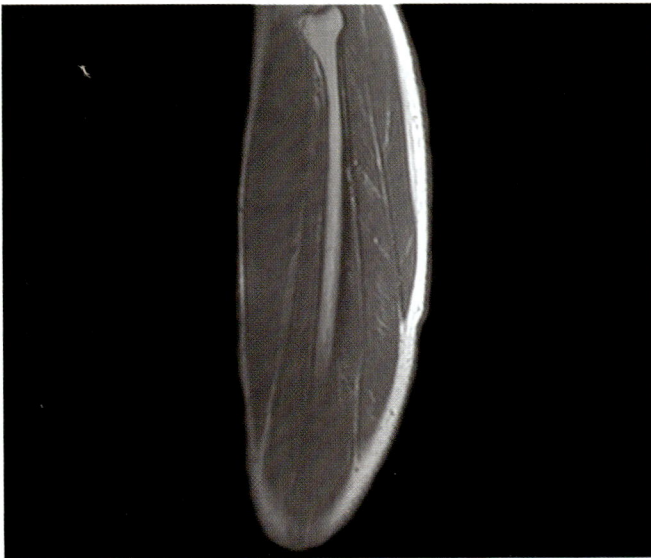

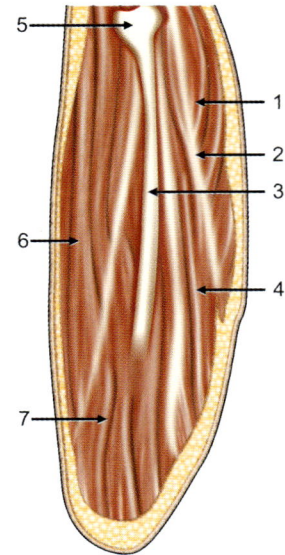

Figure 16.23

1. Gastrocnemius, lateral head
2. Soleus
3. Fibula
4. Flexor hallucis longus
5. Fibula, head
6. Tibialis anterior
7. Extensor hallucis and digitorum longus

Figure 16.24

1. Gastrocnemius, lateral head
2. Soleus
3. Fibula
4. Extensor hallucis and digitorum longus
5. Peroneus longus and brevis

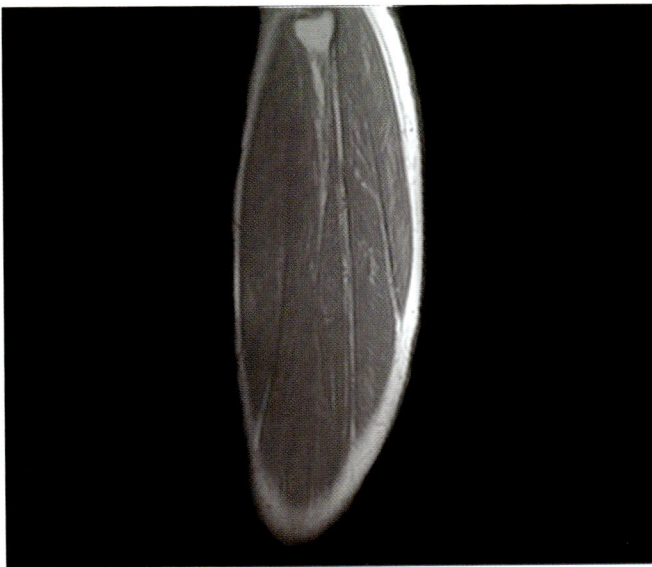

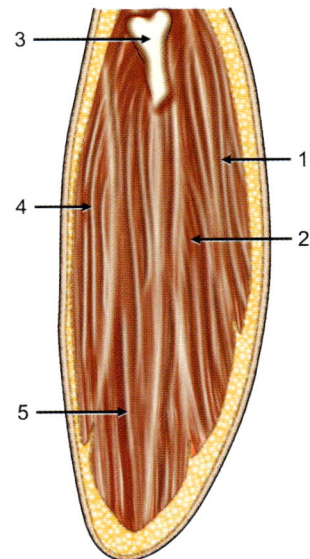

CHAPTER 17

Knee

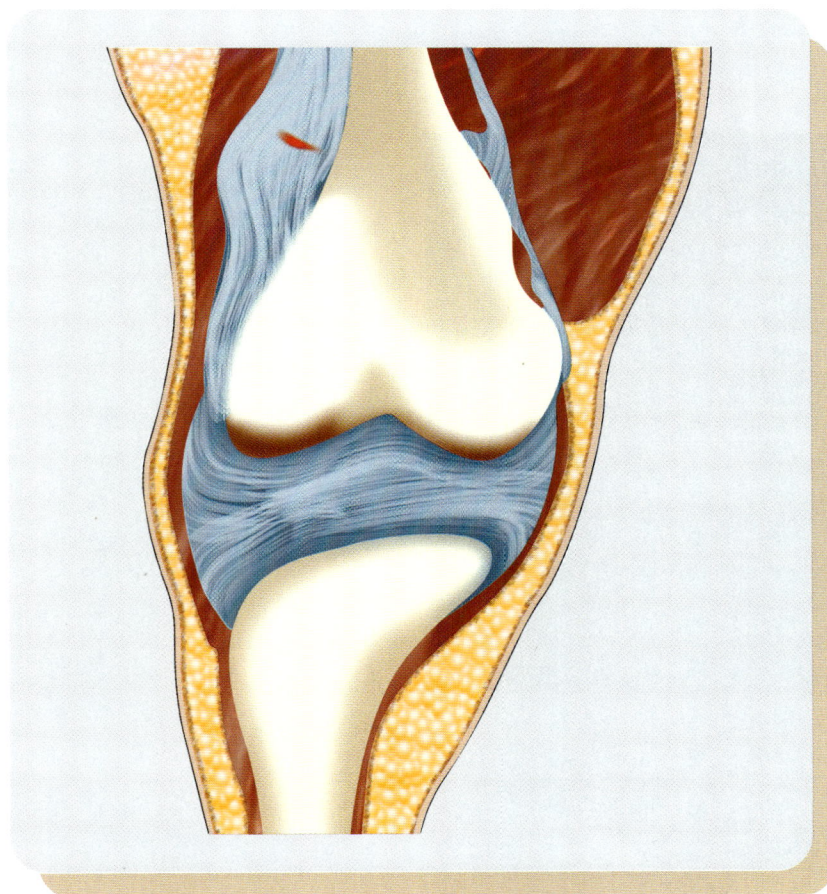

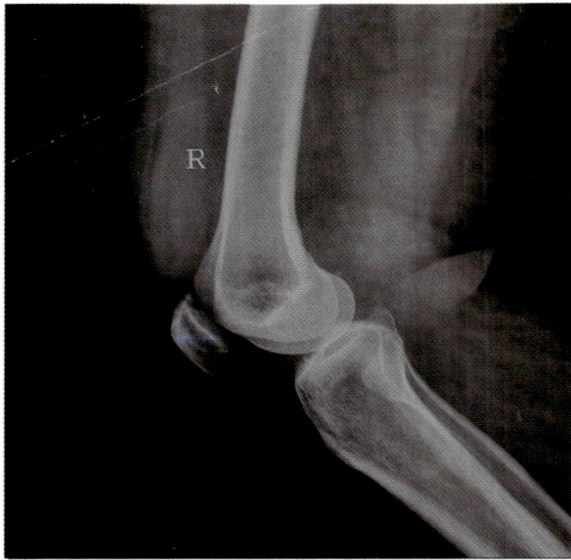

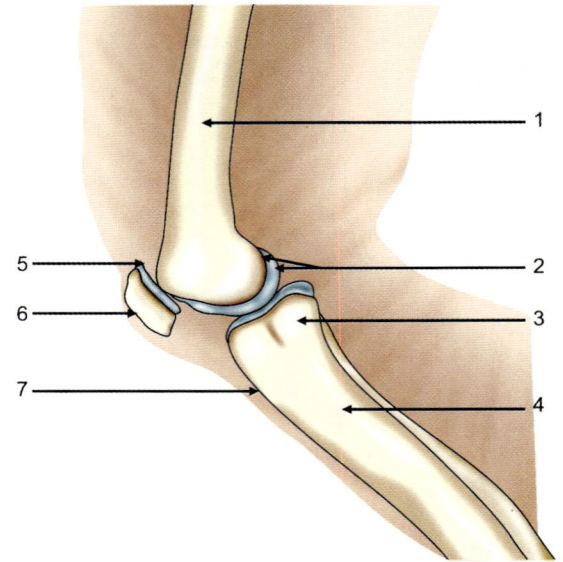

Figure 17.1

1. Femur	5. Patello-femoral joint
2. Femoral condyles	6. Patella
3. Fibula, head	7. Tibial tuberosity
4. Tibia	

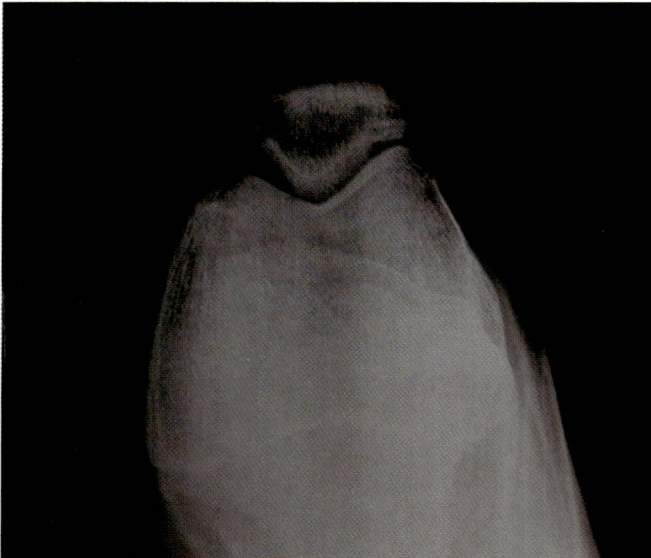

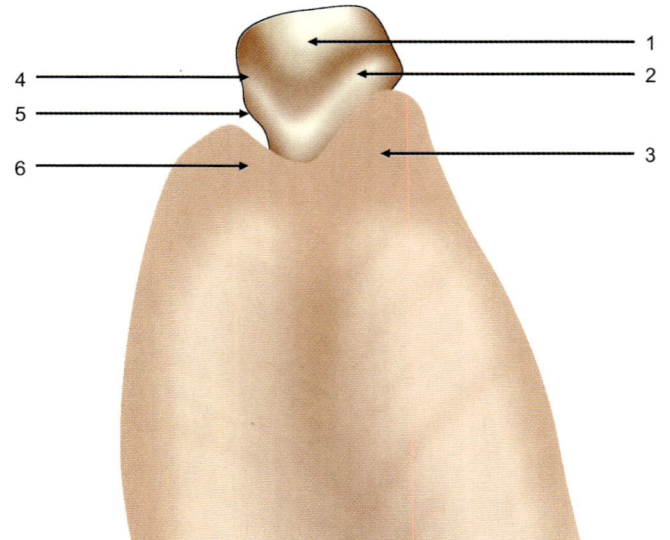

Figure 17.2

1. Patella	4. Medial patellar facet
2. Lateral patellar facet	5. Patellofemoral joint
3. Lateral femoral condyle	6. Medial femoral condyle

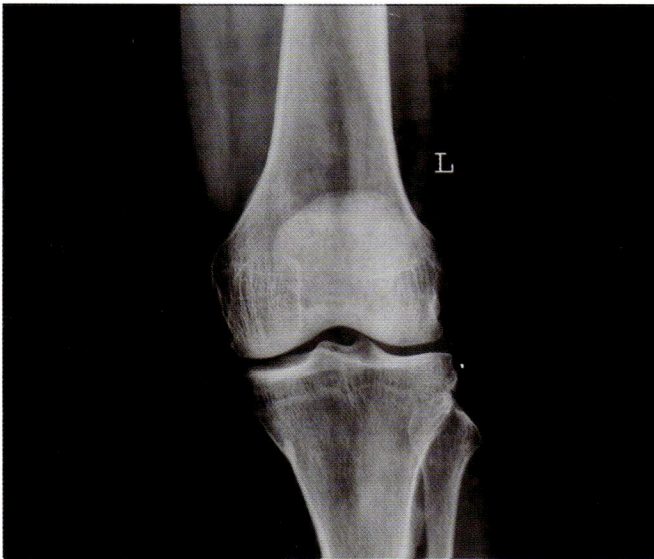

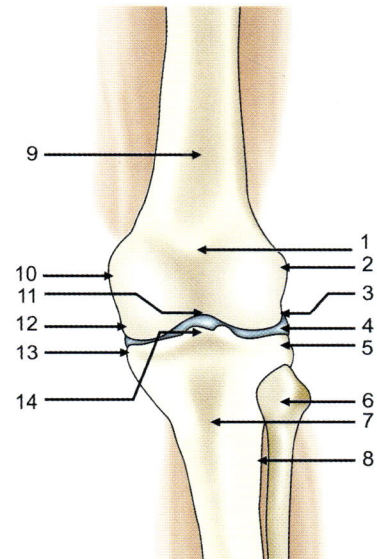

Figure 17.3

1. Patella	6. Fibular head	11. Intercondylar fossa
2. Lateral femoral epicondyle	7. Tibia	12. Medial femoral condyle
3. Lateral femoral condyle	8. Interosseous membrane	13. Medial tibial condyle
4. Joint space	9. Femur	14. Tibial tubercle
5. Lateral tibial condyle	10. Medial femoral epicondyle	

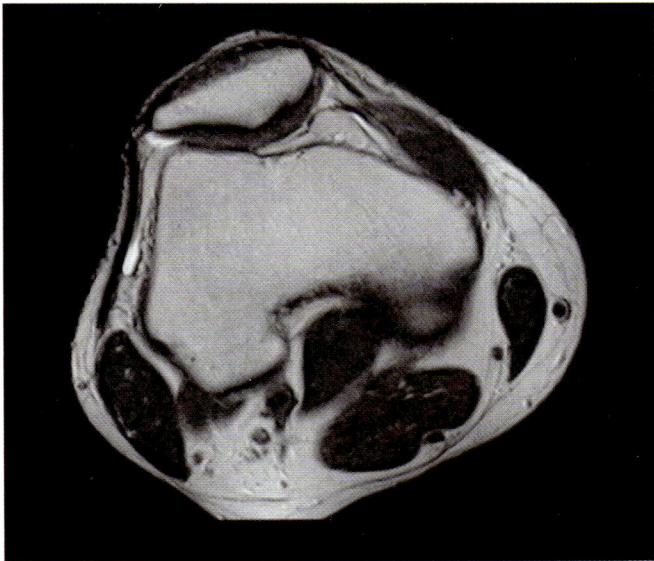

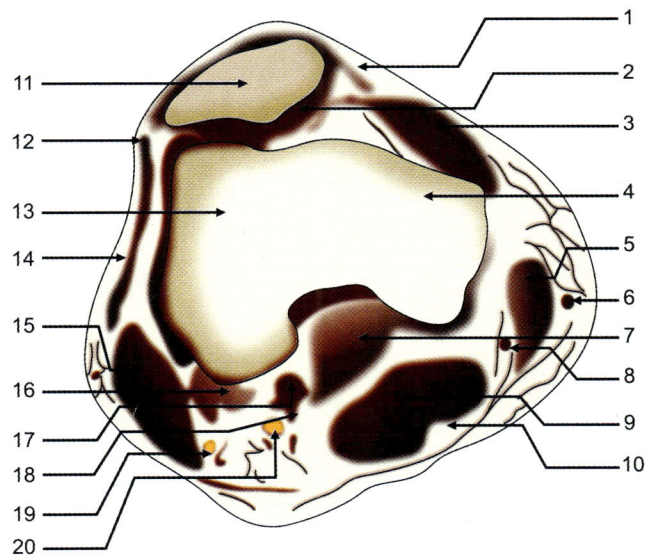

Figure 17.4

1. Medial patellar retinaculum	8. Gracilis	15. Biceps
2. Articular cartilage	9. Semimembranosus	16. Gastrocnemius lateral head
3. Vastus medialis	10. Semitendinosus tendon	17. Popliteal artery
4. Medial femoral condyle	11. Patella	18. Popliteal vein
5. Sartorius	12. Lateral patellar retinaculum	19. Common peroneal nerve
6. Great saphenous vein	13. Lateral femoral condyle	20. Tibial nerve
7. Gastrocnemius, medial head	14. Ilio-tibial tract	

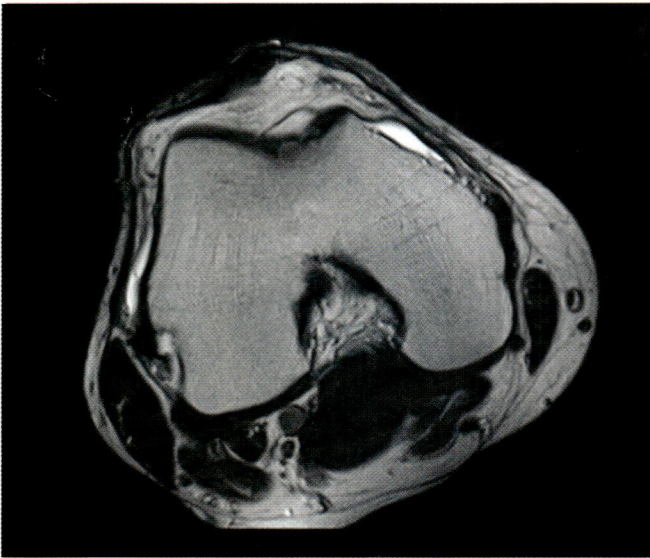

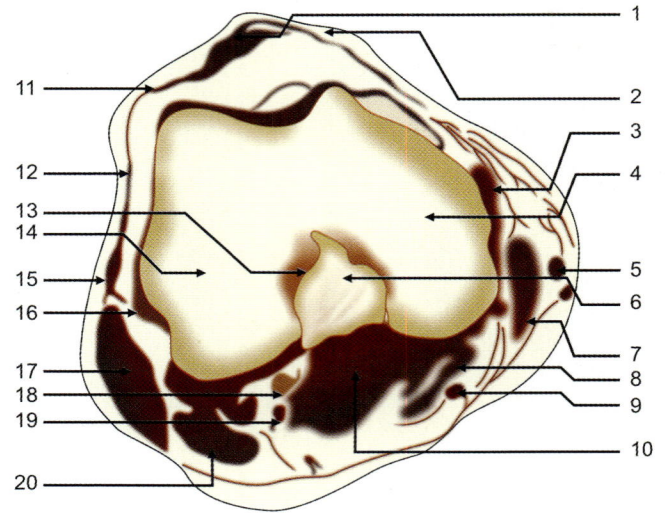

Figure 17.5

1. Patellar ligament	8. Semimembranosus	15. Lateral collateral ligament
2. Medial patellar retinaculum	9. Semitendinosus tendon	16. Popliteus tendon
3. Medial collateral ligament	10. Gastrocnemius, medial head	17. Biceps
4. Medial femoral condyle	11. Lateral patellar retinaculum	18. Popliteal artery
5. Great saphenous vein	12. Iliotibial tract	19. Popliteal vein
6. Intercondylar notch	13. Anterior cruciate ligament	20. Gastrocnemius, lateral head
7. Sartorius	14. Lateral femoral condyle	

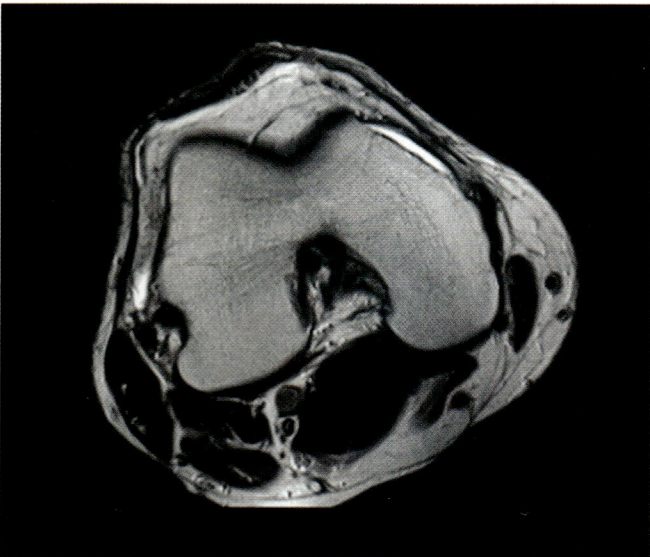

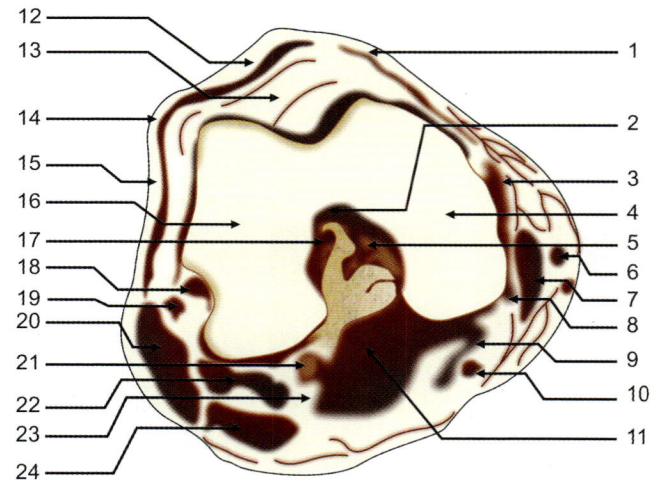

Figure 17.6

1. Medial patellar retinaculum	9. Semimembranosus	17. Anterior cruciate ligament
2. Intercondylar notch	10. Semitendinosus tendon	18. Popliteus tendon
3. Medial collateral ligament	11. Gastrocnemius, medial head	19. Lateral collateral ligament
4. Medial femoral condyle	12. Patellar ligament	20. Biceps
5. Posterior cruciate ligament	13. Infrapatellar fat	21. Popliteal artery
6. Great saphenous vein	14. Lateral patellar retinaculum	22. Plantaris
7. Sartorius	15. Ilio-tibial tract	23. Tibial nerve
8. Gracilis	16. Lateral femoral condyle	24. Gastrocnemius, lateral head

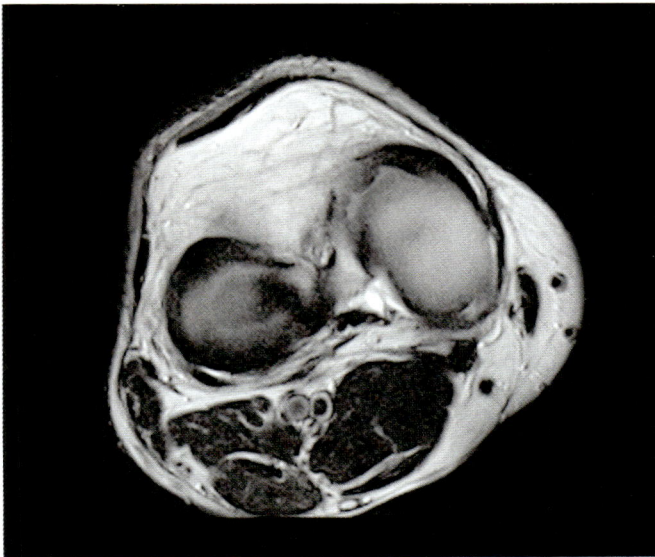
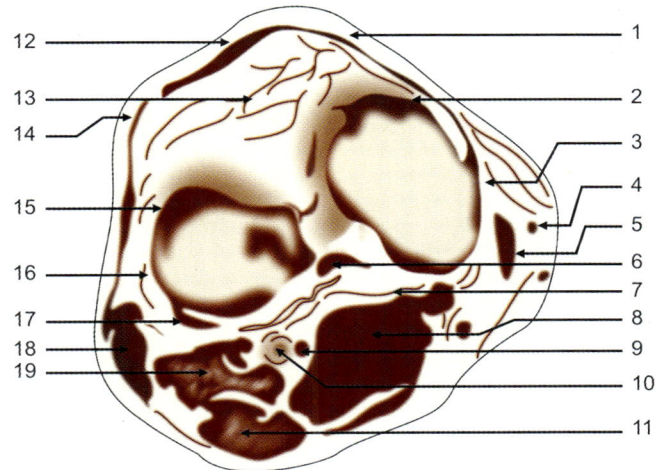

Figure 17.7

1. Medial patellar retinaculum	8. Gastrocnemius, medial head	15. Lateral meniscus
2. Medial meniscus	9. Popliteal vein	16. Lateral collateral ligament
3. Medial collateral ligament	10. Popliteal artery	17. Popliteus tendon
4. Great saphenous vein	11. Gastrocnemius, lateral head	18. Biceps
5. Gracilis	12. Patellar ligament	19. Plantaris
6. Posterior cruciate ligament	13. Infrapatellar Hoffa's fat pad	
7. Posterior joint capsule	14. Lateral patellar retinaculum	

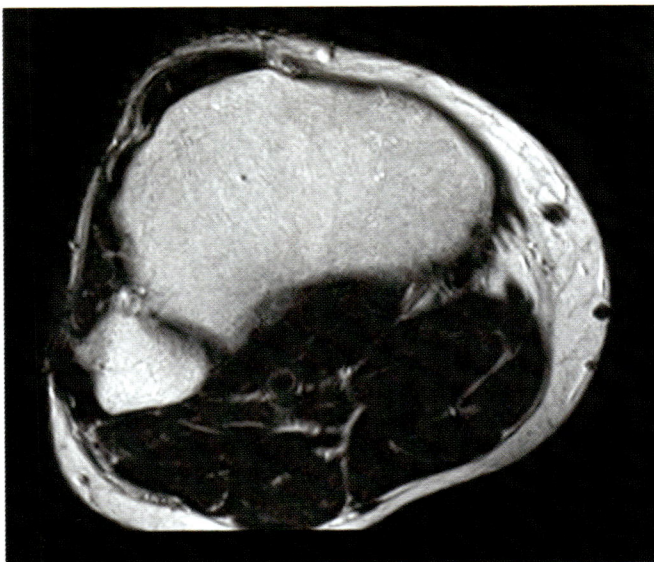
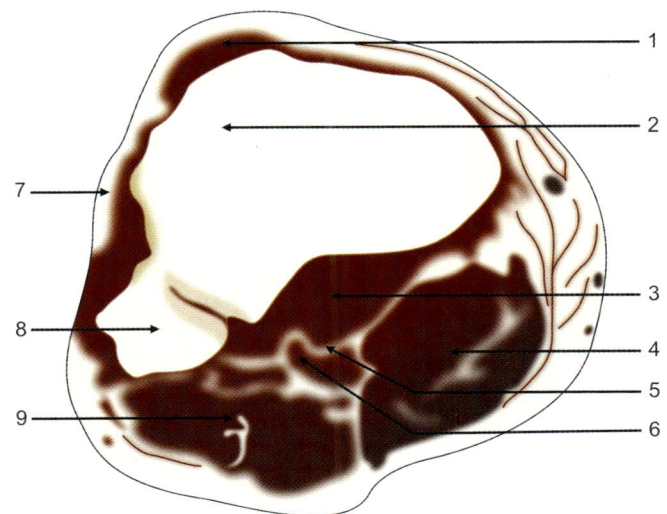

Figure 17.8

1. Patellar ligament	6 Popliteal artery
2. Tibia	7 Iliotibial tract
3. Popliteus	8. Fibula
4. Gastrocnemius medial head	9. Gastrocnemius lateral head
5. Popliteal vein	

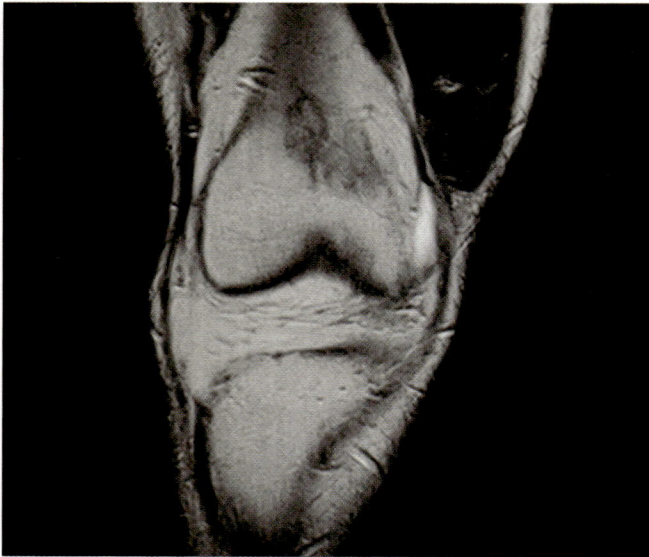
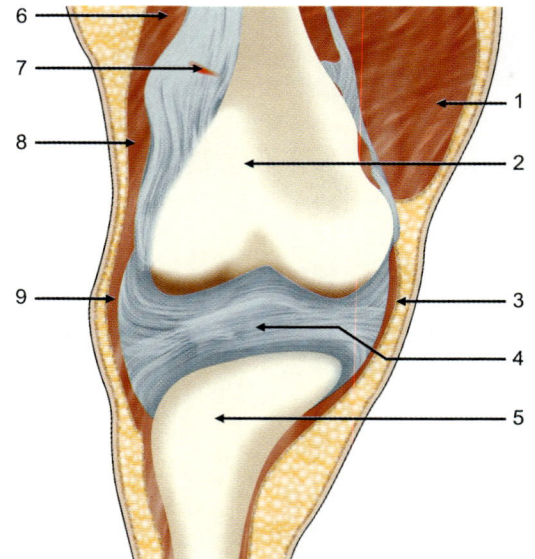

Figure 17.9

1. Vastus medialis	6. Vastus lateralis
2. Femur	7. Superior lateral geniculate artery
3. Medial patellar retinaculum	8. Iliotibial tract
4. Infrapatellar fat	9. Lateral patellar retinaculum
5. Tibia	

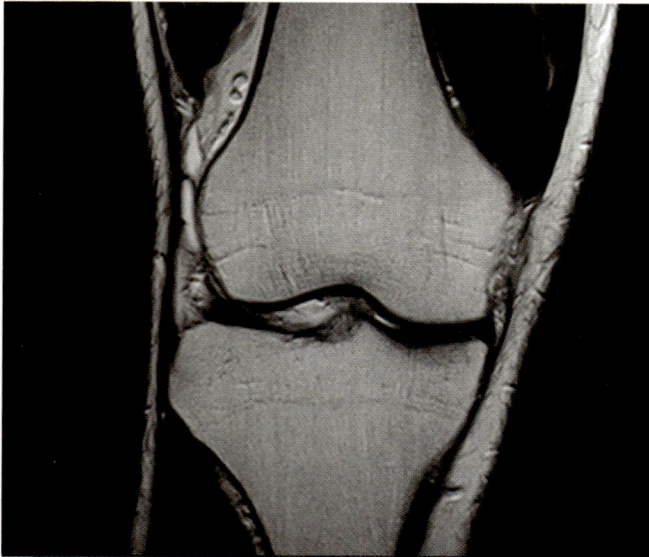
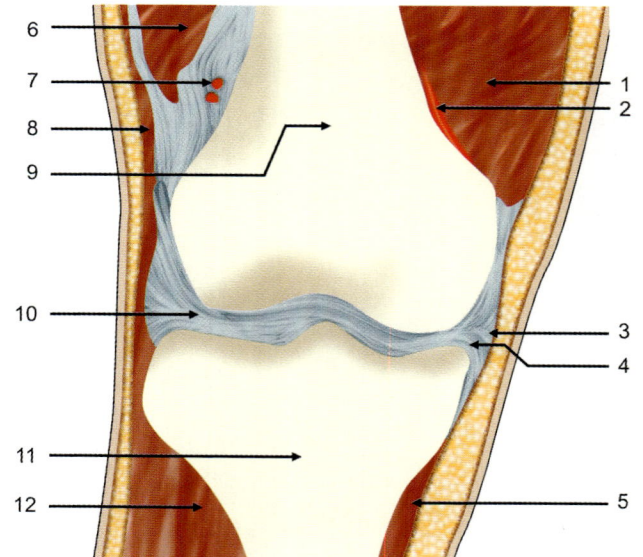

Figure 17.10

1. Vastus medialis	7. Superior lateral genicular artery
2. Superior medial genicular artery	8. Ilio-tibial tract
3. Medial collateral ligament	9. Femur
4. Medial meniscus anterior horn	10. Lateral meniscus, anterior horn
5. Pes anserinus	11. Tibia
6. Vastus lateralis	12. Extensor digitorum longus

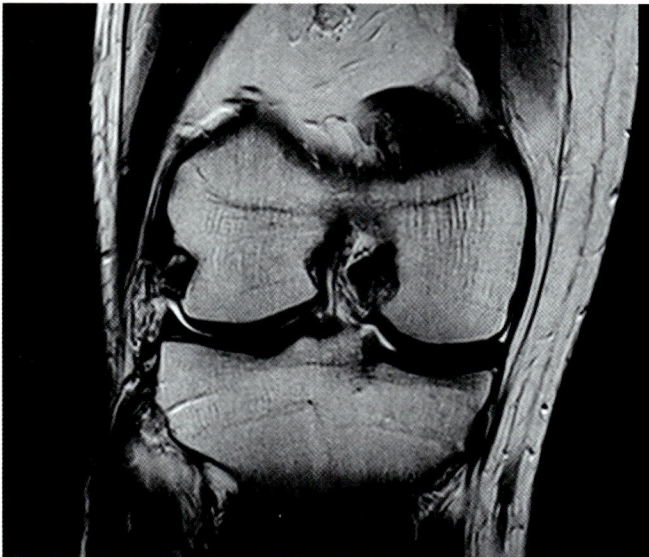

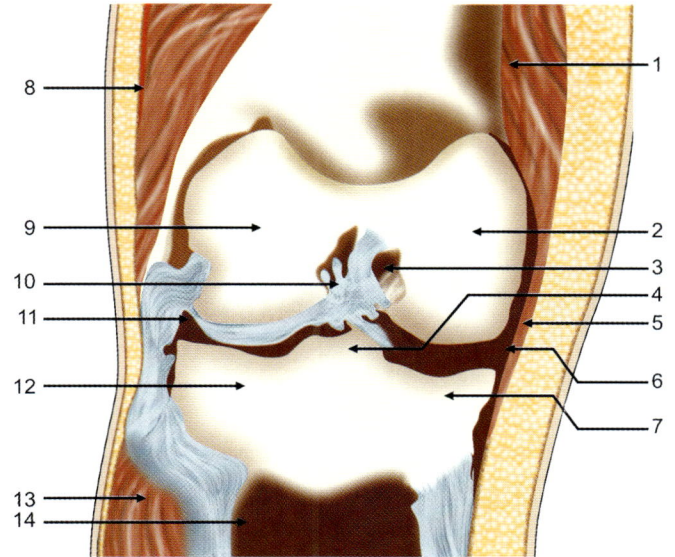

Figure 17.11

1. Vastus medialis	6. Medial meniscus	11. Lateral meniscus
2. Femoral condyle (medial)	7. Tibial condyle (medial)	12. Tibial condyle (lateral)
3. Posterior cruciate ligament	8. Iliotibial tract	13. Extensor digitorum longus
4. Tibial tubercles	9. Femoral condyle (lateral)	14. Tibialis posterior
5. Medial collateral ligament	10. Anterior cruciate ligament	

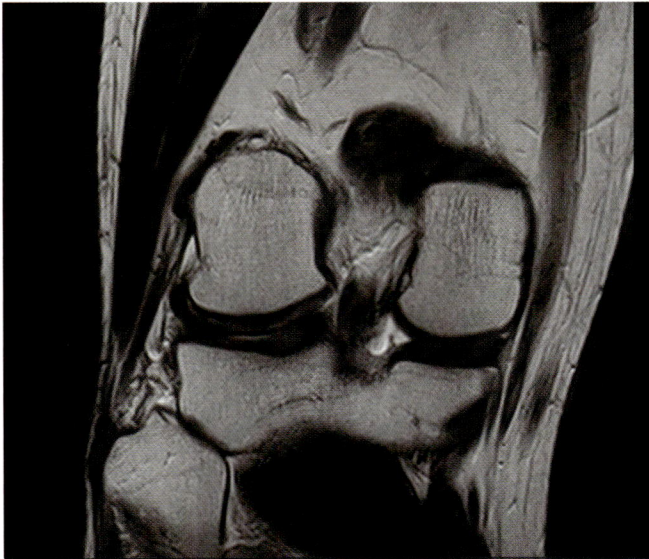

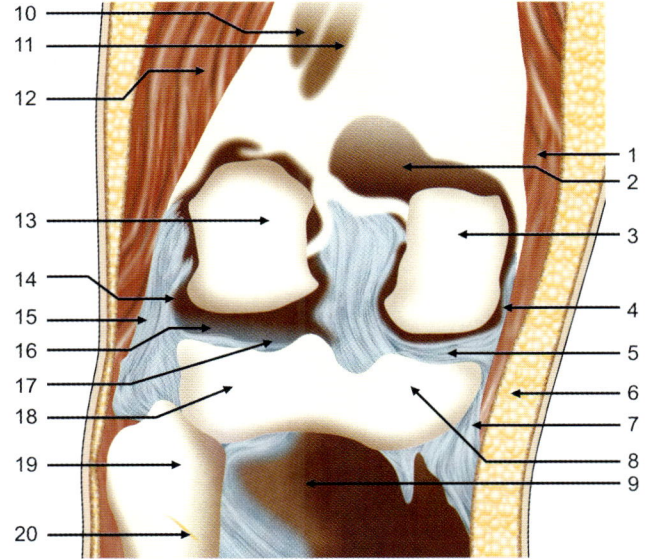

Figure 17.12

1. Sartorius	8. Medial tibial condyle	15. Lateral collateral ligament
2. Gastrocnemius, medial head	9. Popliteus	16. Lateral meniscus
3. Medial femoral condyle	10. Popliteal vein	17. Articular cartilage
4. Medial collateral ligament	11. Popliteal artery	18. Lateral tibial condyle
5. Medial meniscus	12. Biceps femoris	19. Fibula
6. Great saphenous vein	13. Lateral femoral condyle	20. Common peroneal nerve
7. Gracilis tendon	14. Popliteus tendon	

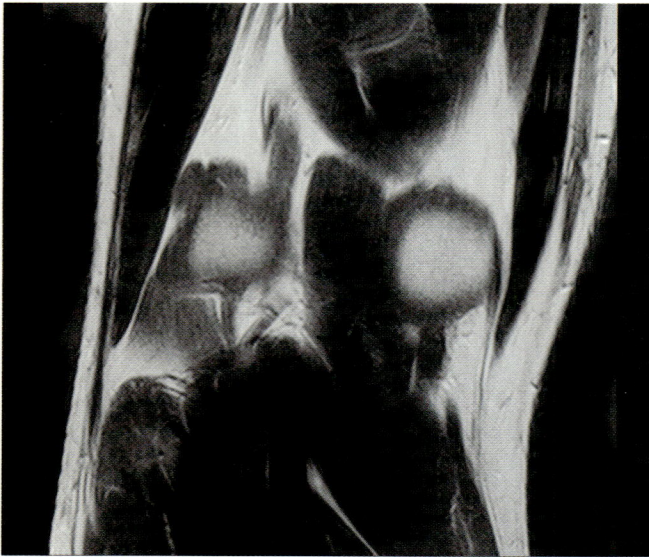

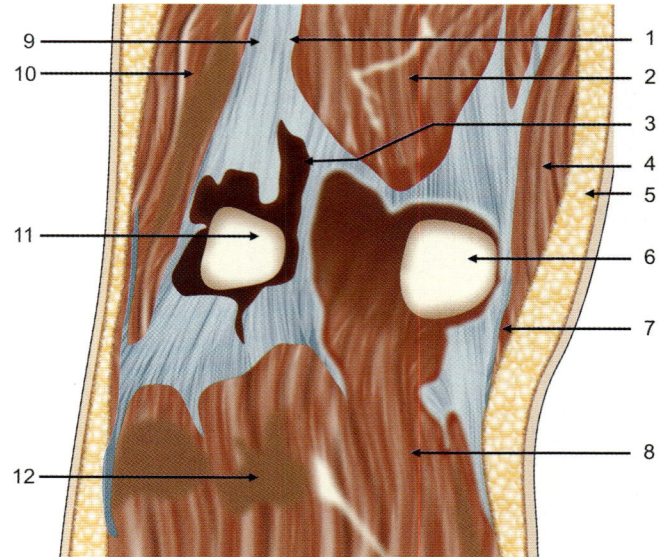

Figure 17.13

1. Tibial nerve	7. Gracilis tendon
2. Semimembranosus	8. Gastrocnemius, medial head
3. Popliteal artery	9. Common peroneal nerve
4. Sartorius	10. Biceps femoris
5. Great saphenous vein	11. Lateral femoral condyle
6. Medial femoral condyle	12. Gastrocnemius, lateral head

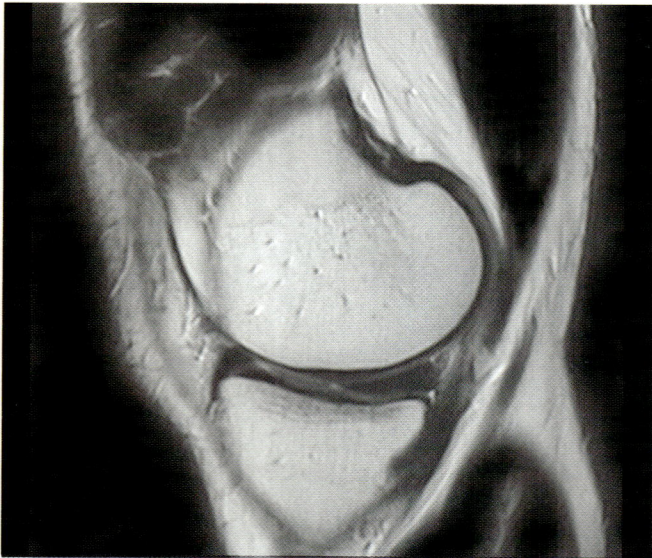

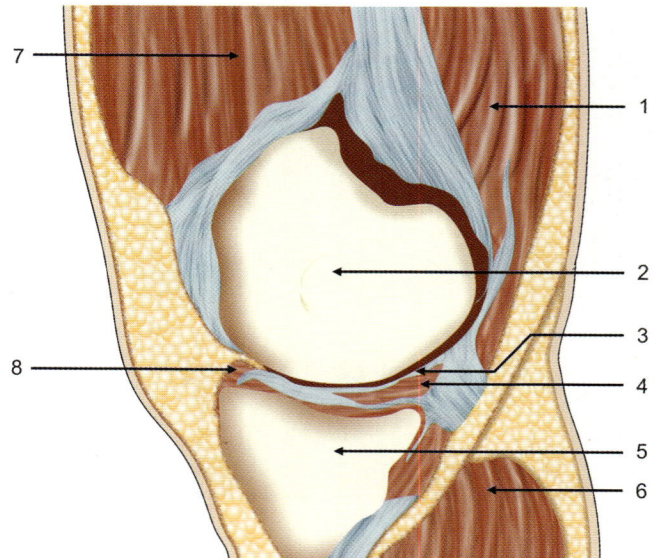

Figure 17.14

1. Semimembranosus	5. Medial tibial condyle
2. Medial femoral condyle	6. Gastrocnemius (medial head)
3. Articular cartilage	7. Vastus medialis
4. Medial meniscus, posterior horn	8. Medial meniscus, anterior horn

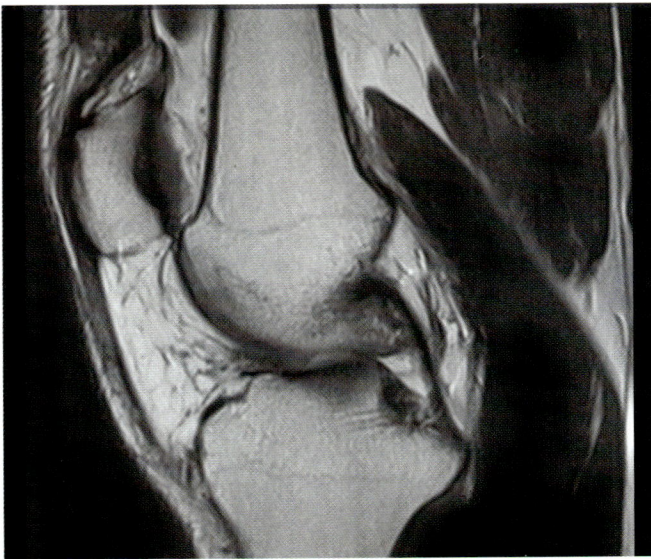

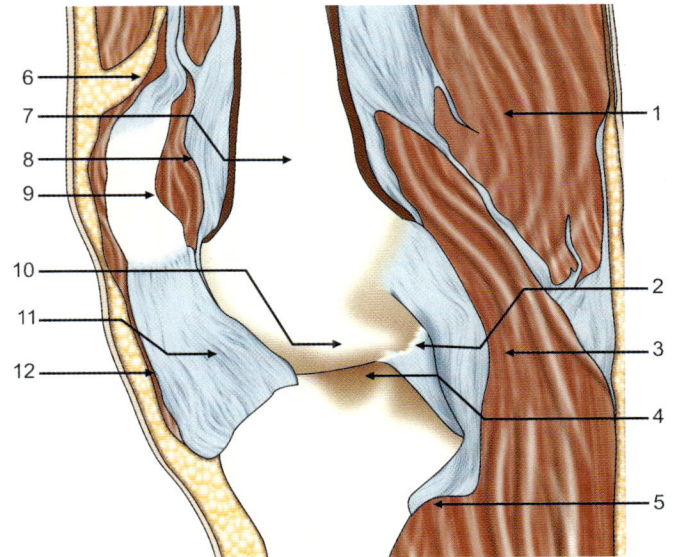

Figure 17.15

1. Semimembranosus	7. Femur
2. Posterior cruciate ligament	8. Articular cartilage
3. Gastrocnemius (medial head)	9. Patella
4. Medial intercondylar eminence	10. Anterior cruciate ligament
5. Popliteus	11. Hoffa's fat pad
6. Quadriceps tendon	12. Patellar ligament

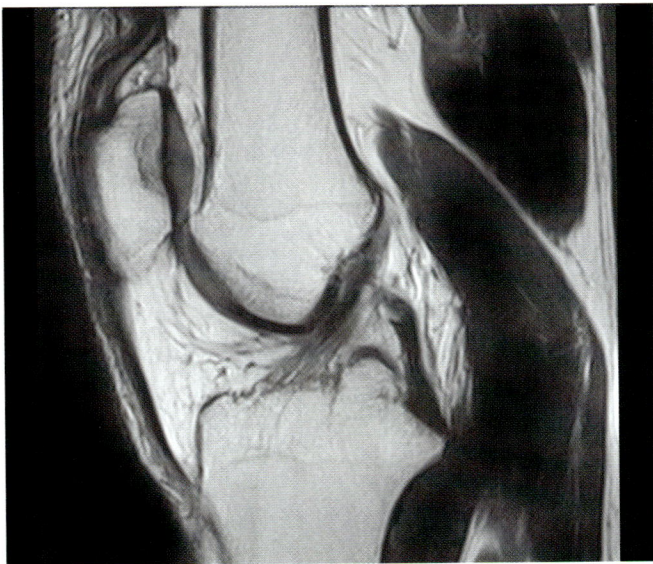

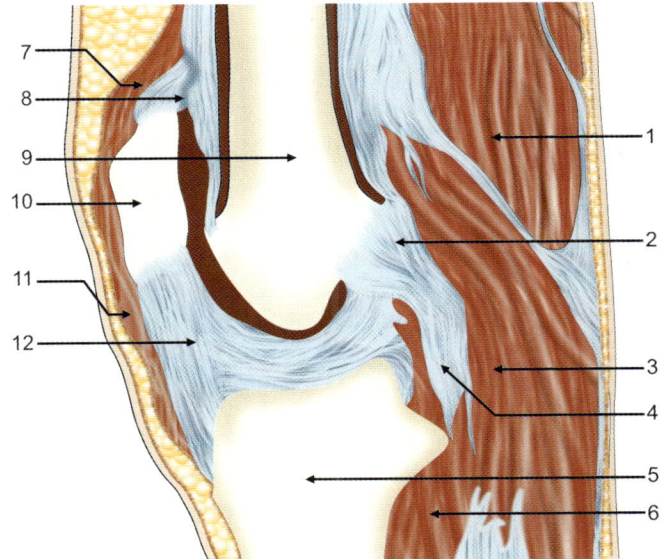

Figure 17.16

1. Semimembranosus	7. Quadriceps tendon
2. Intercondylar shelf	8. Synovial space
3. Gastrocnemius (medial head)	9. Femur
4. Posterior cruciate ligament	10. Patella
5. Tibia	11. Patellar ligament
6. Popliteus	12. Hoffa's fat pad

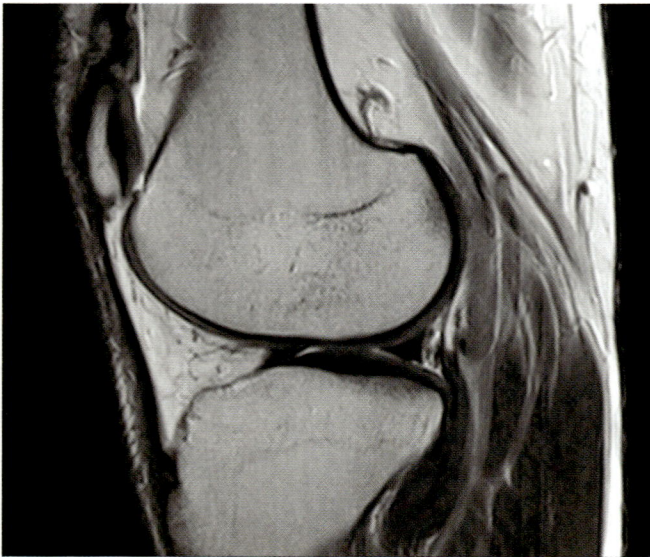

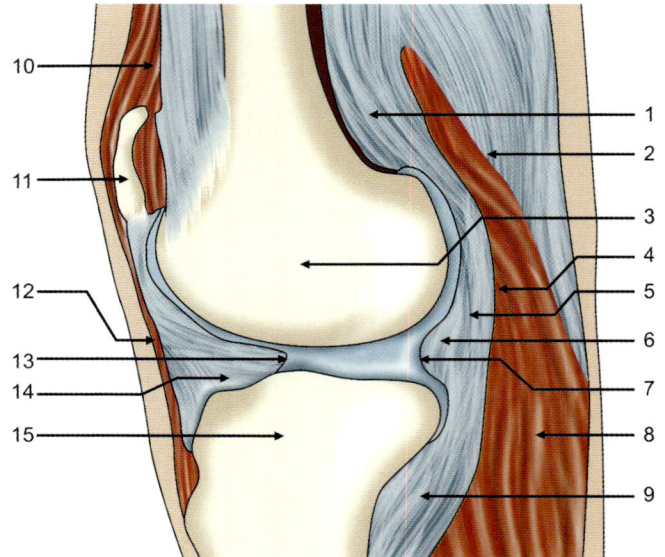

Figure 17.17

1. Superior lateral genicular artery	6. Posterior joint capsule	11. Patella
2. Tibial nerve	7. Lateral meniscus, posterior horn	12. Patellar ligament
3. Femoral condyle (lateral)	8. Gastrocnemius (lateral head)	13. Lateral meniscus, anterior horn
4. Popliteal vein	9. Popliteus	14. Hoffa's fat pad
5. Popliteal artery	10. Quadriceps tendon	15. Tibial condyle (lateral)

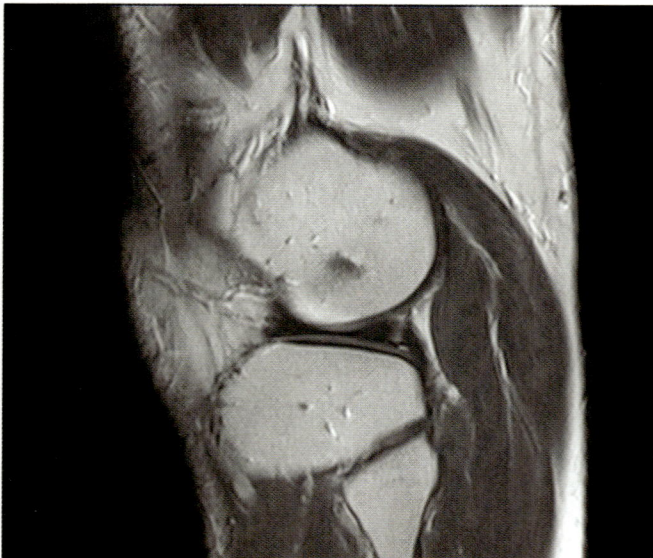

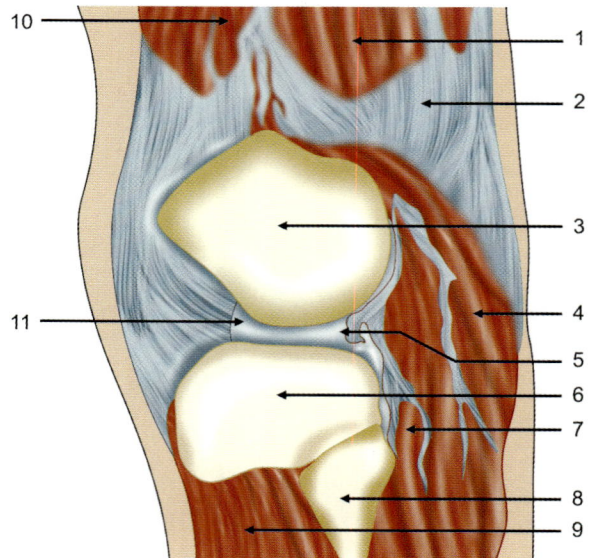

Figure 17.18

1. Biceps femoris	5. Lateral meniscus, posterior horn	9. Tibialis anterior
2. Common peroneal nerve	6. Tibial condyle (lateral)	10. Vastus lateralis
3. Femoral condyle (lateral)	7. Popliteus	11. Lateral meniscus, anterior horn
4. Gastrocnemius (lateral head)	8. Fibula	

CHAPTER 18

Ankle and Foot

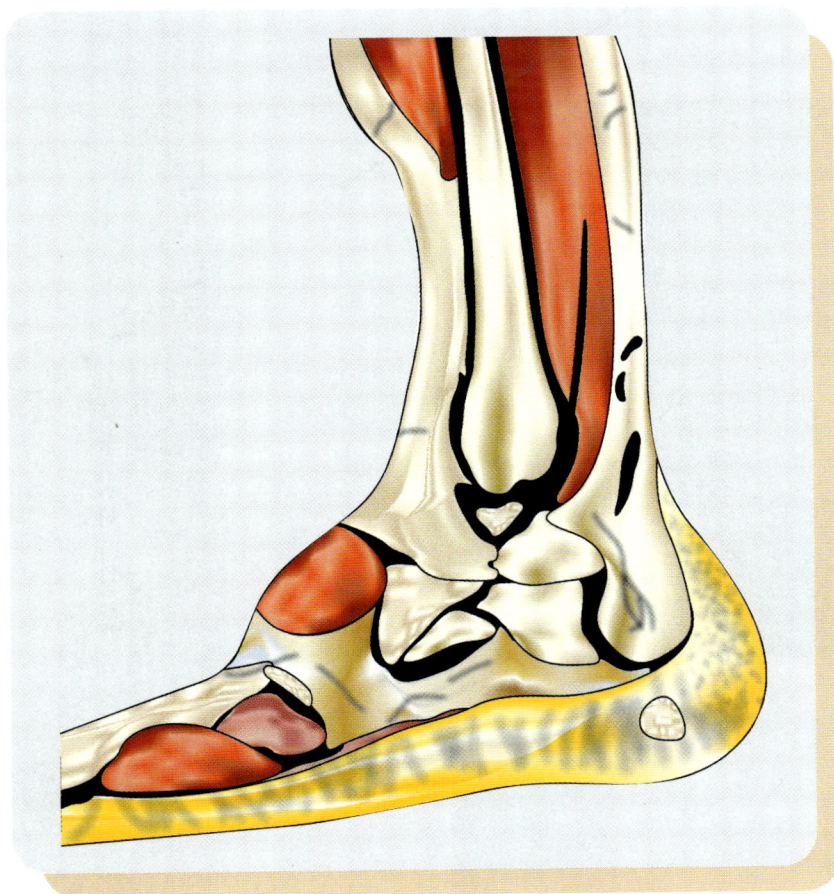

X-RAY FIGURES

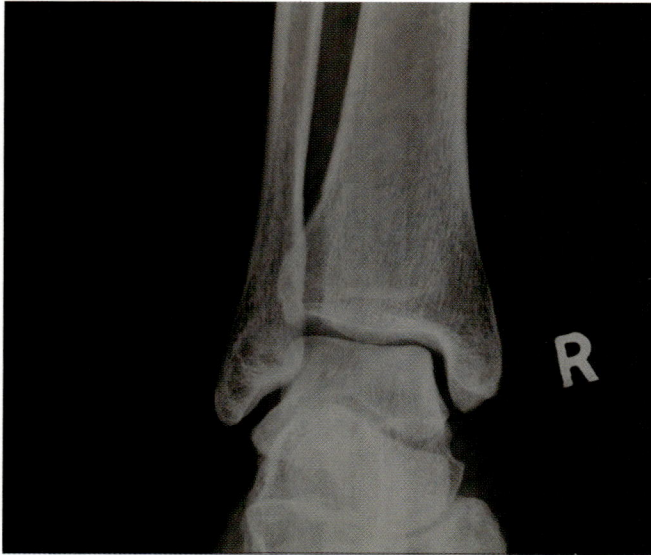

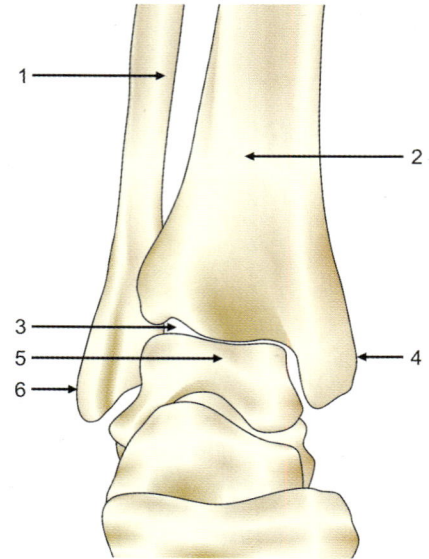

Figure 18.1

1. Fibula
2. Tibia
3. Tibiotalar joint space
4. Medial malleolus
5. Talus
6. Lateral malleolus

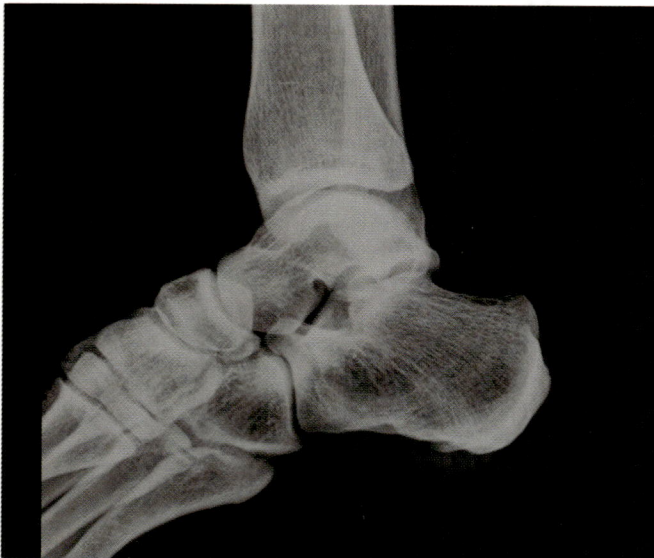

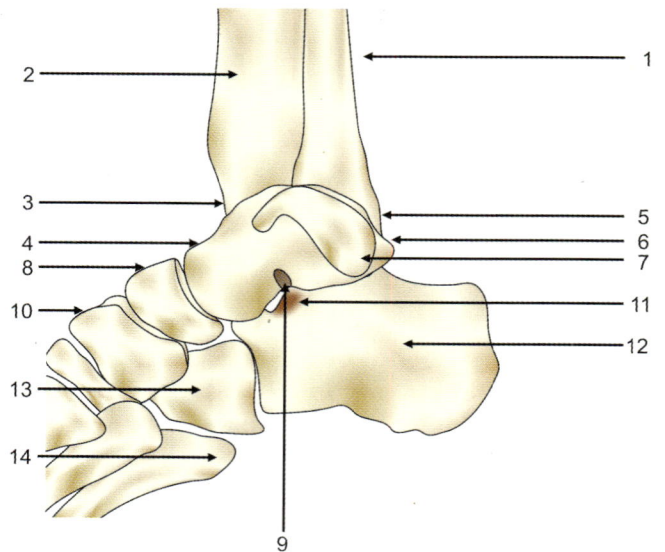

Figure 18.2

1. Fibula
2. Tibia
3. Medial malleolus
4. Head of talus
5. Lateral malleolus
6. Lateral tubercle of talus
7. Medial tubercle of talus
8. Navicular
9. Sinus tarsi
10. Lateral cuneiform
11. Sustentaculum tali
12. Calcaneus
13. Cuboid
14. Base of fifth metatarsal

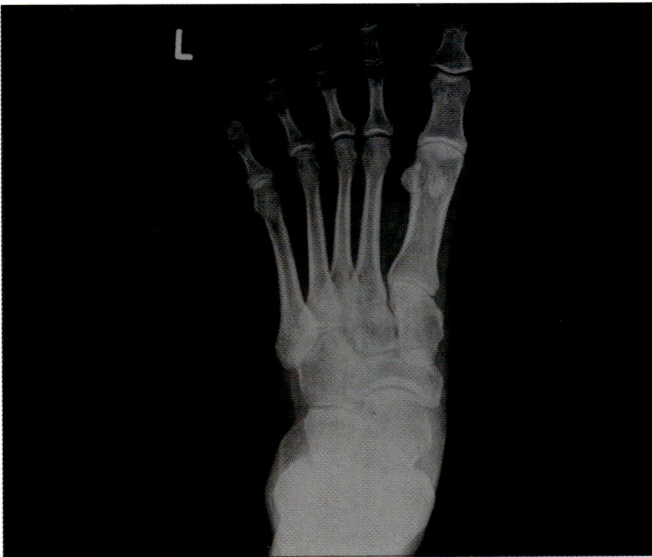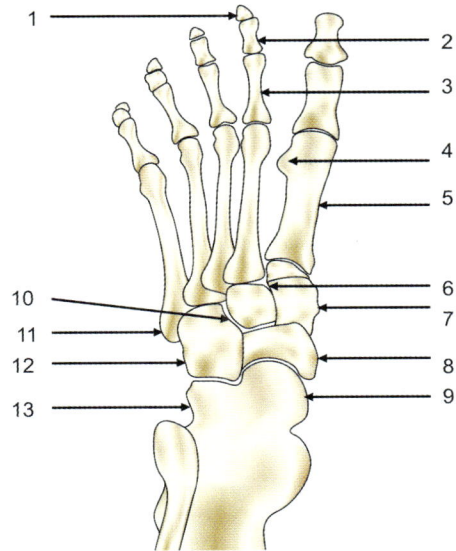

Figure 18.3

1. Distal phalanx of second toe
2. Middle phalanx of second toe
3. Proximal phalanx of second toe
4. Sesamoid bone
5. First metatarsal
6. Intermediate cuneiform
7. Medial cuneiform
8. Navicular
9. Talus
10. Lateral cuneiform
11. Tuberosity of base of fifth metatarsal
12. Cuboid
13. Calcaneus

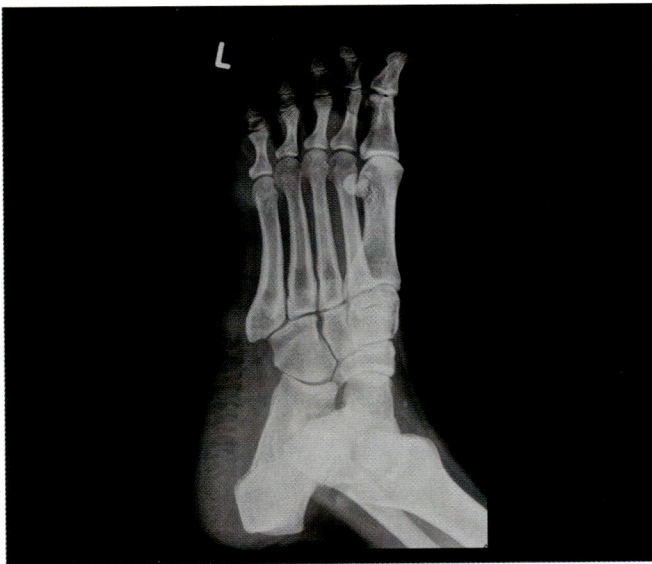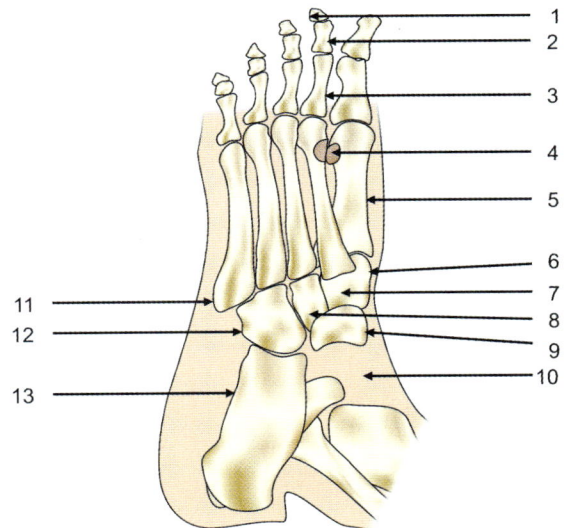

Figure 18.4

1. Distal phalanx of second toe
2. Middle phalanx of second toe
3. Proximal phalanx of second toe
4. Sesamoid bone
5. First metatarsal
6. Medial cuneiform
7. Intermediate cuneiform
8. Lateral cuneiform
9. Navicular
10. Talus
11. Tuberosity of base of fifth metatarsal
12. Cuboid
13. Calcaneus

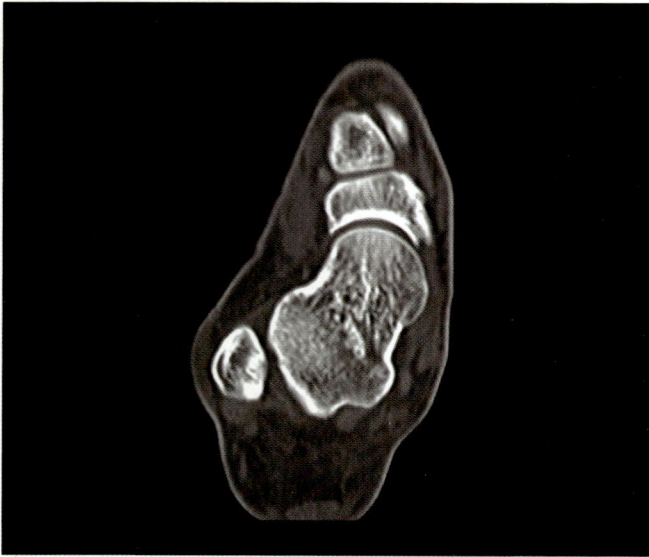

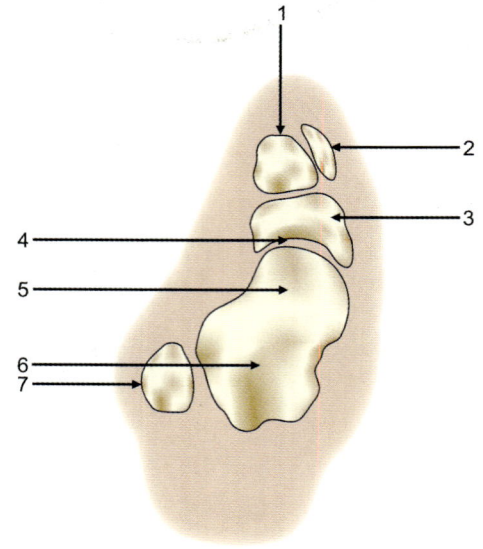

Figure 18.5

1. Intermediate cuneiform
2. Medial cuneiform
3. Navicular
4. Talonavicular joint
5. Head of talus
6. Talus, body
7. Lateral malleolus

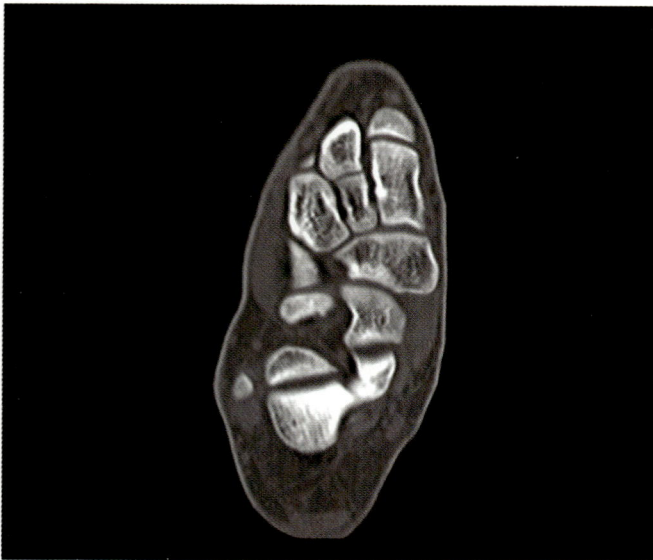

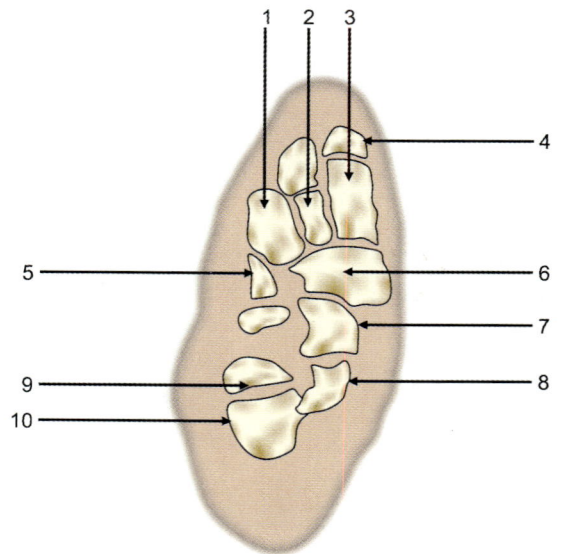

Figure 18.6

1. Lateral cuneiform
2. Intermediate cuneiform
3. Medial cuneiform
4. Base, first metatarsal
5. Cuboid
6. Navicular
7. Talus, head
8. Sustentaculum
9. Talus, posterior facet
10. Calcaneus

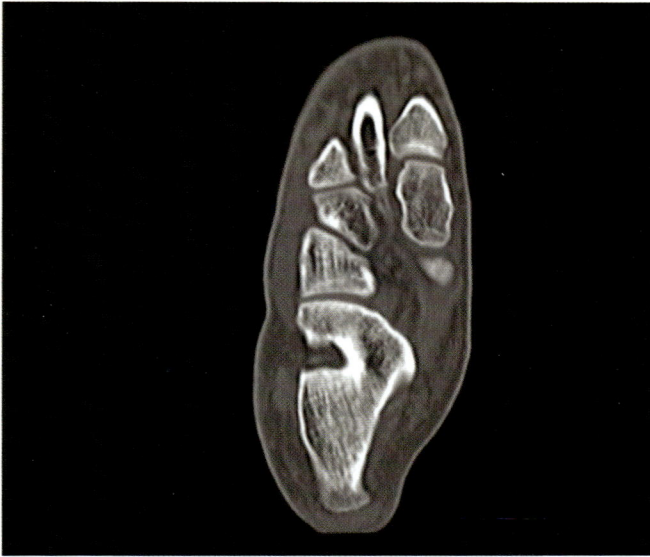

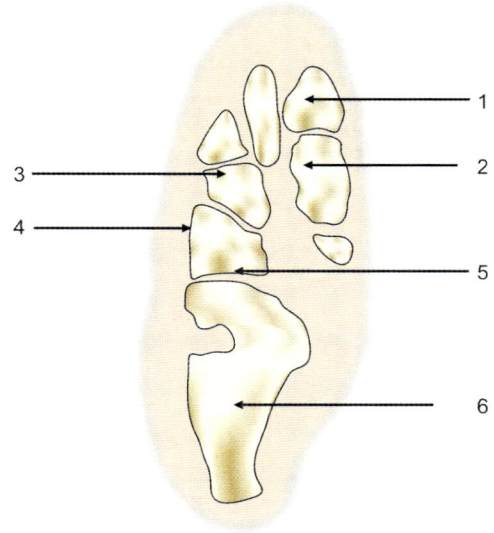

Figure 18.7

1. First metatarsal
2. Medial cuneiform
3. Lateral cuneiform
4. Cuboid
5. Calcaneocuboid joint
6. Calcaneus

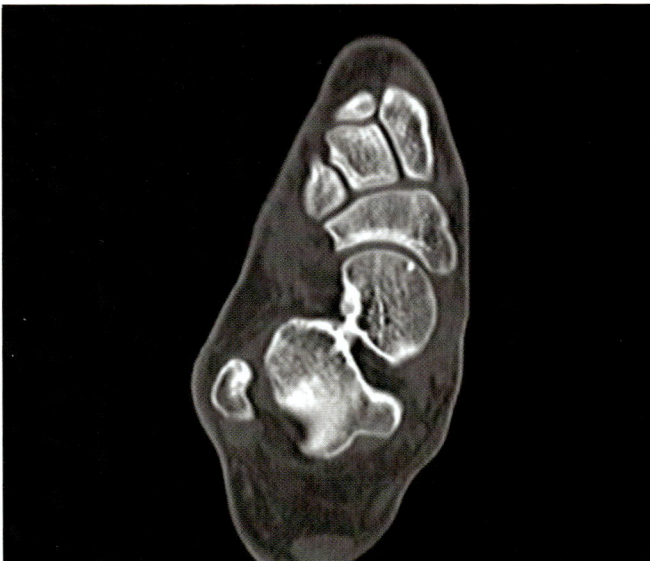

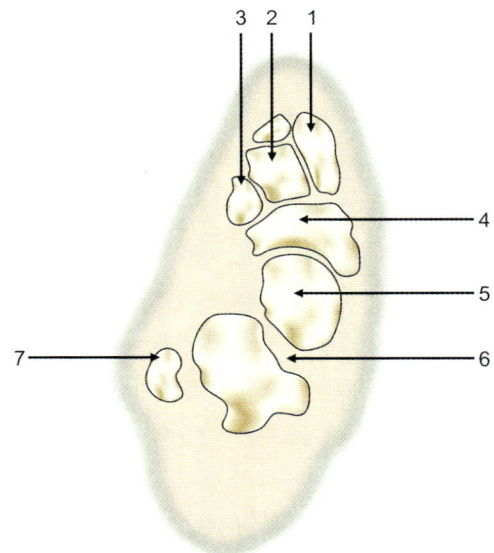

Figure 18.8

1,2,3. Cuneiform
4. Navicular
5. Head, talus
6. Tarsal sinus
7. Lateral malleolus

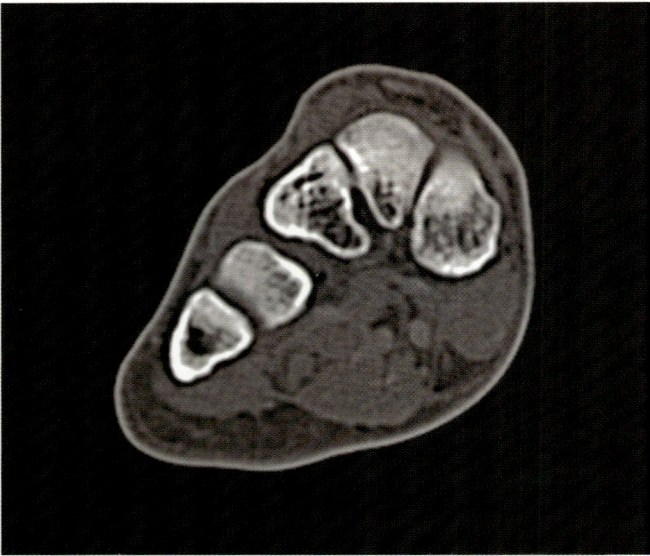

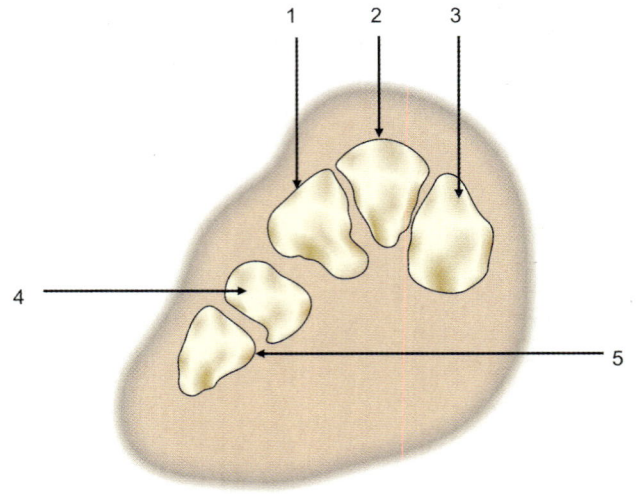

Figure 18.9

1. Lateral cuneiform
2. Intermediate cuneiform
3. Medial cuneiform
4. Cuboid
5. Fifth metatarsal

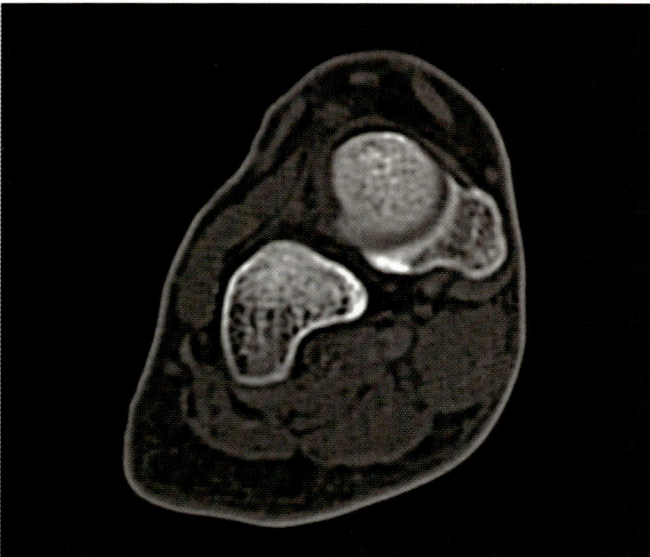

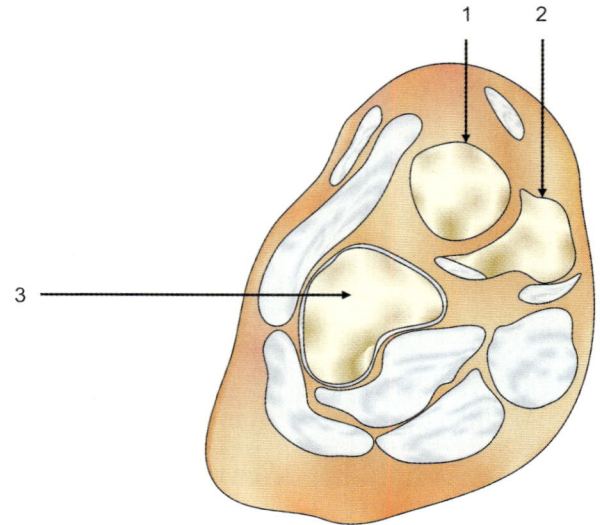

Figure 18.10

1. Talus, head
2. Navicular
3. Cuboid

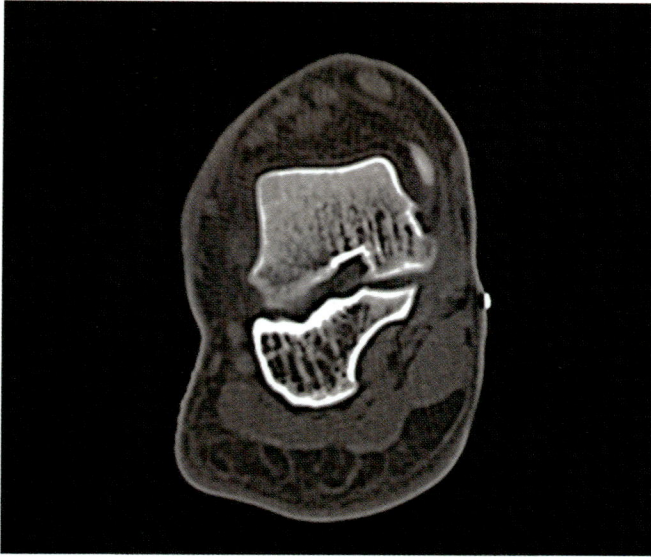

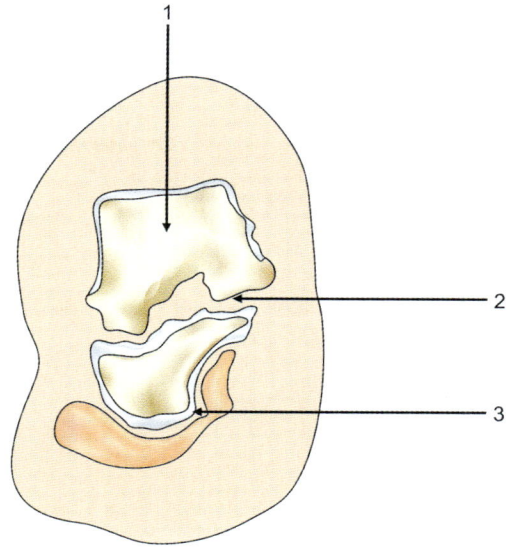

Figure 18.11

1. Talus
2. Middle facet subtalar joint
3. Calcaneus

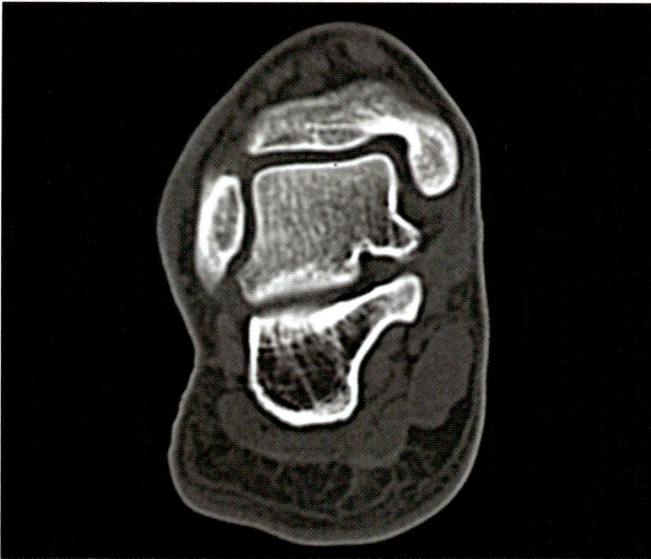

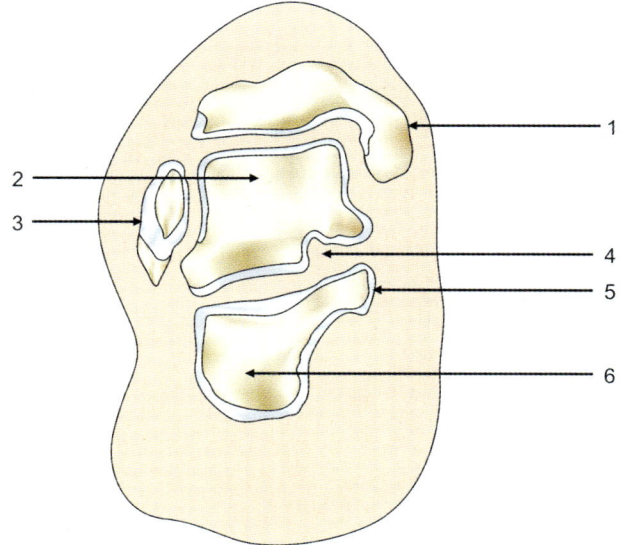

Figure 18.12

1. Medial malleolus
2. Talus, body
3. Lateral malleolus
4. Tarsal sinus
5. Sustentaculum tali
6. Calcaneus

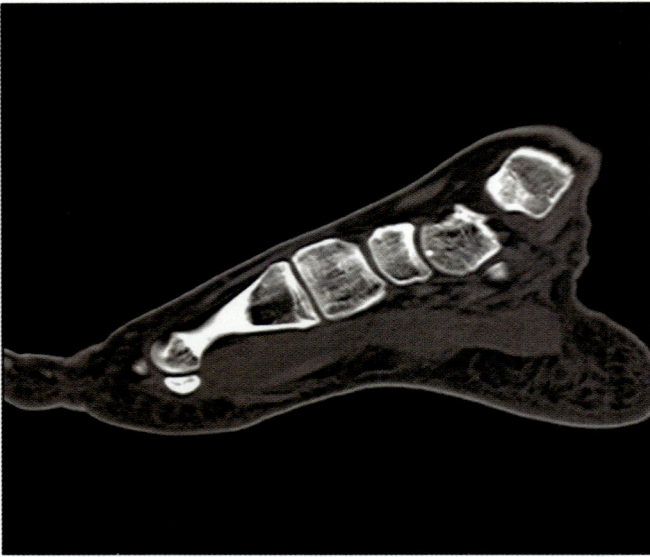

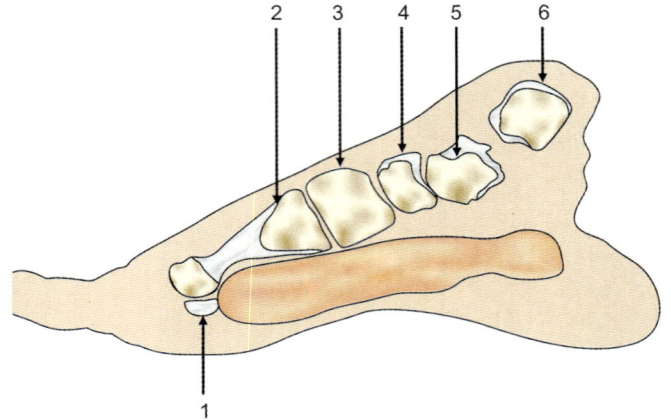

Figure 18.13

1. Sesamoid bone
2. First metatarsal
3. Medial cuneiform
4. Navicular
5. Talus
6. Medial malleolus

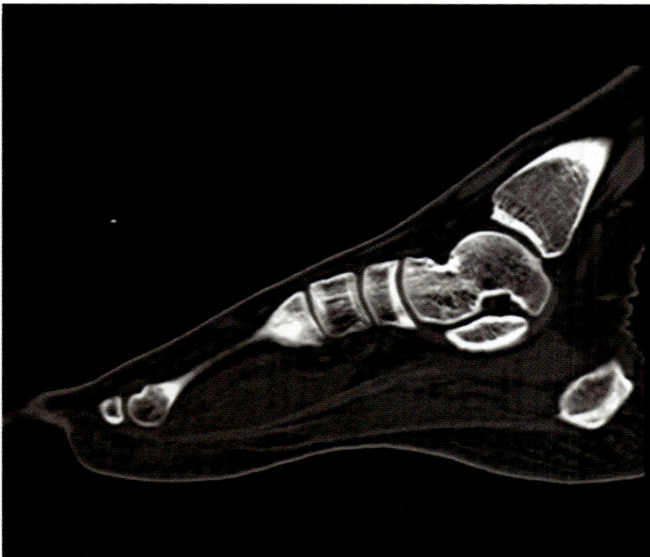

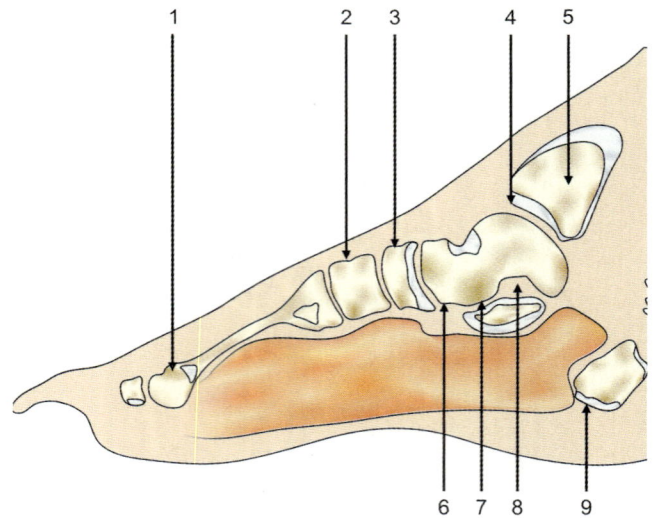

Figure 18.14

1. Second metatarsal
2. Intermediate cuneiform
3. Navicular
4. Ankle joint
5. Tibia
6. Talus, head
7. Medial subtalar joint
8. Tarsal sinus
9. Calcaneus

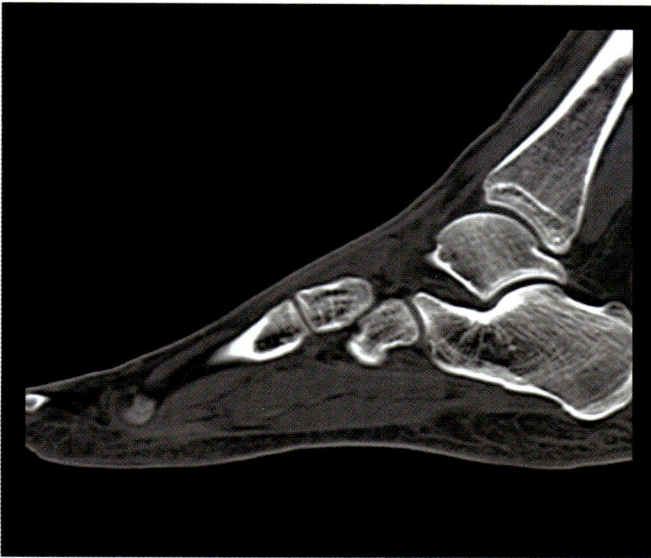
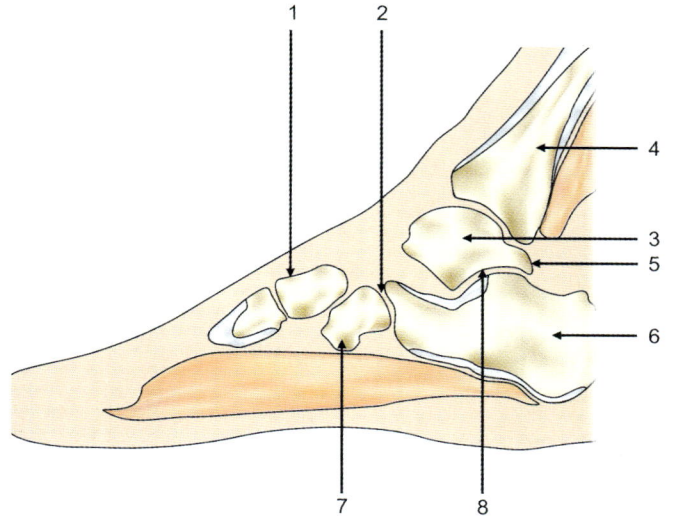

Figure 18.15

1. Lateral cuneiform	5. Lateral talar tubercle
2. Calcaneocuboid joint	6. Calcaneus
3. Talar dome	7. Cuboid
4. Tibia	8. Posterior subtalar joint

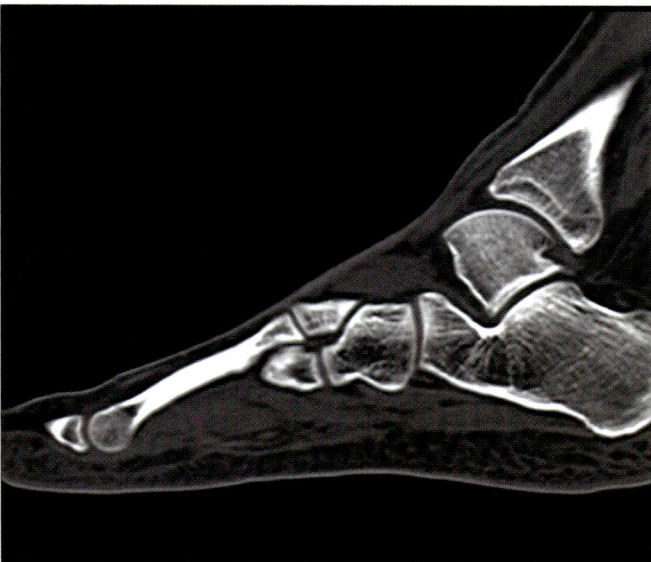
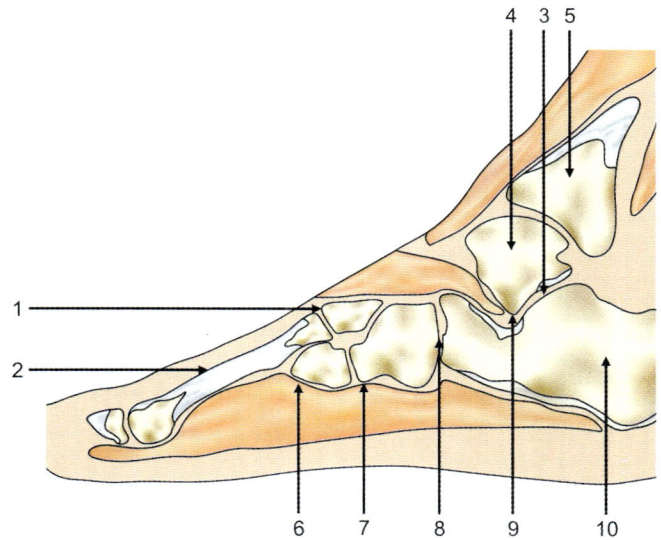

Figure 18.16

1. Lateral cuneiform	6. Fourth metatarsal
2. Third metatarsal	7. Cuboid
3. Posterior subtalar joint	8. Calcaneocuboid joint
4. Talar dome	9. Lateral process, talus
5. Tibia	10. Calcaneus

ANKLE JOINT

Axial Images

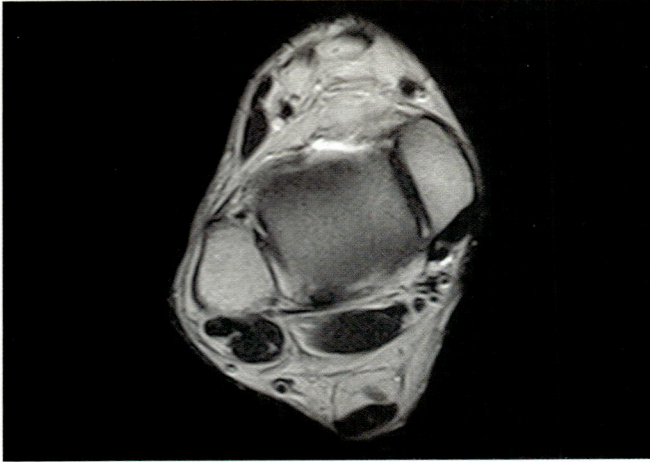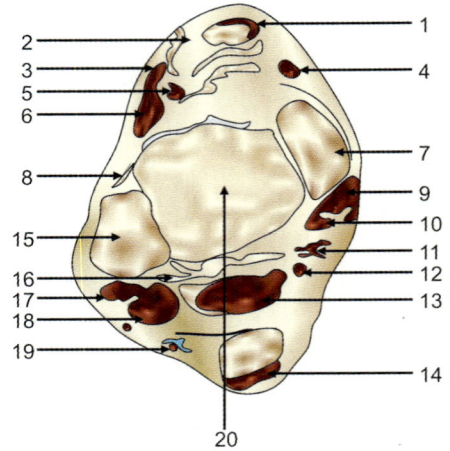

Figure 18.17

1. Tibialis anterior tendon	8. Anterior tibiofibular ligament	15. Lateral malleolus
2. Extensor hallucis longus	9. Tibialis posterior tendon	16. Post tibiofibular ligament
3. Extensor digitorum longus	10. Flexor digitorum longus tendon	17. Peroneus longus
4. Great saphenous vein	11. Posterior tibial artery	18. Peroneus brevis
5. Anterior tibial artery	12. Tibial nerve	19. Lesser saphenous vein
6. Peroneus tertius	13. Flexor hallucis longus	20. Tibiotalar joint
7. Medial malleolus	14. Achilles tendon	

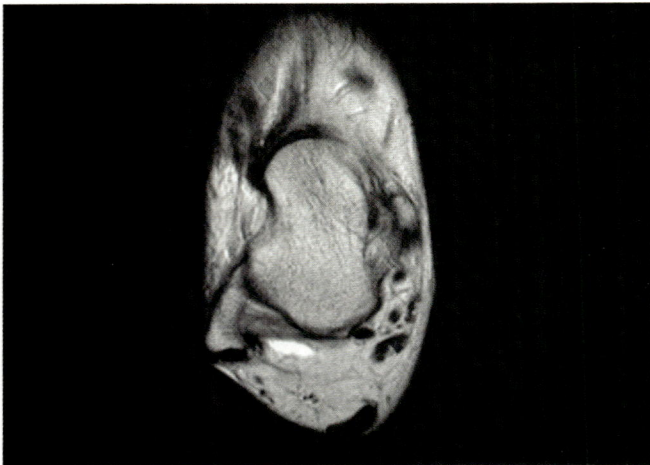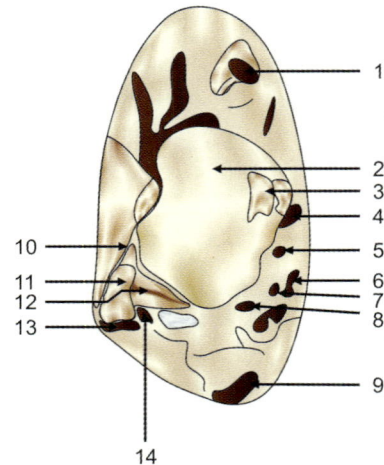

Figure 18.18

1. Tibialis anterior tendon	6. Posterior tibial artery	11. Lateral malleolus
2. Talus	7. Tibial nerve	12. Posterior talofibular ligament
3. Deltoid ligament	8. Flexor hallucis longus tendon	13. Peroneus longus
4. Tibialis posterior tendon	9. Achilles tendon	14. Peroneus brevis
5. Flexor digitorum longus	10. Anterior talofibular ligament	

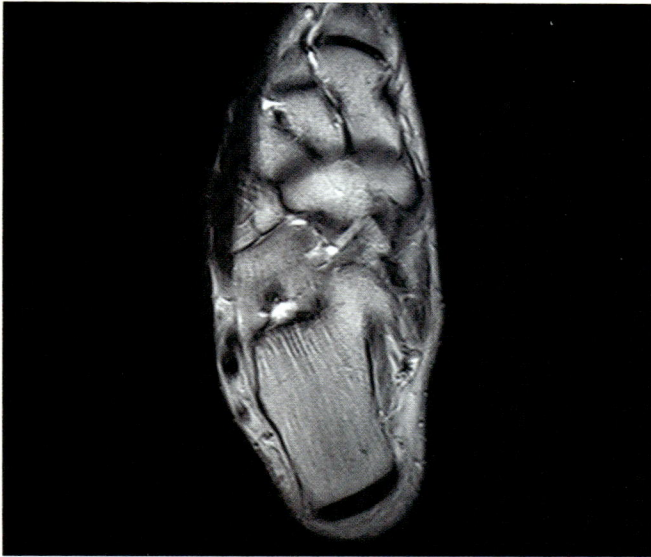

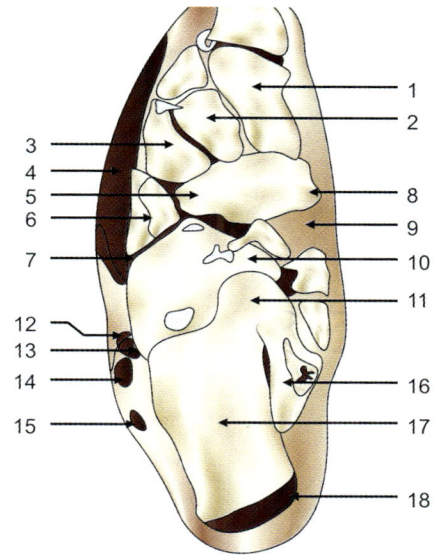

Figure 18.19

1. Medial cuneiform	7. Calcaneocuboid joint	13. Calcaneofibular ligament
2. Intermediate cuneiform	8. Navicular	14. Peroneus longus
3. Lateral cuneiform	9. Tibialis posterior	15. Lesser saphenous vein
4. Extensor digitorum brevis	10. Calcaneonavicular (spring) ligament	16. Quadratus plantae
5. Talus, head	11. Sustentaculum tali	17. Calcaneus
6. Cuboid	12. Peroneus brevis	18. Achilles tendon

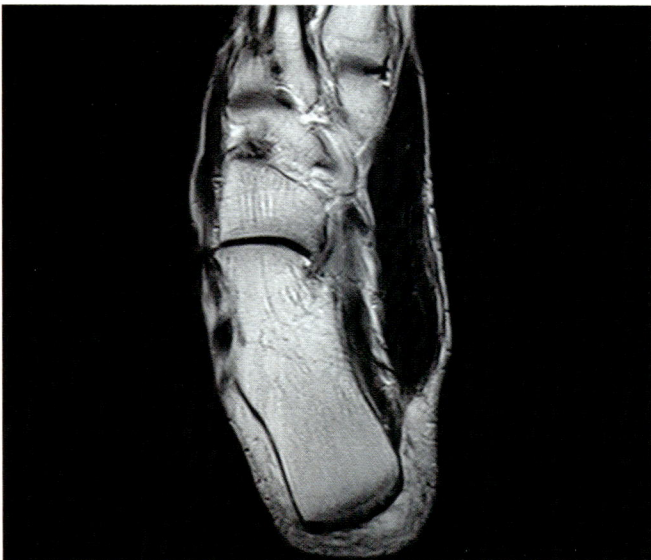

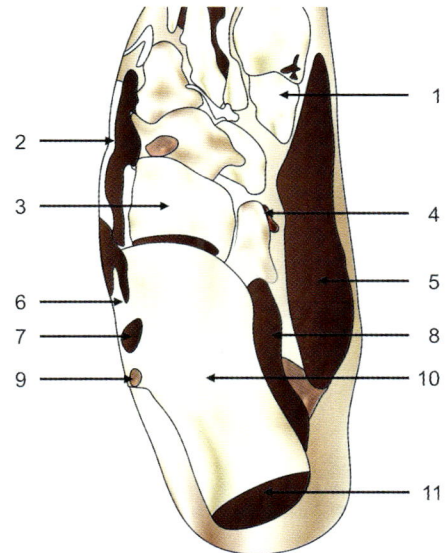

Figure 18.20

1. Medial cuneiform	7. Peroneus longus
2. Extensor digitorum brevis	8. Quadratus plantae
3. Cuboid	9. Calcaneofibular ligament
4. Flexor hallucis longus tendon	10. Calcaneus
5. Abductor hallucis	11. Calcaneal tuberosity
6. Peroneus brevis	

Coronal Images

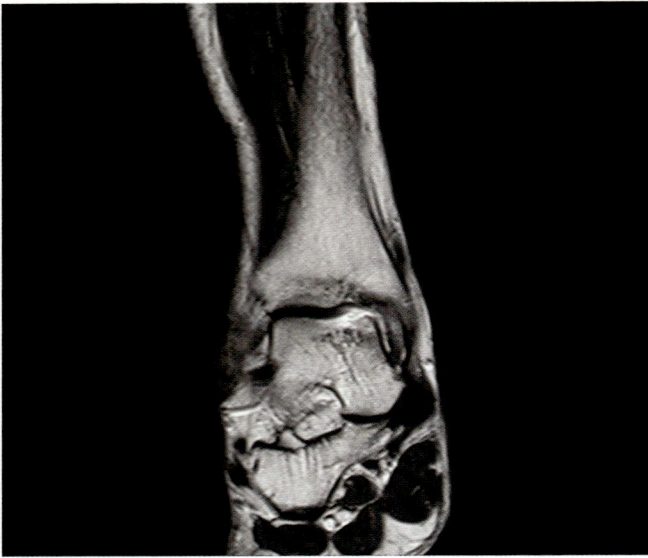
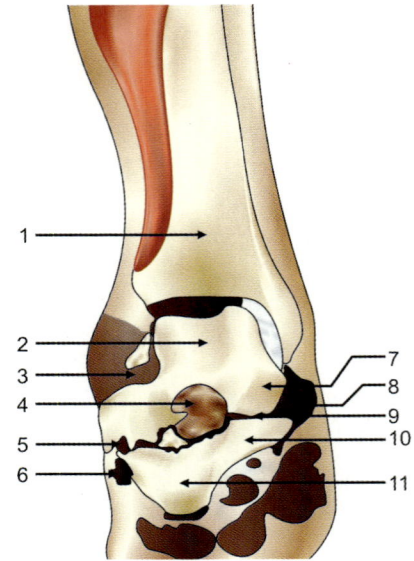

Figure 18.21

1. Tibia	5. Peroneus brevis	9. Middle subtalar joint
2. Talus	6. Peroneus longus	10. Sustentaculum tali
3. Anterior talofibular ligament	7. Middle facet of talus	11. Calcaneum
4. Tarsal sinus	8. Tibialis posterior	

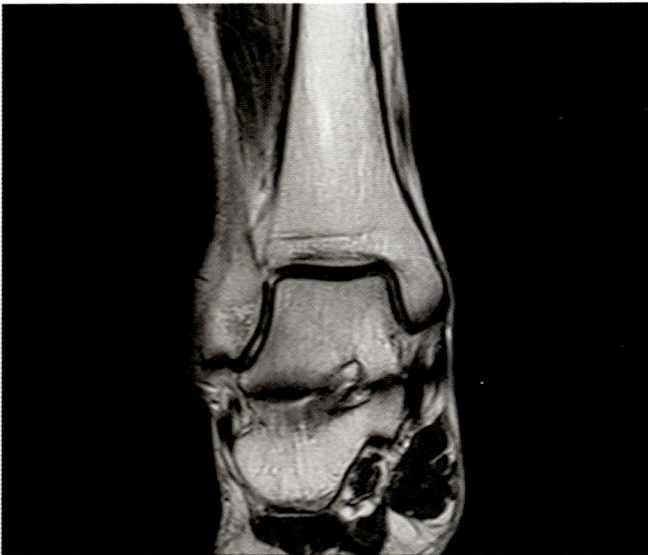
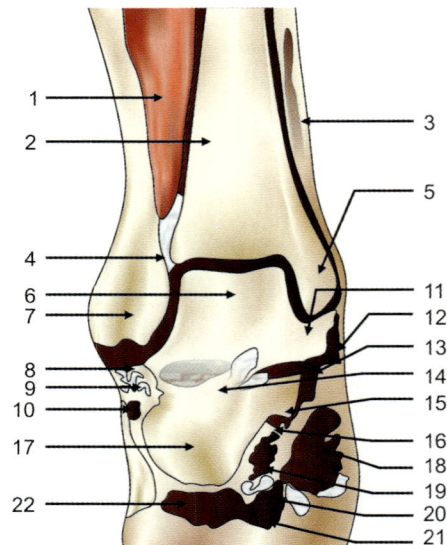

Figure 18.22

1. Extensor hallucis and digitorum longus	8. Calcaneofibular ligament	16. Flexor hallucis longus tendon
2. Tibia	9. Peroneus brevis	17. Calcaneus
3. Great saphenous vein	10. Peroneus longus	18. Abductor hallucis
4. Anterior tibiofibular ligament	11. Deltoid ligament (deep)	19. Quadratus plantae
5. Medial malleolus	12. Tibialis posterior tendon	20. Flexor digitorum brevis
6. Talus, body	13. Flexor digitorum longus tendon	21. Plantar aponeurosis
7. Lateral malleolus	14. Interosseous ligament	22. Abductor digiti minimi
	15. Sustentaculum tali	

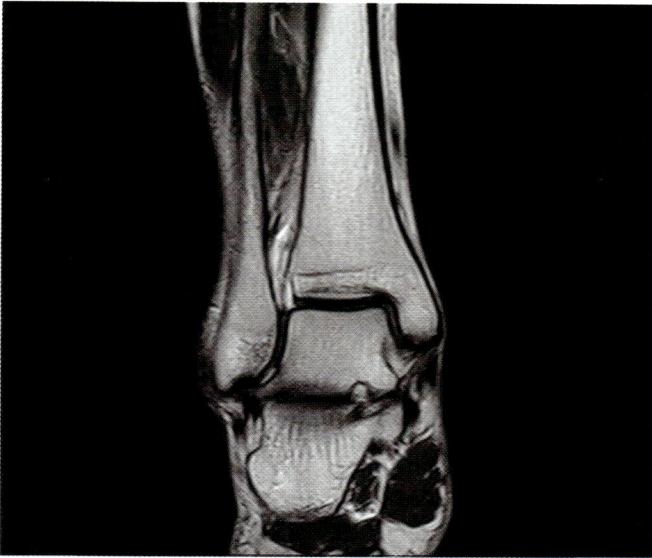

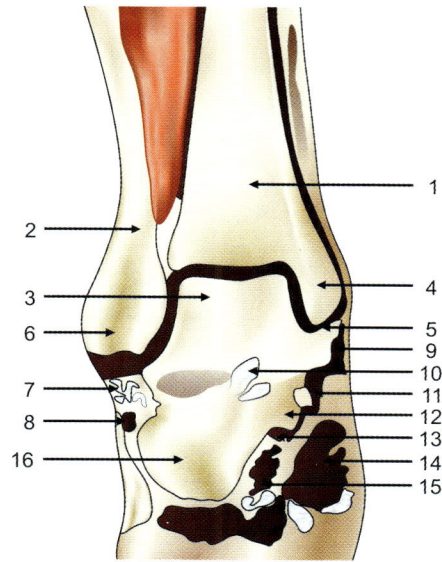

Figure 18.23

1. Tibia	7. Peroneus brevis	13. Flexor hallucis longus
2. Fibula	8. Peroneus longus	14. Abductor hallucis
3. Talus, body	9. Tibialis posterior	15. Quadratus plantae
4. Medial malleolus	10. Tarsal sinus	16. Calcaneus
5. Deltoid ligament	11. Flexor digitorum longus	
6. Lateral malleolus	12. Sustentaculum tali	

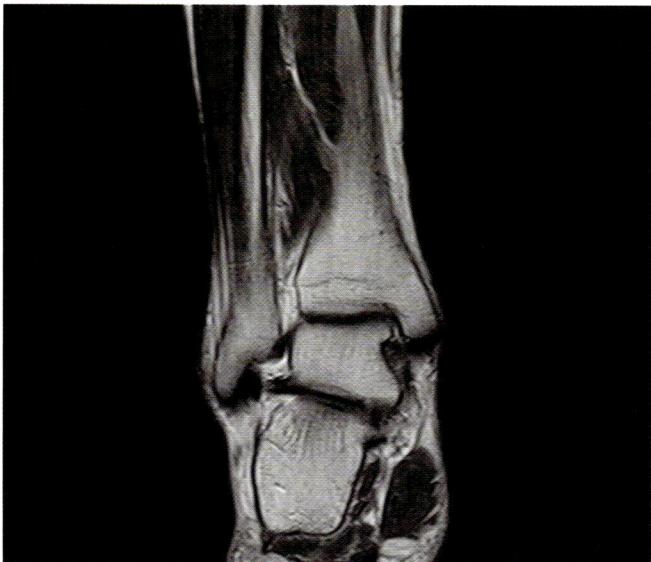

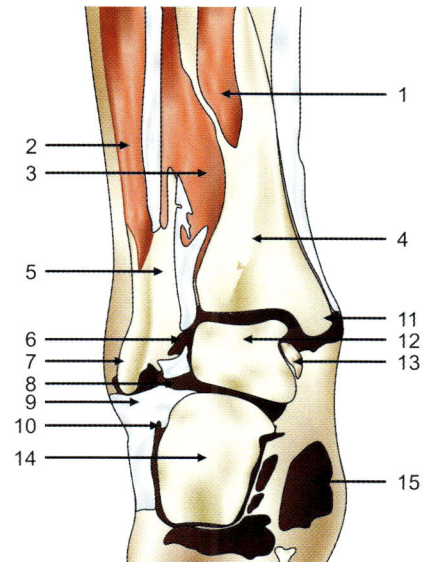

Figure 18.24

1. Tibialis posterior	6. Posterior tibiofibular ligament	11. Medial malleolus
2. Peroneus longus and brevis	7. Lateral malleolus	12. Talus
3. Flexor hallucis longus	8. Posterior talofibular ligament	13. Deltoid ligament
4. Tibia	9. Peroneus longus	14. Calcaneus
5. Fibula	10. Calcaneofibular ligament	15. Abductor hallucis

Sagittal Images

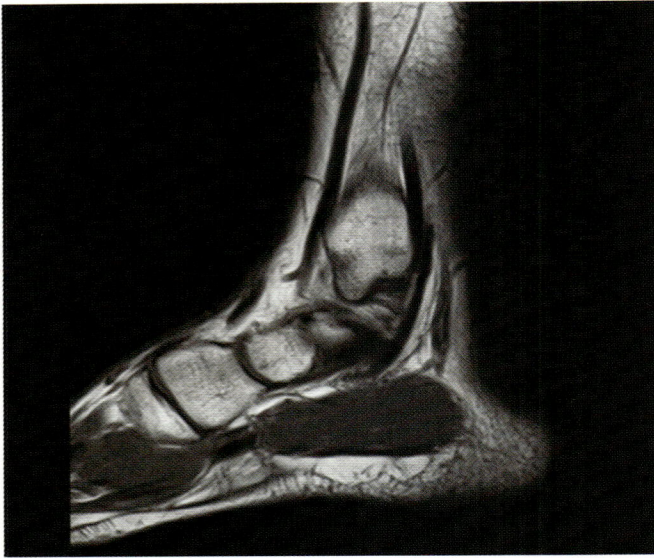

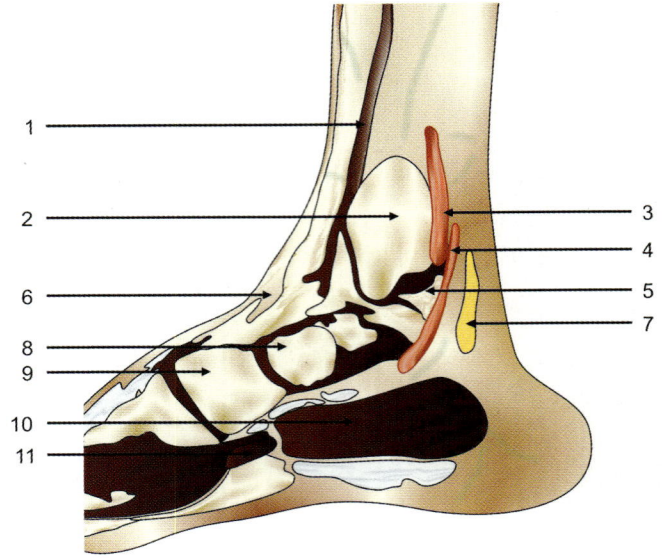

Figure 18.25

1. Great saphenous vein	5. Deltoid ligament	9. Medial cuneiform
2. Medial malleolus	6. Tibialis anterior tendon	10. Abductor hallucis
3. Tibialis posterior tendon	7. Posterior tibial artery and nerve	11. Flexor hallucis longus tendon
4. Flexor digitorum longus	8. Navicular bone	

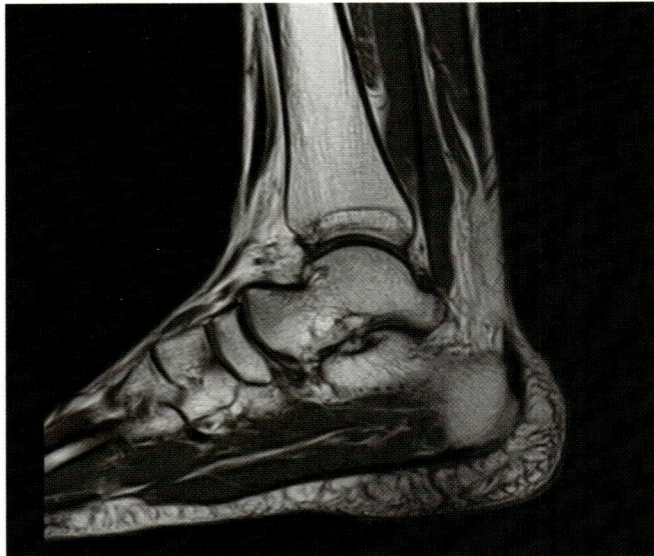

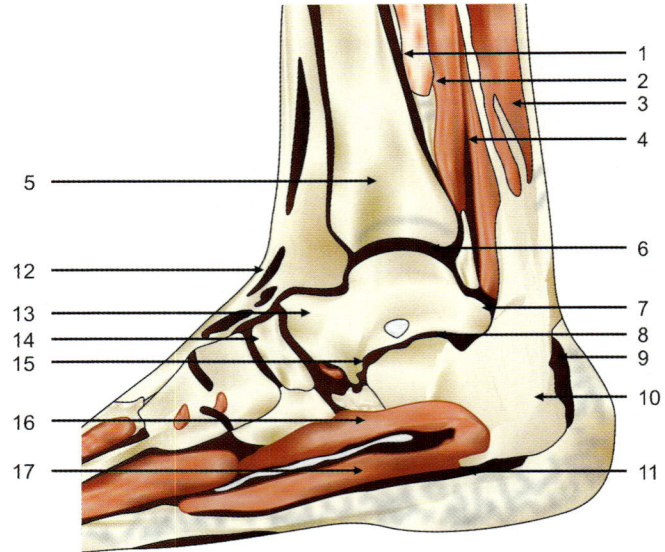

Figure 18.26

1. Tibialis posterior	7. Lateral talar tubercle	13. Head, talus
2. Flexor digitorum longus	8. Interosseous ligament	14. Navicular
3. Soleus	9. Achilles tendon	15. Medial subtalar joint
4. Flexor hallucis longus	10. Calcaneum	16. Quadratus plantae
5. Tibia	11. Plantar aponeurosis	17. Flexor digitorum brevis
6. Ankle joint	12. Tibialis anterior tendon	

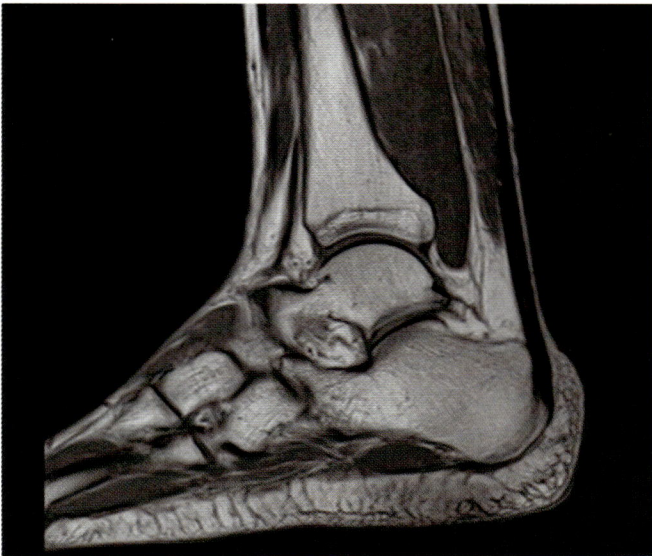

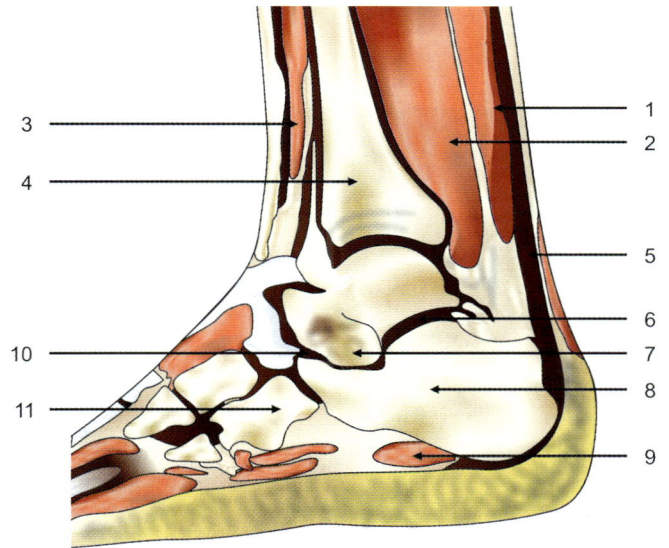

Figure 18.27

1. Soleus	7. Tarsal sinus
2. Long flexor muscles	8. Calcaneum
3. Tibialis anterior	9. Abductor digiti minimi
4. Tibia	10. Anterior subtalar joint
5. Achilles tendon	11. Cuboid
6. Posterior subtalar joint	

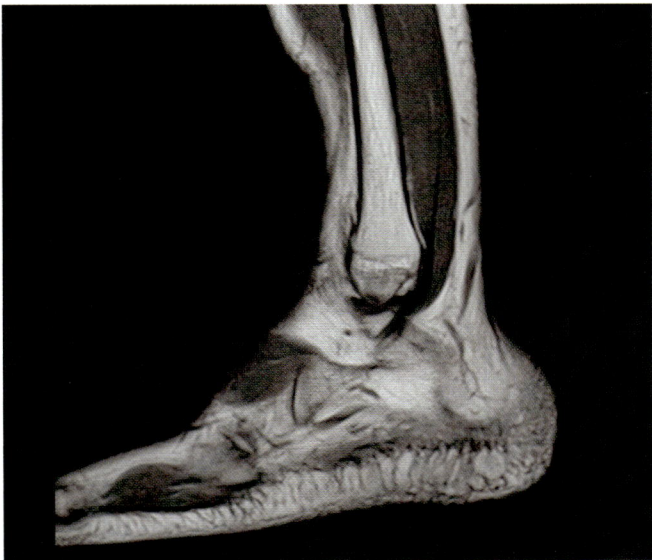

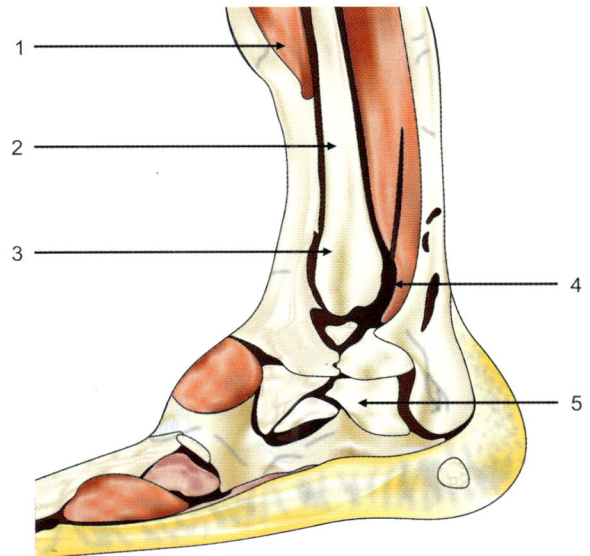

Figure 18.28

1. Extensor digitorum longus
2. Fibula
3. Lateral malleolus
4. Peroneus longus tendon
5. Calcaneum

FOOT

Axial Images

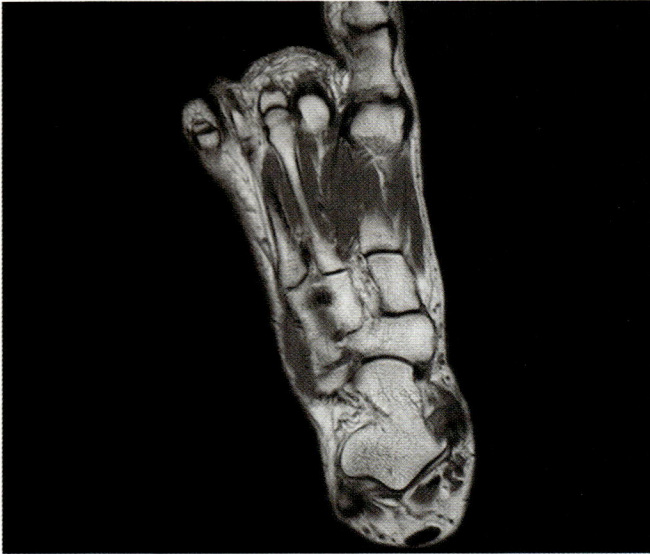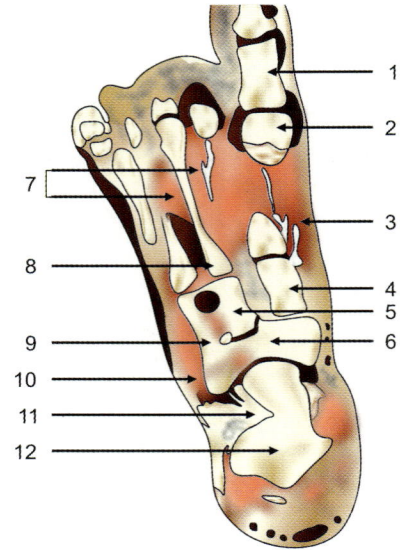

Figure 18.29

1. Proximal phalanx	5. Lateral cuneiform	9. Cuboid
2. First metatarsal	6. Navicular	10. Extensor digitorum brevis
3. Abductor hallucis	7. Dorsal interosseous muscles	11. Tarsal sinus
4. Medial cuneiform	8. Third metatarsal	12. Talus

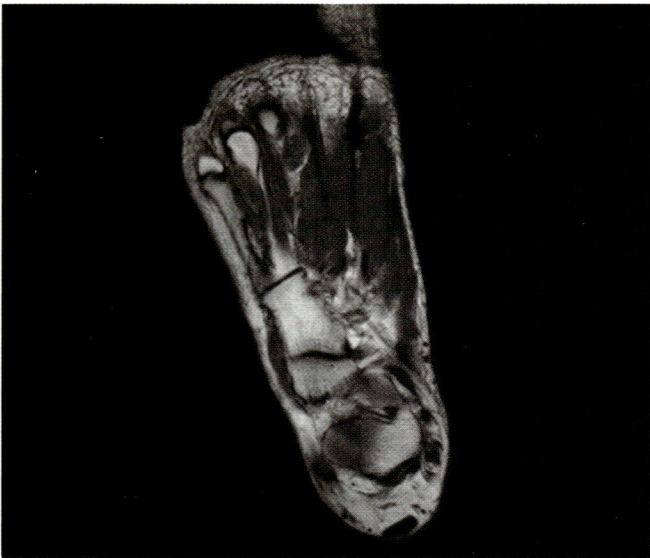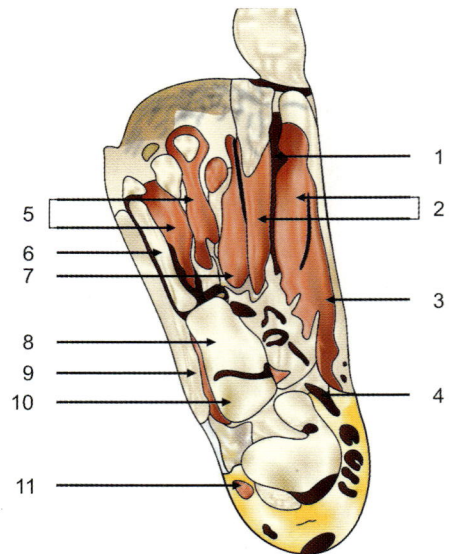

Figure 18.30

1. Flexor hallucis longus tendon	5. Plantar interosseous muscles	10. Calcaneus
2. Flexor hallucis brevis (medial, lateral heads)	6. Fifth metatarsal	11. Peroneal tendons
3. Abductor hallucis	7. Adductor hallucis	
4. Flexor digitorum longus tendon	8. Cuboid	
	9. Extensor digitorum brevis	

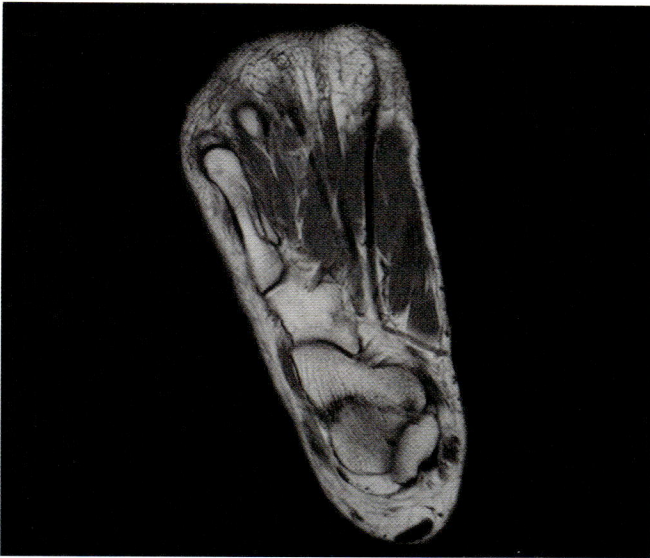
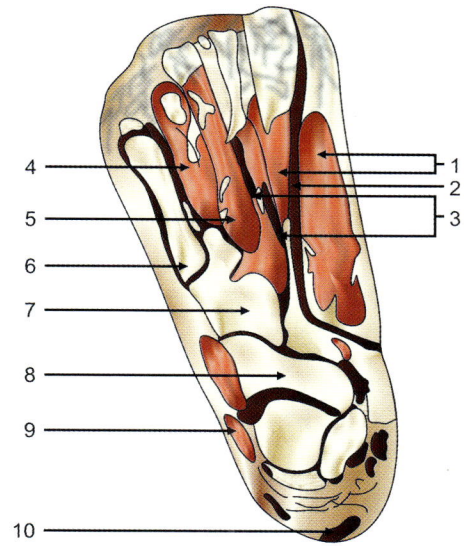

Figure 18.31

1. Flexor hallucis brevis (medial, lateral heads)	6. Fifth metatarsal base
2. Flexor hallucis longus tendon	7. Cuboid
3. Flexor digitorum longus tendons	8. Calcaneus
4. Plantar interosseous muscles	9. Peroneal tendons
5. Adductor hallucis (oblique head)	10. Achilles tendon

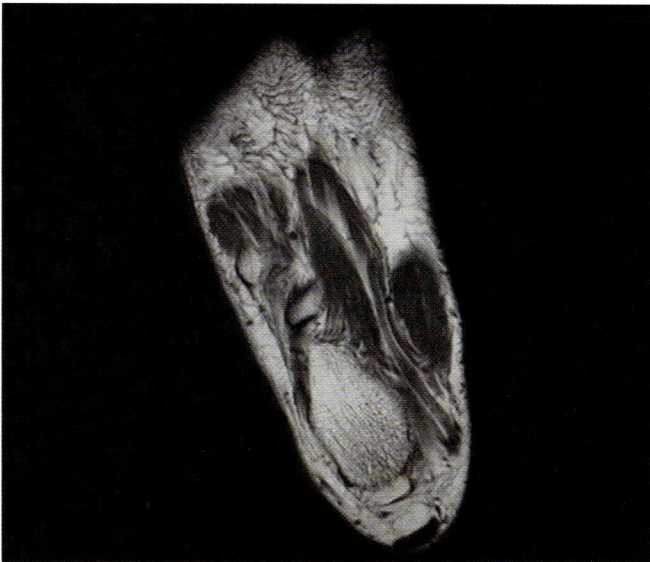
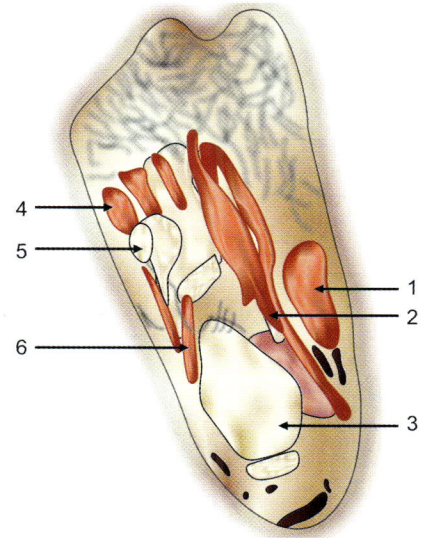

Figure 18.32

1. Quadratus plantae	4. Flexor digiti minimi
2. Flexor digitorum brevis	5. Fifth metatarsal tuberosity
3. Calcaneal tuberosity	6. Abductor digiti minimi

Coronal Images

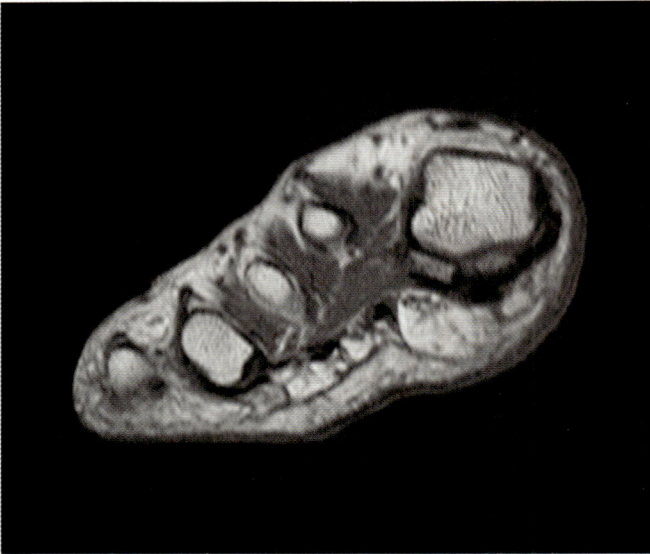

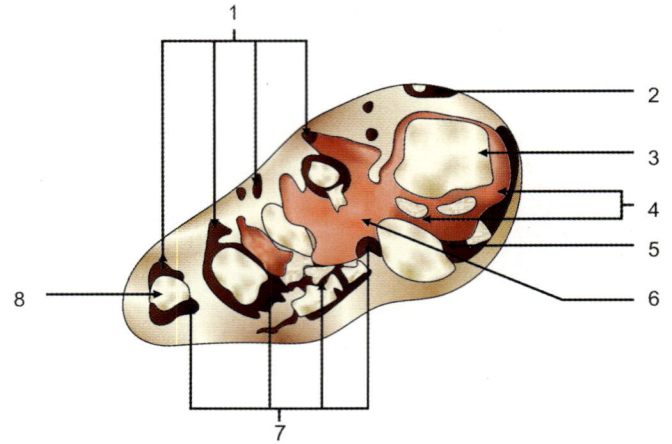

Figure 18.33

1. Short and long extensor tendons, digits
2. Extensor tendon, great toe
3. Great toe
4. Flexor hallucis brevis (medial, lateral heads)
5. Flexor hallucis longus tendon
6. Adductor hallucis (transverse head)
7. Short and long flexor tendons, digits
8. Fifth digit

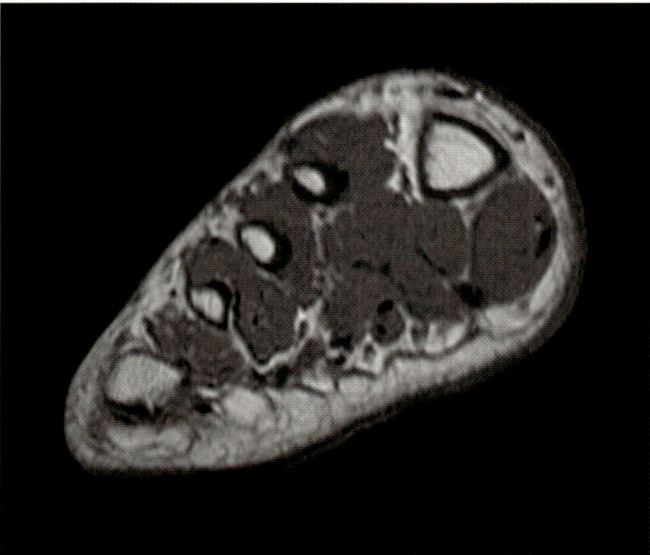

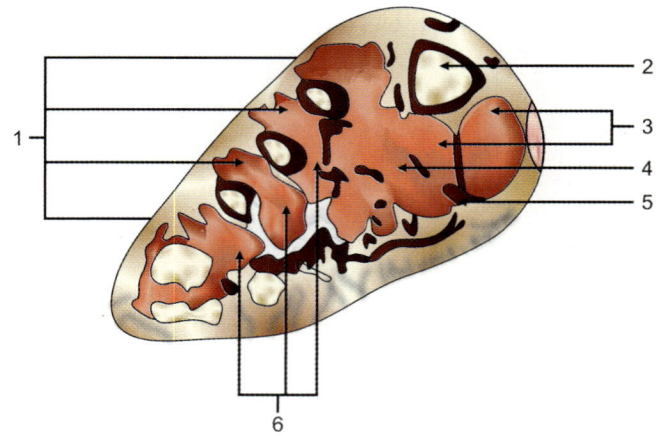

Figure 18.34

1. Dorsal interosseous muscles
2. First metatarsal
3. Flexor hallucis brevis (medial, lateral heads)
4. Adductor hallucis (oblique head)
5. Flexor hallucis longus tendon
6. Plantar interosseous muscles

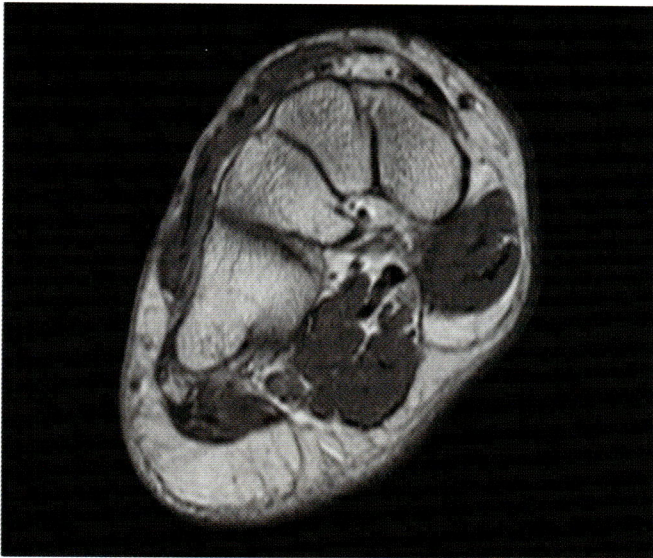
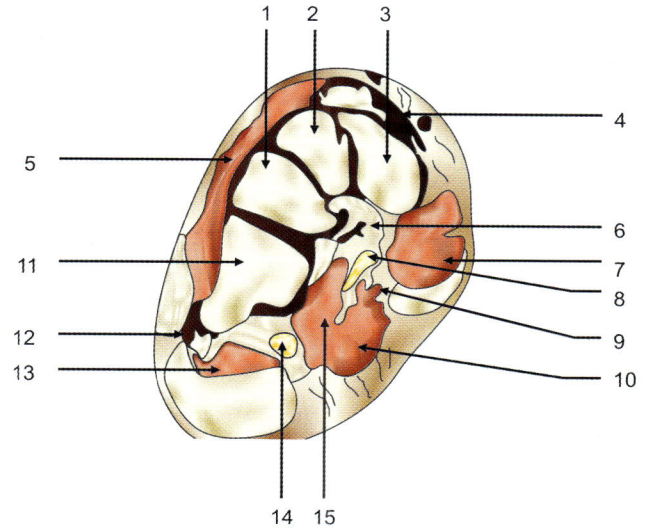

Figure 18.35

1. Lateral cuneiform
2. Intermediate cuneiform
3. Medial cuneiform
4. Extensor hallucis longus tendon
5. Short extensor tendons
6. Flexor hallucis brevis tendon
7. Abductor hallucis muscle
8. Flexor hallucis longus tendon
9. Medial plantar artery, nerve
10. Flexor digitorum brevis
11. Cuboid
12. Peroneus brevis tendon
13. Abductor digiti minimi
14. Lateral plantar artery, nerve
15. Quadratus plantae

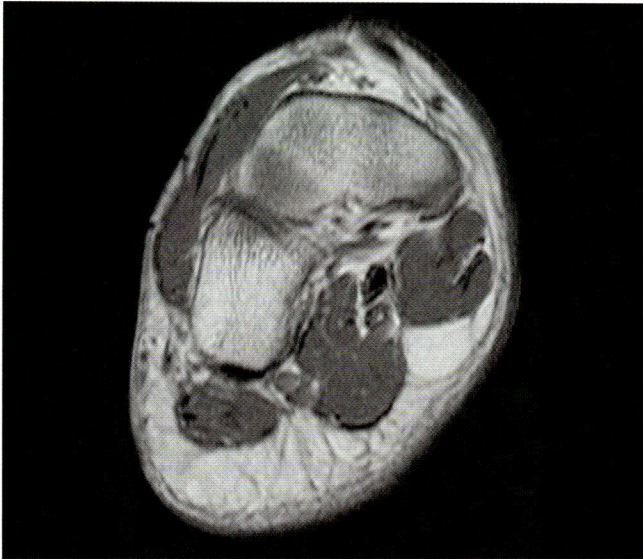
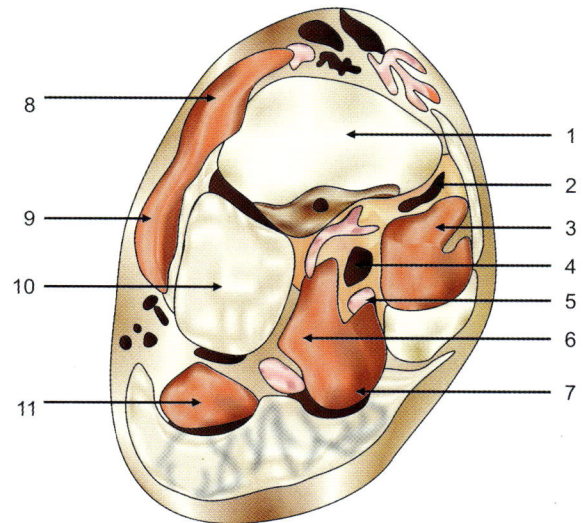

Figure 18.36

1. Navicular
2. Tibialis posterior tendon
3. Abductor hallucis
4. Flexor hallucis longus tendon
5. Medial plantar artery, nerve
6. Quadratus plantae
7. Flexor digitorum brevis
8. Extensor digitorum longus
9. Extensor digitorum brevis
10. Cuboid
11. Abductor digiti minimi

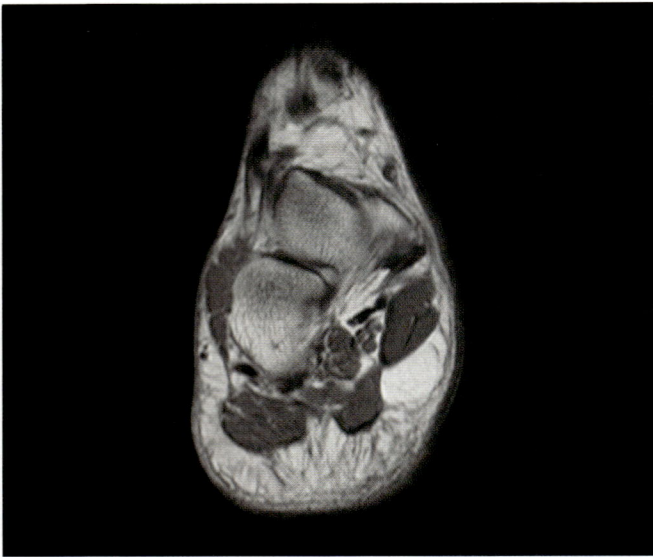

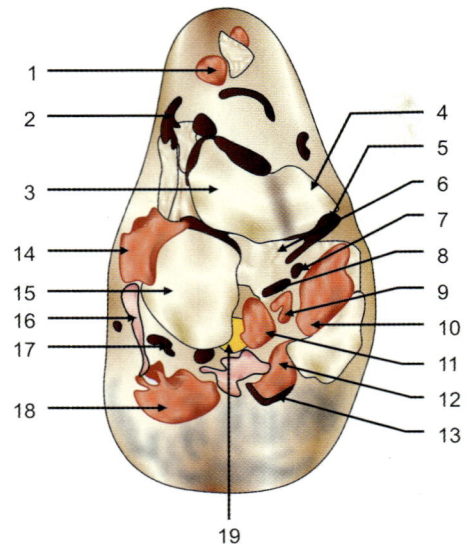

Figure 18.37

1. Extensor hallucis longus	7. Flexor digitorum longus tendon	14. Extensor digitorum brevis
2. Extensor digitorum longus	8. Flexor hallucis longus tendon	15. Calcaneus
3. Talus	9. Medial plantar artery, nerve	16. Peroneus brevis
4. Navicular tuberosity	10. Abductor hallucis	17. Peroneus longus
5. Tibialis posterior tendon	11. Quadratus plantae	18. Abductor digiti minimi
6. Plantar calcaneonavicular (spring) ligament	12. Flexor digitorum brevis	19. Lateral plantar artery, nerve
	13. Plantar aponeurosis	

Sagittal Images

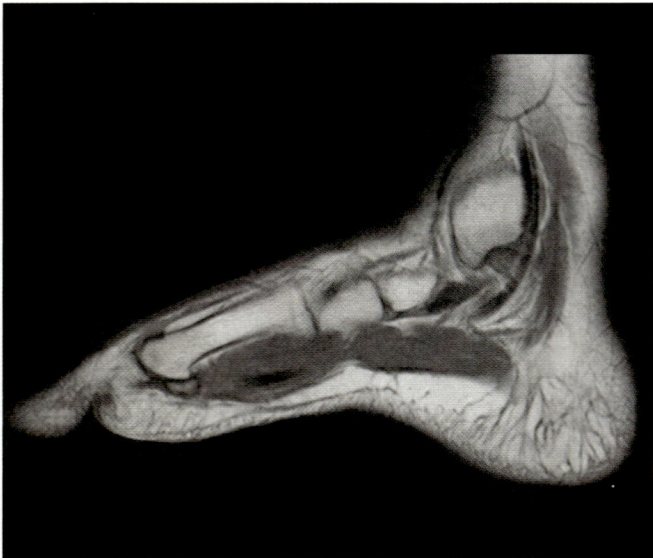

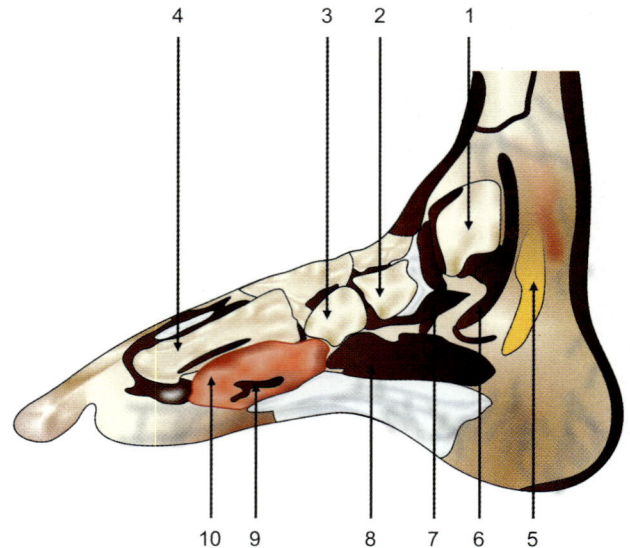

Figure 18.38

1. Medial malleolus	5. Posterior tibial artery nerve	9. Flexor hallucis longus tendon
2. Navicular	6. Flexor digitorum longus tendon	10. Flexor hallucis brevis
3. Medial cuneiform	7. Tibialis posterior tendon	
4. First metatarsal	8. Flexor digitorum brevis	

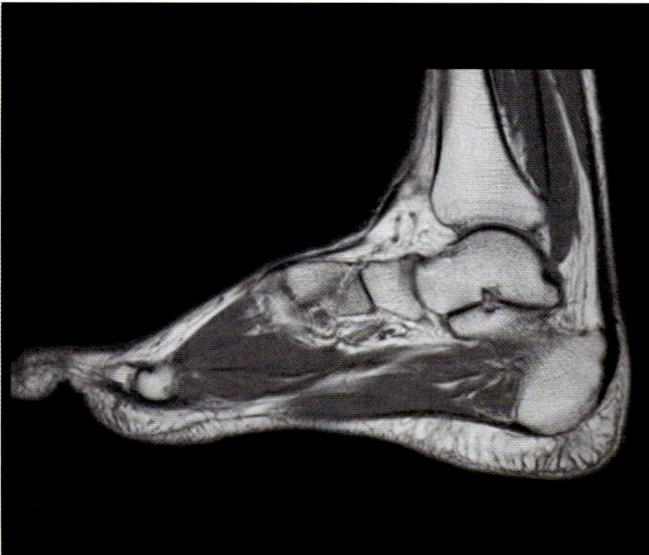

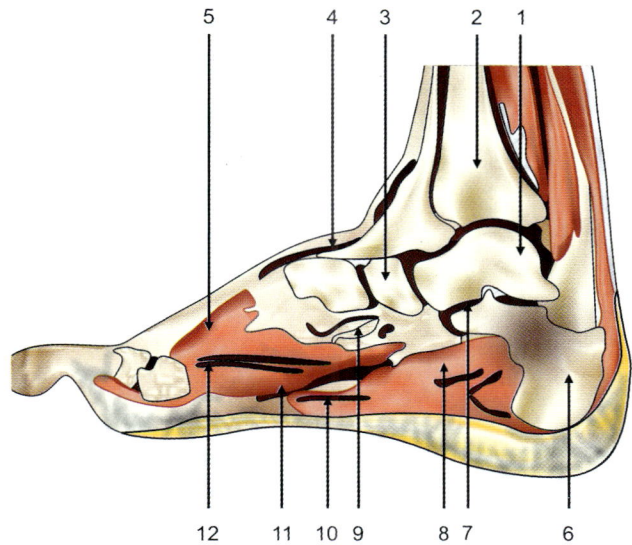

Figure 18.39

1. Talus	7. Medial subtalar joint
2. Tibia	8. Quadratus plantae
3. Navicular	9. Medial plantar artery
4. Tibialis anterior tendon	10. Flexor digitorum brevis
5. Dorsal interosseous muscle	11. Flexor hallucis longus tendon
6. Calcaneus	12. Adductor hallucis

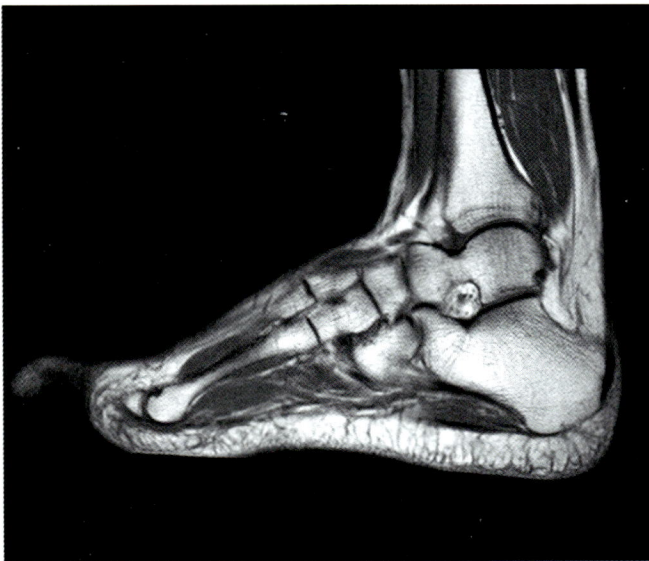

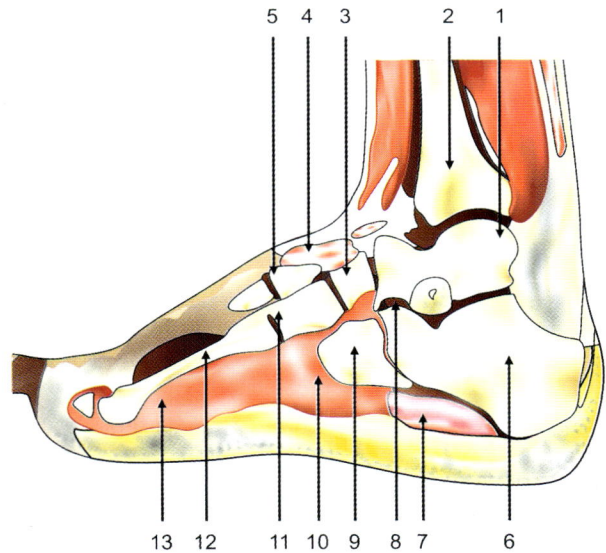

Figure 18.40

1. Talus	6. Calcaneus	11. Lateral cuneiform
2. Tibia	7. Abductor digiti minimi	12. Third metatarsal
3. Navicular	8. Anterior subtalar joint	13. Interosseous muscle
4. Extensor hallucis longus	9. Cuboid	
5. Intermediate cuneiform	10. Peroneus longus tendon	

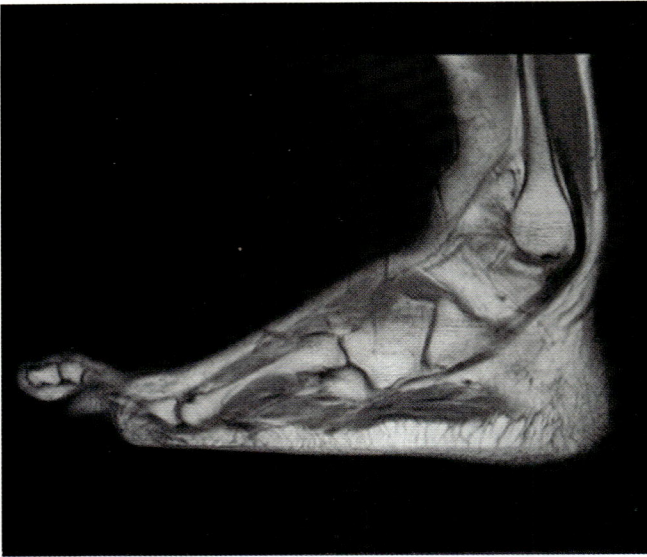

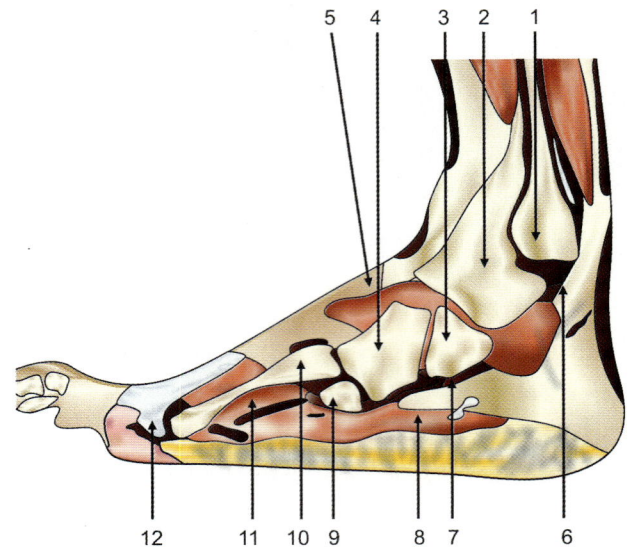

Figure 18.41

1. Lateral malleolus	7. Peroneus longus tendon
2. Talus	8. Abductor digiti minimi
3. Calcaneus	9. Fifth metatarsal
4. Cuboid	10. Fourth metatarsal
5. Extensor digitorum brevis	11. Lumbrical and plantar interosseous
6. Peroneal tendon	12. Proximal phalanx, fifth toe

CHAPTER 19

Lower Extremity Vessels

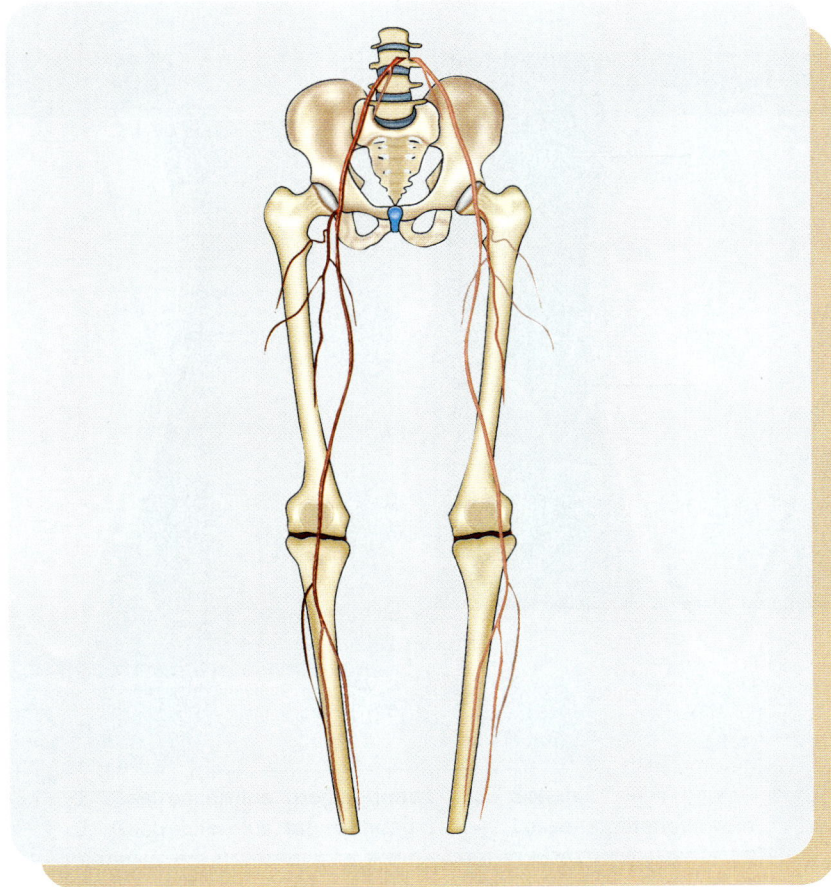

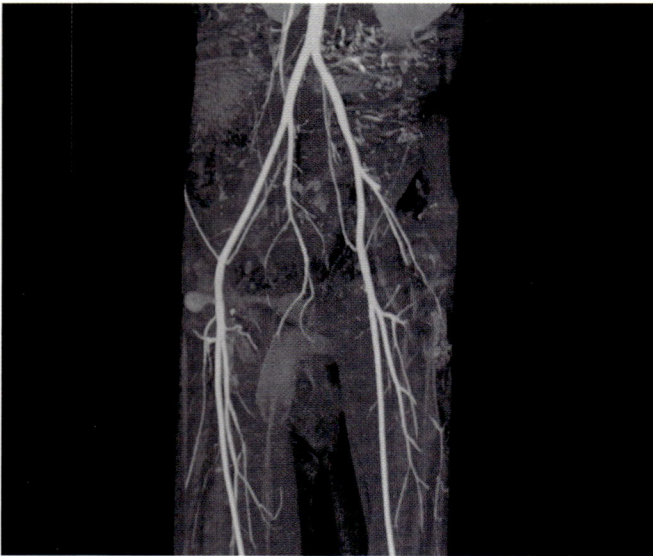

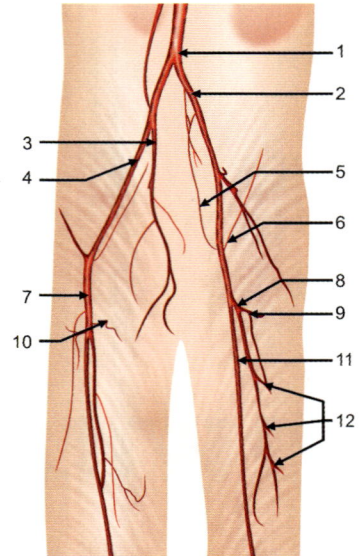

Figure 19.1

1. Aorta	5. Superficial inferior epigastric artery	9. Lateral circumflex artery
2. Common iliac artery	6. Superficial circumflex epigastric artery	10. Medial circumflex artery
3. Internal iliac artery	7. Common femoral artery	11. Superficial femoral artery
4. External iliac artery	8. Profunda femoral artery	12. Muscular branches

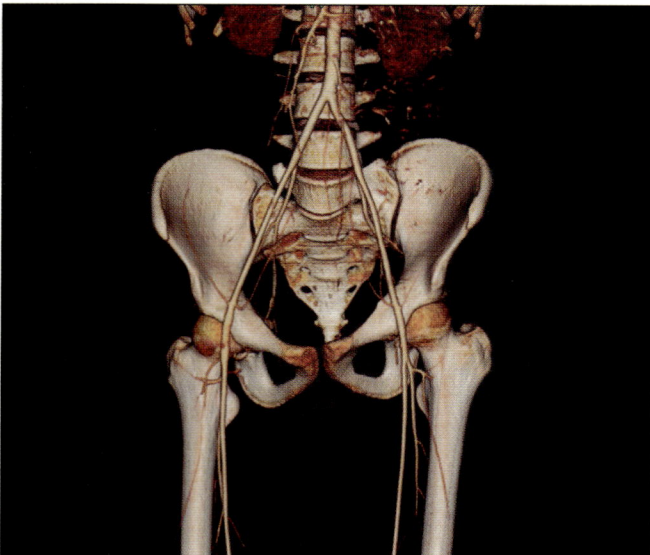

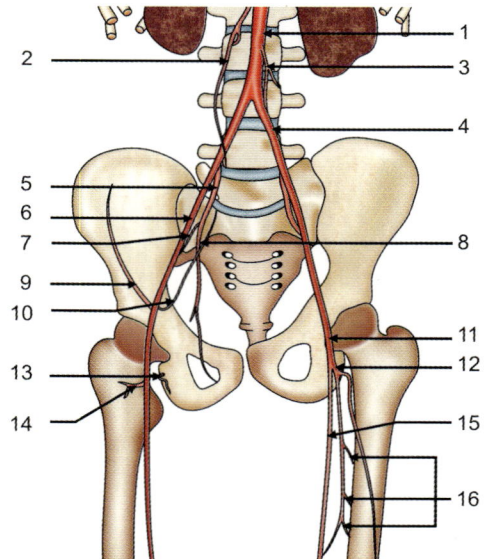

Figure 19.2

1. Aorta	7. Interior iliac, anterior division	13. Medial circumflex artery
2. Superior mesenteric artery	8. Posterior division	14. Lateral circumflex artery
3. Inferior mesenteric artery	9. Superficial circumflex epigastric artery	15. Superficial femoral artery
4. Common iliac artery	10. Superficial inferior epigastric artery	16. Muscular branches
5. Internal iliac artery	11. Common femoral artery	
6. External iliac artery	12. Profunda femoral artery	

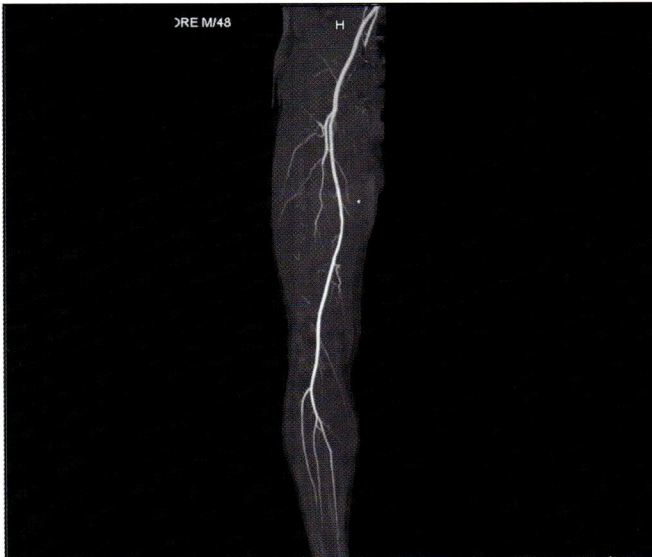

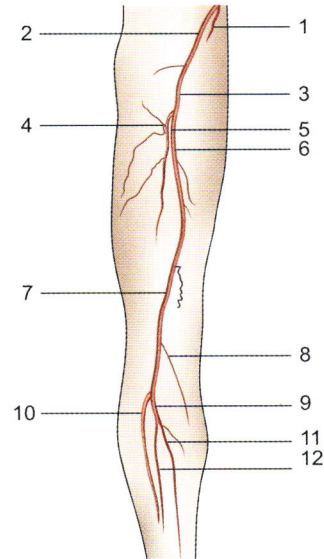

Figure 19.3

1. Internal iliac artery	5. Profunda femoral artery	9. Tibioperoneal trunk
2. External iliac artery	6. Superficial femoral artery	10. Anterior tibial artery
3. Common femoral artery	7. Popliteal artery	11. Posterior tibial artery
4. Lateral circumflex artery	8. Genicular branch	12. Peroneal artery

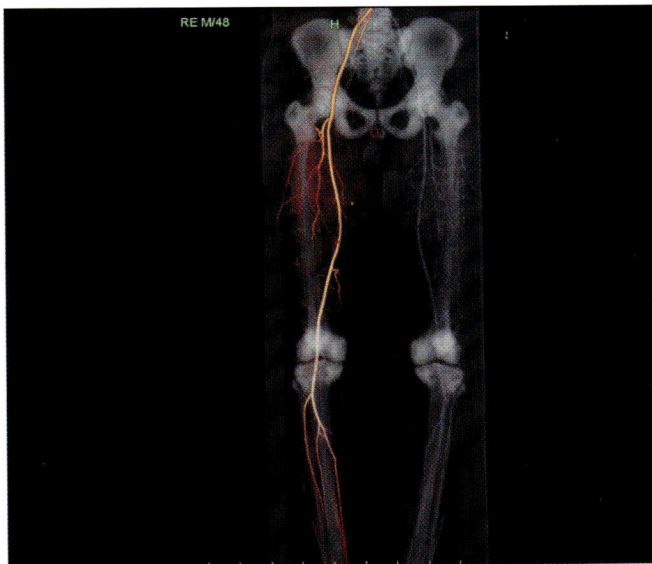

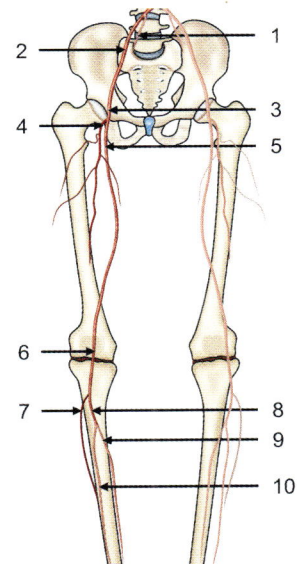

Figure 19.4

1. Internal iliac artery	5. Superficial femoral artery	9. Posterior tibial artery
2. External iliac artery	6. Popliteal artery	10. Peroneal artery
3. Common femoral artery	7. Anterior tibial artery	
4. Profunda femoral artery	8. Tibioperoneal trunk	

Index